Thoracic
Radiology

Thoracic Radiology

Editors

John D. Newell, Jr., M.D.

Associate Professor
Department of Radiology
University of Colorado Health Sciences Center
Denver, Colorado;
and Department of Radiology
National Jewish Center
for Immunology and Respiratory Medicine
Denver, Colorado

Robert D. Tarver, M.D.

Associate Professor
Department of Radiology
Indiana University Medical Center;
and Department of Radiology
Wishard Memorial Hospital
Indianapolis, Indiana

RAVEN PRESS   NEW YORK

Raven Press, Ltd., 1185 Avenue of the Americas, New York, New York 10036

© 1993 by Raven Press, Ltd. All rights reserved. This book is protected by
copyright. No part of it may be reproduced, stored in a retrieval system, or
transmitted, in any form or by any means, electronic, mechanical, photocopying,
recording, or otherwise, without prior written permission of the publisher.

Made in the United States of America

Library of Congress Cataloging-in-Publication Data

Thoracic radiology/editors, John D. Newell Jr., Robert D. Tarver.
      p. cm.
    Includes bibliographical references and index.
    ISBN 0-88167-983-6
    1. Chest—Radiography. I. Newell, John D. II. Tarver, Robert D.
    [DNLM: 1. Thoracic Radiography. WF 975 T487]
RC941.T5 1993
617.5′40757—dc20
DNLM/DLC
for Library of Congress   92-49207
                                                       CIP

The material contained in this volume was submitted as previously
unpublished material, except in the instances in which some of the illustrative
material was derived.

Great care has been taken to maintain the accuracy of the information
contained in this volume. However, neither Raven Press nor the editors can be
held responsible for errors or for any consequences arising from the use of the
information contained herein.

9 8 7 6 5 4 3 2 1

To our wives and children,

Dawn, Robert, and Paige
Karen and Matt

Contents

Contributing Authors

Caroline Chiles, M.D. *Associate Professor, Department of Radiology, Medical College of Virginia, Box 470, Richmond, Virginia 23298*

Dewey J. Conces, Jr., M.D. *Associate Professor, Department of Radiology, Indiana University Medical Center, University Hospital X-64, 926 West Michigan Street, Indianapolis, Indiana 46223*

Janette D. Durham, M.D. *Assistant Professor, Department of Radiology, University of Colorado Health Sciences Center, Campus Box A030, 4200 East Ninth Avenue, Denver, Colorado 80262*

Robert W. Holden, M.D. *Professor and Chairman, Department of Radiology, Indiana University Medical Center, University Hospital X-64, 926 West Michigan Street, Indianapolis, Indiana 46223*

David A. Lynch, M.D. *Assistant Professor, Department of Radiology, University of Colorado Health Sciences Center, Campus Box A030, 4200 East Ninth Avenue, Denver, Colorado 80262*

John T. Mail, M.D. *Department of Radiology, Saint Francis Hospital Center, 1600 Albany Beach Grove, Indianapolis, Indiana 46107*

John D. Newell, Jr., M.D. *Associate Professor, Department of Radiology, University of Colorado Health Sciences Center, 1400 Jackson Street, Denver, Colorado 80206; and Director of Radiology, National Jewish Center for Immunology and Respiratory Medicine, Denver, Colorado 80206*

Robert D. Tarver, M.D. *Associate Professor, Department of Radiology, Indiana University Medical Center; and Department of Radiology, Wishard Memorial Hospital, 1001 West Tenth Street, Indianapolis, Indiana 46202*

W. Richard Webb, M.D. *Professor in Residence, Department of Radiology, University of California, San Francisco, 505 Parnassus Avenue, Box 0628, San Francisco, California 94143-0628*

Preface

This book on thoracic radiology focuses on common areas of clinical practice in diagnosing diseases of the thorax using modern imaging techniques. It highlights the areas of thoracic radiology that are considered most important based on the editors' and contributors' experience in this subspecialty of radiology.

The book is for those interested in a concise discussion of the core practice of thoracic radiology, including radiology residents, practicing clinical radiologists, internal medicine specialists, pulmonologists, and cardiothoracic surgeons.

The book is divided into ten chapters. Chapter 1 describes the technical aspects of thoracic imaging focusing on conventional radiology and computed tomography. Pulmonary infections and bronchogenic carcinomas are discussed in chapters 2 and 3, respectively. Emphysema and bronchiectasis are covered in chapter 4 and the radiology of interstitial lung disease is reviewed in chapter 5. Pulmonary thromboembolic disease is covered in chapter 6, followed by a discussion in chapter 7 of normal anatomy and diseases affecting the chest wall and pleura. Finally, chapters 8, 9, and 10 cover imaging of the thoracic aorta, ICU radiology and interventional radiology. We consider these ten topics to be the most essential in thoracic radiology.

John D. Newell Jr., M.D., F.C.C.P.
Robert D. Tarver, M.D.

Thoracic
Radiology

Thoracic Radiology, edited by
J.D. Newell, Jr., and R.D. Tarver,
Raven Press, Ltd., New York © 1993.

CHAPTER 1

Thoracic Imaging Techniques

John D. Newell, Jr.

Twenty years ago the thoracic radiologist relied on conventional radiographic techniques as the primary tools for radiologic diagnosis. In this chapter we will discuss the imaging techniques that are most often used by the thoracic radiologist today. Conventional radiographic techniques have advanced considerably over the last 20 years and now computed tomography (CT), magnetic resonance imaging (MRI), and digital radiology are complementing the traditional techniques in almost every department of radiology. There are additional radiologic techniques used to diagnose and treat diseases of the thorax, and these include nuclear scintigraphy, angiography, interventional techniques, and ultrasonography. These latter methods will be discussed in upcoming chapters where appropriate.

CONVENTIONAL RADIOGRAPHY

The importance of obtaining properly exposed and reproducible chest radiographs cannot be overemphasized. In 1980 there were approximately 63,135,000 chest radiographic examinations performed in the United States (1). This represents 45 percent of all conventional radiologic studies. If one were to estimate a cost of $72 per examination (a conservative estimate), the chest radiography business is a 4.4 billion dollar a year industry in the United States alone.

There are four main components of a chest radiographic system: x-ray generator, x-ray tube, grid, and screen-film system. The x-ray generator should be a three-phase, 12-pulse unit or multipulse unit with a power rating of 100 kW. The generator should have a peak kilovoltage (kVp) rating of 150 and a maximum

current rating of 1000 ma. The x-ray generator should be capable of a minimum exposure time of 2 msec. The x-ray tube should have a 100 kW capacity, and the anode should rotate at least 10,000 rpm. A 12° anode angle and a 0.6 mm focal spot size are recommended. A focal spot size of no larger than 1.5 mm should be used for high-quality work. There should be adequate collimation of the x-ray tube, and the intrinsic filtration of the tube and collimator should be at least 2.5 mm of aluminum. An additional 0.35 mm of copper filtration should be added to give a total equivalent filtration of 18.5 mm of aluminum if 140–150 kVp techniques are going to be used. A high-quality aluminum interspaced grid should be used. This device is placed between the patient and the x-ray recording system to eliminate some of the scattered radiation coming from the patient. In our experience, the best grid has been a stationary grid with a 12:1 grid ratio with at least 100 grid lines/inch. The 12:1 grid is especially important when using the Kodak (Rochester, NY) Insight HC film-screen combination. The grid should be focused at 72 inches, the standard distance between the x-ray tube and the patient. A phototiming system should be used to obtain automatically the optimum film density in any radiographic exposure. The phototiming detector is usually a set of three discrete phosphorus plates that are embedded in a Lucite block, which is behind the grid and screen-film combination. There are some systems that use an ion chamber detector that is positioned in front of the film-screen combination and behind the grid. The phototiming system should be capable of controlling exposures down to 2 msec in length.

The x-ray detection system and image display system are one in the same thing in conventional radiography. This remarkable device is, of course, the x-ray film. The film is loaded between two rare earth phosphors in modern systems that enable very low exposure levels for a frontal radiograph, approximately 10 mR. This is possible because of the great amount of photon amplification that occurs from an x-ray passing through the phosphor

---

J. D. Newell, Jr.: Department of Radiology, University of Colorado Health Sciences Center; and National Jewish Center for Immunology and Respiratory Medicine, Denver, Colorado 80206.

that then emits light in the visible spectrum, and to the great sensitivity of rare earth film in absorbing the x-rays and the visible light that reaches the film. There is an emulsion present on each side of modern chest radiographic film so that the film is exposed on both sides. This dual emulsion feature of thoracic radiographic film also increases the sensitivity of the detection process. There has been considerable technical advancement in the manufacture of rare earth phosphors and their corresponding films. The phosphor-film combination is referred to as a screen-film combination.

Eastman Kodak recently introduced a very innovative film-screen combination that they call their Insight HC system. This advanced asymmetrical Insight intensifying screen system has an ultrathin, very high resolution phosphor layer as the front screen and a standard resolution rear screen. The phosphor layers luminesce at different intensities when struck by x-rays. As a result, the two sides of the film generate two different radiographic images that are summed together. The film that is used in this system has two emulsions, with one optimized for the front phosphor and one optimized for the rear phosphor. There are two anticrossover layers between the two emulsions so there is no print-through phenomena (Fig. 1). The disadvantage to this design is that the film must be placed in the cassette with the right film emulsion next to the corresponding screen phosphor. It is important to realize that, in order to create a good radiographic image of the thorax, the subject contrast must be lowered since there is a wide range of densities in the chest (e.g., air-containing lung, soft tissue-containing cardiomediastinal structures, and the bony structures of the chest wall, shoulder girdle, and spine). This is achieved by using a somewhat higher kVp that will decrease subject contrast and by using a wide latitude screen-film combination such as the Insight HC system. The higher the kilovoltage used, the wider the latitude or decreased subject contrast. This makes pulmonary nodules stand out from adjacent ribs. Unfortunately, calcium-containing nodules are not seen as well, and the sharpness of the entire radiographic image decreases with increased kVp for a variety of reasons. The decreased sharpness makes the evaluation of interstitial densities within the thorax more difficult, which has been another objection to the

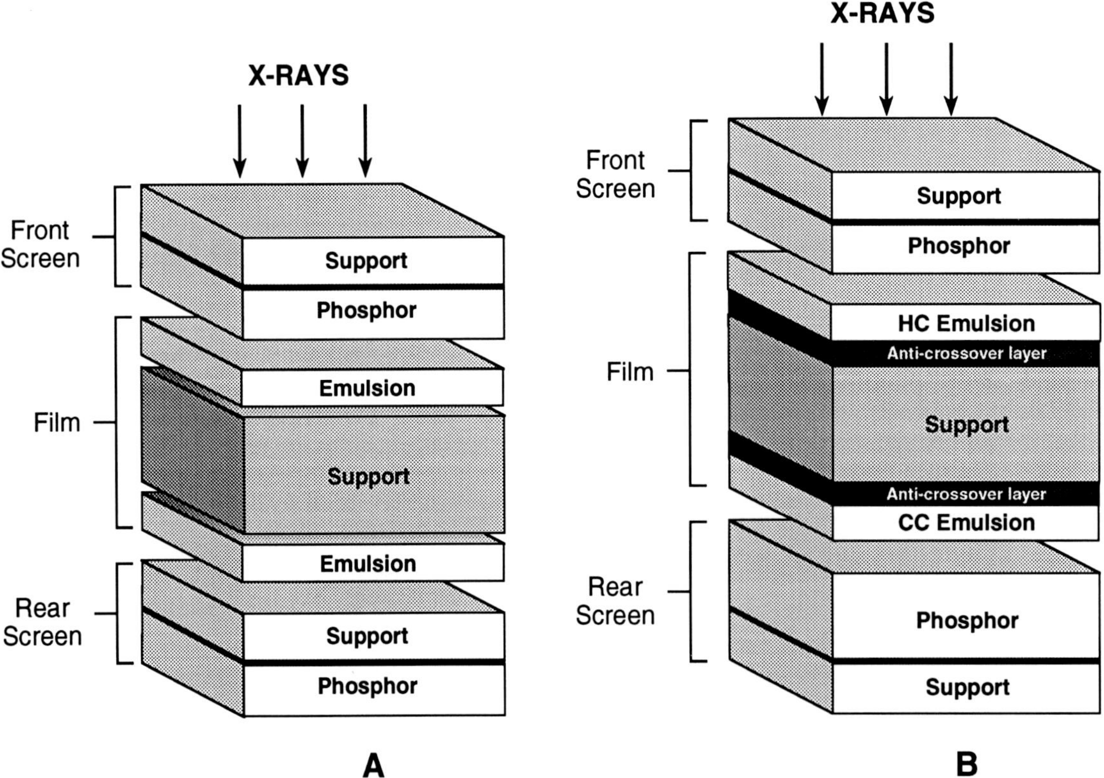

FIG. 1. An older symmetrical design, with light crossover, of film screen systems (*left*) and the newer asymmetrical design, without light crossover, of the Insight HC system (*right*). Note the different phosphors and film emulsions with the Insight HC system. The anticrossover layers are very important in the Insight HC system, because they isolate the front and back film emulsions from each other.

high kilovoltage techniques. The Insight HC screen-film combination can produce a final image of the thorax with relatively sharp anatomic detail and sufficient latitude using 110–125 kVp. This is the current kilovoltage range that is used for conventional radiography of the thorax in most institutions.

A dedicated chest radiographic unit is used in departments where a large number of chest radiographic examinations are done. A dedicated chest radiographic unit is available from several manufacturers, including General Electric, Siemens, and Picker. This unit combines the x-ray generator, x-ray tube, grid, phototimer, and screen-film combinations with an additional x-ray tube alignment device and an automatic film loading and developing system that greatly increases the throughput of patients and also improves the consistency between examinations done on the same patient. This type of dedicated chest radiography equipment is highly recommended to any department that is doing a lot of radiographic examinations of the thorax.

The four main elements in good thoracic radiographic technique are patient positioning, degree of inspiration, and proper film exposure to achieve an optimal film density. The patient is generally positioned in the frontal and lateral projections, with the x-ray beam transversing the patient from posterior to anterior (PA) in the frontal view and from right to left in the lateral view. These projections are referred to as the standard PA and left lateral radiographs, and are generally obtained on most patients referred for thoracic radiography. It is important to position patients consistently from one examination to another so that consistent measurements of the heart and any other normal or abnormal structures within the thorax can be made. The radiograph should normally be exposed after the patient has been instructed to take a full breath, but before the patient's glottis closes. This will put the patient's lung volume near total lung capacity. It is very important to ensure good inspiratory effort if serial examinations are going to be reviewed for any significant changes. The final element of a good plain radiographic examination is the proper exposure of the film to achieve an optimal film density. The use of a modern screen-film system like the one described previously will greatly aid in obtaining a good radiographic examination of the thorax. This can generally be achieved by using 110–125 kVp and a phototimer to adjust the film density so that the optical density over the lung zones is approximately 1.6. This will generally allow a mediastinal optical density of 0.7 or greater to be obtained. This will enable the physician to see detail in the mediastinum that might be missed using a different kVp and a different screen-film combination (Fig. 2).

PORTABLE CHEST RADIOGRAPHY

Thoracic radiographic examinations can also be obtained on patients who are too sick to come to the radiol-

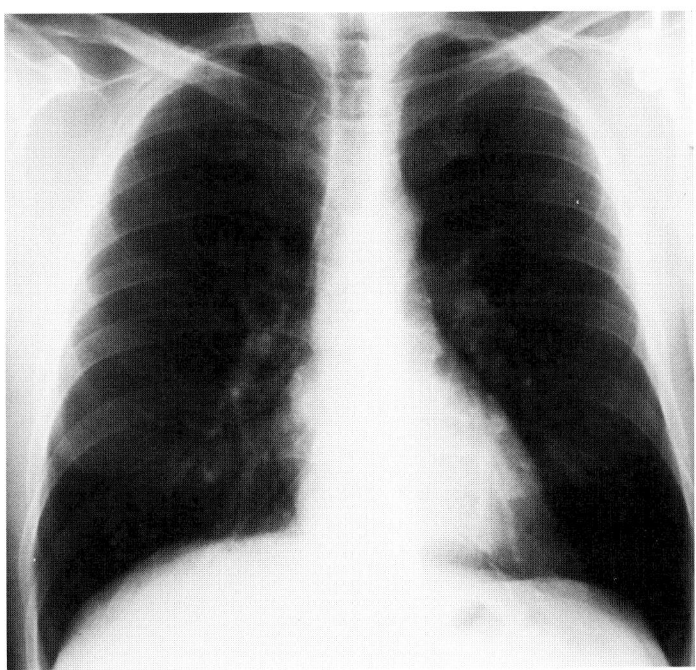

FIG. 2. PA chest radiograph from a normal subject using the Insight HC film-screen combination. The examination was obtained using a phototimer and 125 kVp. This film illustrates the advantages of a wide latitude screen-film combination in conventional chest radiography.

ogy department. This is done using a portable, battery-powered x-ray generator and x-ray tube system. A portable screen-film system can be used to obtain reasonably high-quality studies. The Kodak Insight HC system, described previously, with a new laser-produced flexible grid that is integrated into the cassette is the newest grid film-screen system available. The overall film quality is usually not as good using portable radiography compared with examinations done in the department. Because a high-quality grid is not used, the x-ray tube focal spot size is not as small as on the nonportable systems, and the patient is generally examined at less than 72 inches focal film distance, which decreases sharpness in the image. The latest generation of portable x-ray imagers are quite mobile, with self-propelled sustained speeds of up to 2.5 mph. They have very flexible positioning of the x-ray tube available. The generators are capable of producing kilovoltages that are equivalent to 110 kVp, with exposure times as short as 2 msec. The new portable generators use a new technology called medium frequency output, which is equivalent to, or better than, a three-phase, 12-pulse generator. The new computerized portable radiographic units are capable of storing up to 144 separate programs of x-ray exposure.

The technical factors on portable radiographic examinations vary considerably, depending on what x-ray tube to film distance can be achieved and whether the patient is capable of voluntarily controlling his or her respirations. The most common position is either the supine or upright frontal projection with the patient as near to full inspiration as possible. The x-ray beam passes through the patient from anterior to posterior so that there may be considerable magnification of the heart compared to a PA radiograph. Additional distortion may be introduced because of varying distances that are used to obtain the radiograph (40–72 inches). The supine positioned film is generally harder to interpret than an upright film. The technical factors that are used will vary depending on the physical size of the patient along with the factors previously mentioned. A phototiming unit is generally not available for use in these examinations, and one must measure the thickness of the patient's chest and refer to a technique chart to compute the proper kVp, ma, and exposure time to use with any given patient to achieve a film density of 1.6 over the lung zones. In our experience, we recommend using 100 kVp with as short an exposure as possible at 72 inches with the patient in an upright frontal position and at full inspiration.

DIGITAL RADIOGRAPHY

An important concept in digital radiography of the chest is that the recording or detection system is quite different from a conventional radiographic image detection system. The image recording system and image display system have been decoupled from one another in modern digital radiography systems (Fig. 3). This enables manipulation of the digital image after it is recorded and before it is displayed. The digital image can be optimized before it is recorded on film or displayed on a cathode ray tube (CRT) display.

There are several digital techniques that have been used to create digital radiographic systems. These techniques include scan projection radiography, digital video fluoroscopy, digitization of wide latitude film, and imaging plates using photostimuable phosphors (2). The most promising system at this time is the imaging plate system using photostimuable phosphors. This system is referred to as a computed radiographic system (CRS) and is currently being developed independently by multiple companies. The heart of the system is a europium-activated barium fluorohalide compound that is distributed across a large plate providing an area detector for diagnostic x-rays. This area detector is referred to as an imaging plate (IP). The IP is being manufactured in various sizes to suit different clinical radiological examinations. The imaging plate size is available in 36 cm × 36 cm and 36 cm × 43 cm sizes for adult thoracic digital radiography work.

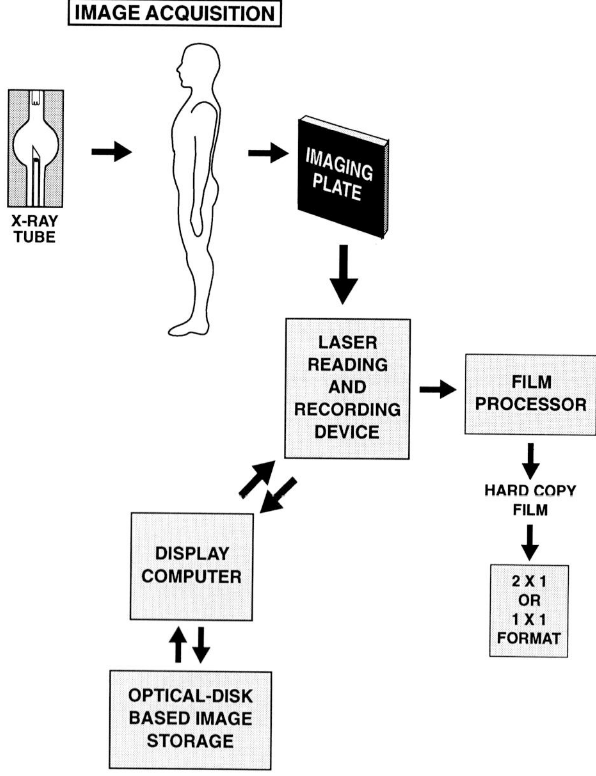

COMPUTED RADIOGRAPHY SYSTEM

FIG. 3. The basic components of a digital radiography system illustrating the concept of decoupling the image detection system from the image display medium.

The IP is exposed to diagnostic x-rays and a latent image is stored in the IP photostimuable phosphors. Subsequently, the latent image is read from the phosphors by using a laser scanning device, and the light that is reemitted by the phosphor is proportional to the number of x-rays that were absorbed there. This light is absorbed by a photomultiplier tube and subsequently converted to a digital image by using an analog-to-digital converter. A current commercial system has a maximum spatial resolution of 2.5 lp/mm. This is equivalent to about a 1760 × 1760 line image resolution on a 36 cm × 36 cm IP. This appears to be the minimum resolution necessary for a digital radiography system if it is going to replace conventional screen-film detection systems (3). A recent study examining the detection of the visceral pleural line in patients with a pneumothorax concluded that there was no significant difference between conventional and digital radiographic films in their ability to detect pneumothoraces (4). The issue of how well digital radiographic films will compete with newer conventional radiographic films such as the Insight HC system described previously is not known at this time.

The recorded CRS image can be computer-enhanced and displayed on a CRT display or output onto a sheet of single emulsion film that is typically 36 cm × 25 cm in size. Two images are output on this film that are each one-fourth of the area of the original 36 cm × 36 cm IP. The one image is processed so that it appears similar to a conventional chest radiograph. The second image is processed so that the edges of objects within the image are much sharper, and this presumably will aid in the detection of subtle abnormalities not seen as easily in the first image (Fig. 4). There is considerable research going on at this time to determine the best computer processing algorithms to use in generating digital images for various clinical radiological problems. The CRS images are not routinely interpreted on the CRT displays because the resolution of the current generation of CRT displays is limited to 1024 × 1024 lines, which is not adequate for thoracic radiography. There are also problems in using video terminals to view digital images that have been discussed recently in the radiology literature (4).

A prototypic CRS has been evaluated with over 5000 examinations over a 2-year period (5). This study concluded that the digital system has multiple advantages over conventional radiography systems: image quality is excellent; film density is adjustable independent of x-ray dose, which eliminates repeat examinations; dose is decoupled from the other attributes of image quality; digital archival of the radiographic images is possible; and costs associated with film and repeat radiographic examinations are reduced. Disadvantages include reduced patient throughput (ca. 40 patients/hour) and a smaller final image of the adult thorax to which some physicians might have some initial difficulty adjusting. The spatial resolution is also less than the most advanced film screen systems (e.g., Insight HC). A current CRS system begins at around $250,000. The exact role of digital radiology in ambulatory-type radiographic examinations is not clear

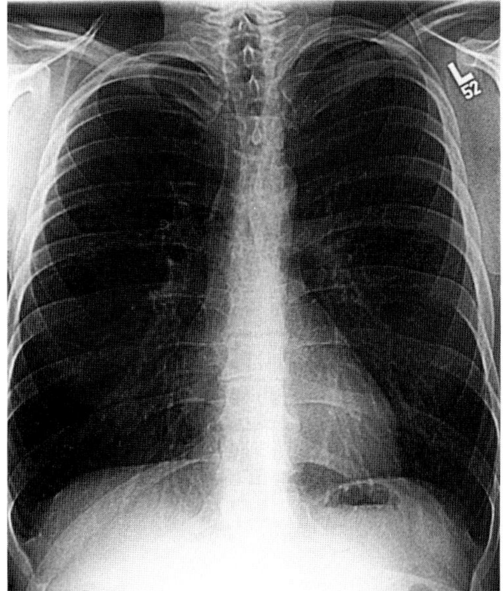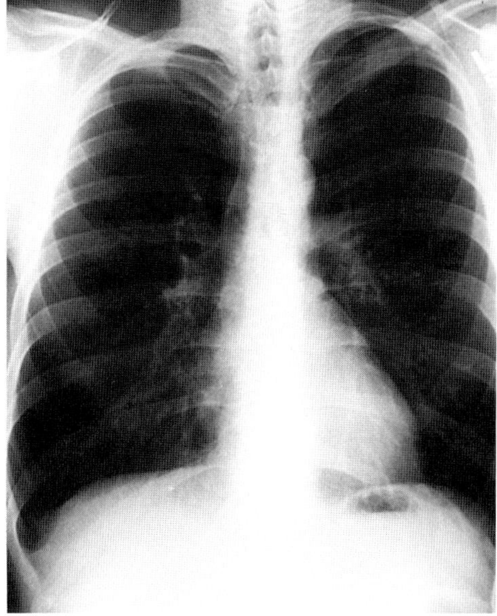

FIG. 4. An example of a digital radiographic image obtained using an imaging plate and subsequently two hard copy films were generated. The image on the *right* is processed by the computer to simulate a conventional radiograph, and the image on the *left* uses a different computer processing scheme to edge-enhance the original image.

at this time. Digital radiography has been most widely applied in the intensive care unit setting.

PORTABLE DIGITAL CHEST RADIOGRAPHY

The same portable x-ray generator and x-ray tube system that are used for conventional portable chest radiography can be used with an IP to obtain digital radiographs of very sick patients who require portable radiography. The IP is substituted for the portable screen-film system, and the contrast and film density can be manipulated by the computer after the IP has been exposed, so that repeat portable examinations can be eliminated to a large degree. The radiographic dose can also be reduced for most applications. The ability to obtain consistent radiographic density on a portable radiograph even when the patient is overexposed or underexposed is the primary benefit that digital radiography offers the radiologist and the patient. The application of digital radiography technology has been most widespread in the intensive care unit setting, and this is the most likely immediate application of the technology for most radiology departments (6,7).

CONVENTIONAL TOMOGRAPHY

Conventional tomography is a technique that is still used in some centers to rapidly clarify the presence or absence of a solitary pulmonary nodule and to classify it as benign or indeterminate. The patients who are referred for conventional tomography for the workup of a possible solitary pulmonary nodule can be divided into five categories (8,9). Twenty percent of the patients referred will have resolved whatever abnormality was identified on the screening chest film. This is demonstrated using conventional fluoroscopy at approximately 80 kVp before any conventional tomograms are obtained. Twenty percent will have an extrapulmonary lesion such as an area of pleural thickening or some bony abnormality that is superimposed on the thorax. This finding is easily identified on conventional tomography. Twenty percent will have characteristic benign calcifications within a granuloma or hamartoma. Twenty percent will have a characteristic shape that suggests that they are either benign lesions or possibly malignant lesions. The final 20 percent will require further study. The additional radiographic evaluations that are usually done at this point involve either transthoracic needle aspiration biopsy of the lesion or quantitative CT analysis of the nodule.

Either linear or complex motion tomography can be used to evaluate and characterize the presence of a solitary pulmonary nodule. The examination is usually performed at a lower kVp (65–75 kVp), which increases the

subject contrast within the pulmonary nodule. This higher subject contrast maximizes the chances of identifying calcification within the lesion. The technique that we recommend for conventional tomography of a solitary pulmonary nodule is as follows: Linear tomography is preferred to complex motion tomography, because of the increased likelihood of identifying calcifications within the nodule on linear rather than complex motion tomography (10). A 15° tomographic arc is used with approximately 0.5-second exposure time using 65–75 kVp. The total exposure is usually ∼25–50 mas. Kodak Lannex regular screens are used along with Kodak OG film. This screen-film combination is a high-contrast system that increases the likelihood of identifying calcifications within the nodule. With the patient in the supine position, 6-mm–thick coronal sections are obtained at 10 mm intervals through the area of the lesion for initial localization. Then, 6-mm–thick coronal sections are obtained at 2 mm intervals through the entire lesion.

Conventional tomography can be used to study the hilum and the mediastinum. The evaluations are usually done in three projections. The technique works best at a higher kVp than the study of pulmonary nodules (e.g., 95–105 kVp), and the use of a trough-shaped x-ray tube filter is also recommended. Kodak Lannex medium screen and the Kodak OC film are recommended for this study. This screen-film system, higher kVp, and the use of a trough filter help to decrease subject contrast, which improves the final tomographic images of the hilum and mediastinum. Slice thickness and slice spacing are usually customized by the radiologist for a particular examination. The routine use of complex motion tomography and 2 mm slice thickness at 5 mm intervals has been satisfactory in my experience. At this time, CT is used instead of conventional tomography for most evaluations of the hilum and mediastinum.

COMPUTED TOMOGRAPHY

CT has revolutionized thoracic imaging since its introduction in the 1970s. The equipment has had a steady evolution, and CT is a very good, noninvasive technique to evaluate diseases affecting the chest wall, pleura, lung parenchyma, mediastinum, pericardium, heart, and aorta. A brief description of CT equipment and CT scanning techniques will follow, including details of the cine-CT scanner.

The current generation of CT scanners, such as those made by General Electric (11,12), have five major components. There is the power distribution unit, high-voltage generator, computer subsystems, operator's console, a remote console, and a table gantry subassembly. The internal scanner geometry that is currently used on the newer slip ring CT scanners and also on the older nonslip-ring CT scanners is either a rotating x-ray tube and rotating set of detectors, or a stationary set of detectors and a rotating x-ray tube. Modern scanners are capable of obtaining a scout view, or digital projection radiograph, that aids in planning any CT examination of the body. The current generation of CT scanners have high-voltage x-ray generators capable of producing images at 80–140 kVp. This can be done using x-ray tube currents between 10–300 ma, depending on the kVp used. The scan field of view should match the size of the patient, typically 35 or 48 cm. The display field of view should again be chosen to match the patient's diameter and also may be reduced further to obtain retargeted high-resolution images of the chest (i.e., a display field of view of 25 cm). The latest generation of slip-ring CT scanners can obtain routine images in 1 second and use a partial or half-scan mode on the order of 0.6 seconds. The scan plane can be varied in thickness from 1.0–10 mm. The 1.0 mm collimation is essential in assessing pulmonary nodules and in obtaining high-resolution images of the lung parenchyma. The standard spatial resolution that is possible on the current generation of CT scanners is approximately 0.78 mm. There are special high-resolution modes that can be used to obtain 0.50 mm of limiting resolution (13,14). A high spatial resolution computer algorithm is essential in assessing diffuse lung disease. The matrix size of the image that is usually used for obtaining thoracic images is 512×512, with a 40 cm field of view that provides a pixel size of 0.78 mm. It is possible to obtain even higher resolution by reprocessing the images using a so-called retargeting procedure that reconstructs a small area of interest that gives increased resolution; in high-resolution CT imaging of the lungs, this retargeted field of view varies between 20–25 cm for optimum work. The retargeted imaging technique provides the most optimal image quality in assessing diffuse lung disease.

Modern CT scanners can display each image as it is obtained or a batch of images can be obtained in a more rapid or dynamic mode with the computer reconstructing the images at the end of the study. Dynamic scanning is helpful if a volume of thorax needs to be examined rapidly after the administration of a bolus of contrast material, such as in the evaluation of the mediastinum or pulmonary hilum for adenopathy and in the assessment of aortic dissection. Dynamic scanning is also useful at one level in assessing aortic dissection, where multiple images are obtained one after another, and the collection of images provides a temporal CT angiogram in the axial plane of the aorta, which is quite helpful in assessing dissection. It is important to deliver any intravenous contrast material in a consistent compact bolus for contrast-enhanced CT examinations. A power injector designed for CT scanning is essential. The amount of contrast delivered is typically 150 ml of an agent containing 240–280 mg of iodine per ml of contrast. The rate of injection is usually set at 1 ml/second, with a scan delay

of 40 seconds. This scan delay will load the patient with 40 ml of contrast prior to obtaining the first CT image. Contrast-enhanced examinations are most useful in assessing pulmonary hilar adenopathy, mediastinal masses, and invasion of the mediastinum by adjacent tumor and aortic disease.

The newer CT systems (e.g., GE 9800 HiSpeed Advantage) use a slip-ring design and provide a new, faster dynamic scanning method known as spiral scanning (Fig. 5). The spiral scans are especially helpful in assessing pulmonary nodules and in providing three-dimensional reconstructions of mediastinal structures, such as the heart and the central airways (13–15). The spiral scanning techniques can examine a volume of anatomy much faster than older dynamic scanning techniques, and this reduces the time of the examinations on critically ill patients and also reduces the total volume of intravenous contrast necessary to complete a given study.

The cine-CT scanner provides an innovative CT scanner geometry, where a scanning electron beam is deflected around a ring of tungsten anodes that emit x-rays and are detected by another set of detectors that are also in the scanner gantry. The cine-CT scanner can obtain images with a scan time as short as 50 msec. The cine-CT scanner is particularly well adapted to examining cardiac patients and trauma or pediatric patients where cardiac, respiratory, or patient motion is a major factor in de-

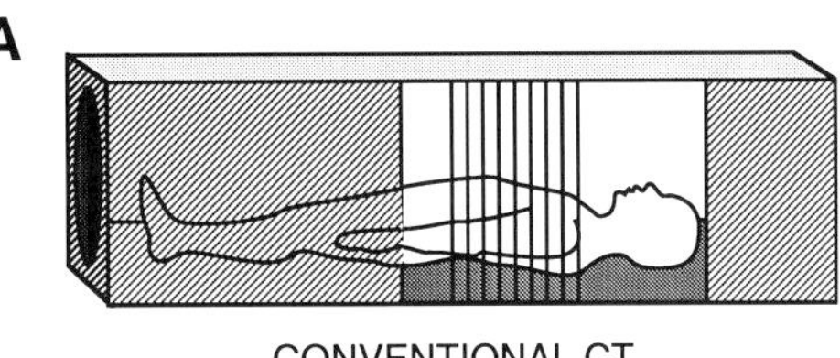

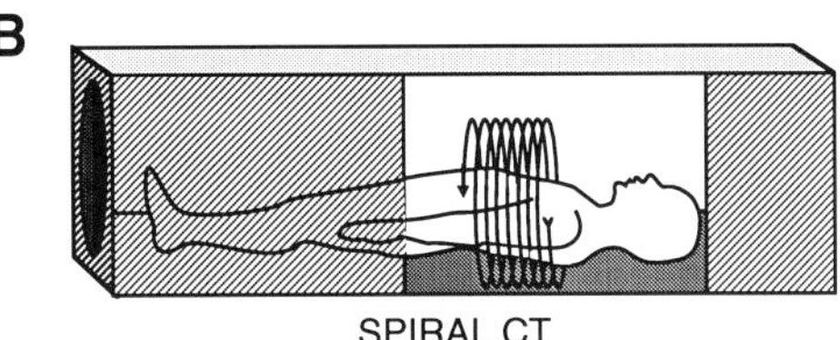

FIG. 5. Conventional CT scanning acquisition is illustrated in (**A**) at the top. The spiral CT scanning technique is shown in (**B**) at the bottom. In spiral scanning the raw image data are obtained continuously using a slip-ring CT scanner and a CT table that moves during the scan acquisition period. There are three important parameters in spiral CT scanning that determine the final image resolution: scan collimation, table speed, and interscan gap or separation. The thinking now is that these should be fairly symmetric (i.e., 10 mm collimation, 10 mm/sec table speed, and 10 mm interval between scans). The scan interval can be varied after the examination is completed, and it is this feature that really aids in evaluating pulmonary nodules retrospectively.

grading the images that might be obtained on a standard CT scanner. The cine-CT scanner design was described in detail in 1984 (16). This scanner consists of an electron beam scan tube, a stationary detector array, and a data acquisition system. The electron beam scan tube assembly comprises an electron gun, which produces electrons that are then accelerated electronically. The electrons are then focused by a set of electromagnetic lenses to impact a circular tungsten target that produces x-rays that are detected by a detector system opposite the tungsten target ring. The system generates approximately 650 ma beam at 125 kVp. The beam is then focused and bent through an angle of 33–37° and swept along the tungsten target mentioned previously through an angle of rotation of approximately 210°. The x-rays emitted from the tungsten target pass through the patient and are detected on the opposite side of the ring. The system can obtain a pair of scans simultaneously by a fan beam of radiation that is generated from the tungsten targets and subsequently collimated into two scans of approximately 8 mm in thickness. Two rings of stationary detectors are above the patient and receive the transmitted fan beam radiation to produce the two simultaneous images. The detector system comprises an array of scintillation crystals that are coupled with photodiode arrays. The signals in the photodiode are subsequently digitized and the digital data are reconstructed by a computer. The scanner can be operated in three modes. The first mode is a rapid sequential mode, where the entire heart can be examined within a single heartbeat. The second is a flow mode, which obtains 50 msec scans that are separated by a longer interscan delay, which is approximately equal to that of one or two R-R intervals. In the flow mode of operation, the scans are cardiac-gated and obtained so that the heart is in diastole. An additional dual section study, where two images are obtained, can be done at one level at the rate of 18 frames/second, or an eight-section volume study encompassing the whole left ventricle can be obtained at a frame rate of 4.5 frames/second. The cine-CT scanner has proved useful in evaluating left and right ventricular functions, myocardial perfusion, coronary artery bypass graft patency, central pulmonary thromboembolism, and upper airway obstruction.

MAGNETIC RESONANCE IMAGING OF THE THORAX

Magnetic resonance proton imaging has provided a new technique to assess the anatomic structures within the thorax and is useful for assessing a variety of disease states in the thorax (17–21). MRI may be used for assessing invasion of the mediastinum and chest wall by tumor. This is particularly helpful in the case of Pancoast tumors and is discussed more by Webb in chapter 3.

MRI is also a valuable tool in assessing aortic dissection and invasion of the pericardium and heart by tumor. However, MRI examination of the thorax is more expensive and more time consuming than CT, and does require high-quality electrocardiographic gating and in some cases respiratory artifact suppression techniques to assess the thoracic anatomy adequately.

MRI of the thorax has been performed using field strengths from 0.06–4.0T. Both permanent magnet and superconducting magnet magnetic resonance imagers can provide quality images of intrathoracic anatomy. The discussion that follows is based on my imaging experience acquired using a 1.5T General Electric (Milwaukee, WI) Signa MR scanner. This device is capable of spin echo and gradient echo imaging. The spin echo techniques with T1-weighted sequences are the best for anatomical detail, and the gradient echo sequences are very helpful in trying to assess flow. This device does provide cardiac gating and respiratory artifact suppression techniques. This machine also offers presaturation to suppress the flow-induced phase artifacts in flowing blood in the heart and great vessels within the thorax. This machine also offers first-order flow motion compensation or velocity compensation that is particularly useful in gradient echo sequences to suppress motion and flow-induced phase artifacts. General Electric and other vendors have very active research programs that are pushing the capabilities of MRI rapidly forward, including the development of echo planar imaging, magnetic resonance angiography, and ultrafast gradient echo imaging.

The techniques that we are going to describe herein are general techniques using both cardiac gating and respiratory artifact suppression for assessing the thorax in the axial and coronal planes. The general magnetic resonance examination of the thorax uses spin echo cardiac-gated and respiratory-compensated axial images using a short TR and a short TE value. The number of excitations used varies from two to four in these studies. The respiratory compensation technique on the GE 1.5T Signa MR scanner provides the best images using four excitations. The imaging time can be reduced by reducing the number of phase-encoding steps to 128. This may be necessary in the long TE, TR techniques. The TR value is set by the heart rate. If the patient's heart rate is 60, the TR value then is 1000 msec. TE values typically range between 20–30 msec, depending on the artifact suppression techniques that are used. Routinely, both presaturation artifact suppression is used with spin echo imaging and flow compensation techniques with gradient echo imaging. The thorax is examined from apex to the diaphragm using 10-mm–thick transaxial spin echo images with short TR and TE values and a 5 mm interslice gap. The entire thorax then is usually examined in ~15 transaxial images. The exam can be extended down below the diaphragm to assess the adrenal glands for enlargement and abnormal signal intensity.

The coronal spin echo examination is also obtained using short TR and short TE techniques. The coronal images are obtained to cover the entire thorax from anterior to posterior. The coronal images are particularly useful in assessing antero-posterior window abnormality, diaphragm abnormality, and thoracic inlet abnormality. The coronal images are obtained with an 8-mm–slice thickness and 4 mm interslice gap.

After the initial spin echo images are obtained, additional magnetic resonance tomograms using spin echo or gradient echo techniques can be used. Gated gradient echo techniques are routinely used in both the axial and oblique sagittal tomographic planes to assess the aorta for aortic dissection and aortic aneurysm formation. The gradient echo images are also routinely obtained to assess abnormality within the pulmonary parenchyma, such as suspected pulmonary arterial venous malformation and carcinoid tumor. Additionally, long TR, TE images may be obtained to distinguish areas of postobstructive pneumonia from tumor. Long TR, TE sequences are also useful in trying to assess the difference between recurrent tumor or persistent tumor in the mediastinum from mediastinal fibrosis following radiation and chemotherapy. There are new fat suppression techniques that are useful again in trying to assess recurrent tumor from fibrosis in the mediastinum. The magnetic resonance contrast agent, gadolinium diethylenetriaminepentaacetic acid, has also been used to try to assess recurrent tumor versus fibrosis in the mediastinum. The recurrent tumor will enhance using gadolinium diethylenetriaminepentaacetic acid, whereas the fibrosis will not.

REFERENCES

1. Johnson JL, Abernathy DI. Diagnostic imaging procedure volume in the United States. *Radiology* 1983;146:851–853.
2. Newell JD, Kelsey CA. Digital radiology of the thorax. In Newell JN, Kelsey CA, eds. *Digital imaging in diagnostic radiology.* New York: Churchill Livingston, 1990.
3. Seeley GW, Newell JD. The use of psychophysical principles in the design of a total digital radiology department. *Radiol Clin North Am* 1985;23:341–348.
4. Elam EA, Rehm K, Hillman BJ, Maloney K, Fajardo LL, McNeill K. Efficacy of digital radiography for the detection of pneumothorax: comparison with conventional chest radiography. *Am J Roentgenol* 1992;158:509–514.
5. Merritt CRB, Matthews CC, Scheinhorn D, Balter S. Digital imaging of the chest. *J Thorac Imaging* 1985;1:1–13.
6. Marglin SI, Rowberg AH, Godwin JD. Preliminary experience with portable digital imaging for intensive care radiography. *J Thorac Imaging* 1990;5:49–54.
7. Sagel SS, Jost RG, Glazer HS. Digital mobile radiography. *J Thorac Imaging* 1990;5:36–48.
8. Muhm JR. Current place of plain-film tomography in chest disease. *J Thorac Imaging* 1985;1:32–38.
9. Huston J, Mujm JR. Solitary pulmonary opacities on plain tomography. *Radiology* 1987;163:481–485.
10. Chassen MH, McCarthy MJ. Pulmonary nodules: detection of calcification by linear and pluridirectional movement in tomographic study. *Radiology* 1985;156:589–592.
11. General Electric Product Datasheet on the CT 9800 Quickscanner System. General Electric Company Medical Systems Group, Milwaukee, WI.
12. General Electric Product Datasheet, B7910JA/JE. CT 9800 Scanner System. General Electric Company Medical Systems Group, Milwaukee, WI.
13. Mayo JR, Webb WR, Gould R, et al. High-resolution CT of the lungs: an optimal approach. *Radiology* 1987;163:507–510.
14. Mayo JR. High resolution computed tomography: technical aspects. *Radiol Clin North Am* 1991;29:1043–1049.
15. Costello P, Anderson W, Blume D. Pulmonary nodule: evaluation with spiral volumetric CT. *Radiology* 1991;179:875–876.
16. Kalender WA, Seissler W, Klotz E, Vock P. Spiral volumetric CT with single-breath-hold technique, continuous transport, and continuous scanner rotation. *Radiology* 1990;176:181–183.
17. Vock P, Soucek M, Daepp M, Kalender WA. Lung: spiral volumetric CT and single breath-hold technique. *Radiology* 1990;176:864–867.
18. Lipton MJ, Higgins CB, Farmer D, Boyd DP. Cardiac imaging with a high speed cine-CT scanner: preliminary results. *Radiology* 1984;152:579–582.
19. Spritzer C, Gamsu G, Sostman HD. Magnetic resonance imaging of the thorax: techniques, current applications, and future directions. *J Thorac Imag* 1989;4:1–18.
20. Swensen SJ, Ehman RL, Brown LR. Magnetic resonance imaging of the thorax. *J Thorac Imag* 1989;4:19–33.
21. White RD, Higgins CB. Magnetic resonance imaging of thoracic vascular disease. *J Thorac Imag* 1989;4:34–50.

Thoracic Radiology, edited by
J.D. Newell, Jr., and R.D. Tarver,
Raven Press, Ltd., New York © 1993.

CHAPTER 2

Pulmonary Infections

Dewey J. Conces, Jr.

Pulmonary infections are a major cause of disease in both hospitalized and nonhospitalized patients, with pneumonia being the sixth leading cause of death in the United States (1). Pneumonias, which account for only 15 percent of nosocomial infections, are the number one cause of death due to hospital-acquired infections (2). The potential fatal outcome of a pulmonary infection leads to a sense of urgency in making a diagnosis when pneumonia is clinically suspected.

When pneumonia is clinically suspected, a chest radiograph is usually obtained to confirm its presence. The chest radiograph will allow identification of an abnormality that is consistent with a pulmonary infection. The radiographic pattern, however, is not specific enough to allow identification of the causative organism (3). Although the radiographic pattern is not specific for the causative organism, it can, when combined with clinical information, allow formation of a list of those organisms that are most likely the cause of the infection. This list will aid in choosing additional diagnostic studies. Antibiotic therapy is usually begun at the time of presentation before the results of specific laboratory tests are available. The list of most likely causative organisms will assist in selecting antibiotics for empiric therapy. The chest radiograph also allows detection of complications resulting from the pneumonia and can be used to monitor the response to antibiotic therapy.

This chapter presents a practical approach to the evaluation of the chest radiograph of a patient with suspected pneumonia. Important clinical information that is essential for optimal interpretation of the radiograph will be presented. Various radiographic patterns and the organisms that cause them will be discussed. Most of the discussion will center on the evaluation of the immunocompetent patient. The assessment of immunocompromised patients with suspected pneumonia will not be covered in depth. Several in-depth discussions of pulmonary infections in the immunocompromised host are available, and the reader is referred to these for further information on this complex group of patients (4–6).

CLINICAL ASPECTS OF PNEUMONIA

A variety of clinical factors need to be considered when evaluating the radiographic findings in a patient with suspected pneumonia. The clinical setting in which the pneumonia develops and the presence of predisposing factors should be considered. The type of clinical presentation provides important clues as to the potential etiologic agents. Unique physical findings may be present that may provide a clue to the offending organism. These clinical findings need to be integrated with the radiographic findings to realize fully the potential information that is contained within the radiograph of the patient with suspected pneumonia.

Acquiring this information requires close communication with the clinical services treating the patient. Close interaction between the referring clinician and the radiologist will optimize the evaluation and initial therapy of the patient.

COMMUNITY-ACQUIRED PNEUMONIA

Pneumonias can be divided into two general categories: community-acquired pneumonia and hospital-acquired or nosocomial pneumonia. Pneumonias that develop outside of the hospital environment are classified as community-acquired pneumonias. This group can be further categorized by the presence of any underlying risk factors. The presence of certain risk factors predisposes the patient to infection from different groups of organisms (Table 1).

D. J. Conces, Jr.: Department of Radiology, Indiana University Medical Center, University Hospital, Indianapolis, Indiana 46223.

TABLE 1. *Underlying conditions in community-acquired pneumonia*

Underlying condition	Usual organisms
None	*Streptococcus pneumoniae*
	Mycoplasma
	Legionella virus
Recent influenza	*Staphylococcus aureus*
	S. pneumoniae
	Hemophilus influenzae
Chronic alcoholism	Gram-negative bacilli
	S. pneumoniae
Aspiration	Mouth anaerobes
Cystic fibrosis	*Pseudomonas*
	S. aureus
Chronic bronchitis	*S. pneumoniae*
	H. influenzae
Old age	*S. pneumoniae*
	S. aureus
Asplenia or hyposplenism	*S. pneumoniae*

Most pneumonias developing in normal adults are due to either *Streptococcus pneumoniae, Mycoplasma pneumoniae, Legionella,* or virus (7). Of this group, *S. pneumoniae* is the most common cause of pneumonia. In recent years the spectrum of organisms causing community-acquired pneumonia has changed, with a decrease in the incidence of *S. pneumoniae* and an increase in other etiologic agents, such as *Chlamydia pneumoniae* (8). Patients with underlying medical conditions are at risk for developing pneumonia from other organisms. Recent infection by influenza is associated with an increased incidence of pneumonia due to *Staphylococcus aureus* (9). *S. pneumoniae* and *Hemophilus influenzae* are also common causes of pneumonia following an influenza infection. Alcoholics are frequently colonized with Gram-negative organisms and are at increased risk of aspiration (10). This results in an increased incidence of Gram-negative bacillary infections, especially those caused by *Klebsiella* (11,12). Individuals with altered consciousness due to seizure disorders, previous strokes, narcotic abuse, or anesthesia are at risk for aspirating pharyngeal secretions with resultant aspiration pneumonia (13). Aspiration pneumonia and the lung abscess that may develop are usually due to anaerobic organisms that normally inhabit the mouth. Poor oral hygiene with resulting periodontitis results in an increased number of mouth anaerobes, with a resultant increased risk of developing aspiration pneumonia (13). Patients with cystic fibrosis are frequently colonized with *Pseudomonas aeruginosa* or *S. aureus* and may develop pneumonia due to these organisms (14). Similarly, patients with chronic bronchitis are often colonized with *H. influenzae* or *S. pneumoniae* (15,16). Pneumonia in these patients frequently represents a progression of the infection from the bronchus to the alveolus. Elderly patients, especially those residing in a nursing home, have an increase in pneumonias due to *S. aureus, S. pneumoniae,* and

Gram-negative bacilli (16–18). Asplenia caused by splenectomy or hyposplenism due to sickle cell disease, amyloidosis, or sarcoidosis predisposes to infection by *S. pneumoniae* (19).

NOSOCOMIAL PNEUMONIA

Hospital-acquired or nosocomial pneumonias are pulmonary infections that develop in hospitalized patients. These pneumonias are caused by a different group of organisms than cause the typical community-acquired pneumonia. The oropharynx of the normal nonhospitalized individual is colonized predominantly by low virulence Gram-positive organisms. Following hospitalization, the population of the oral flora changes. The patient becomes colonized with more virulent, often antibiotic-resistant Gram-negative bacilli (20). Colonization by Gram-negative bacilli increases with the severity of the illness, with colonization rates reaching 73% in critically ill patients. These organisms when aspirated may produce a severe pneumonia. Gram-negative bacilli that commonly cause nosocomial pneumonia include *Pseudomonas, Serratia, Klebsiella, Escherichia coli, Proteus mirabalis, Acinetobacter,* and *Enterobacter* (21). *Legionella* has been associated with point-source outbreaks of hospital-acquired pneumonia (22). The source of these outbreaks is usually a contaminated water source within the hospital. Although Gram-negative bacilli are the most common cause of nosocomial pneumonia, Gram-positive bacteria are responsible for a significant number of hospital-acquired pneumonias. Nosocomial pneumonias are frequently caused by *S. aureus, S. pneumoniae,* and anaerobic bacteria (23). Immunocompromised patients are also susceptible to a large number of opportunistic organisms, including *Aspergillus, Phycomycetes, Pneumocystis,* and cytomegalovirus (4).

A variety of predisposing factors may be found in the hospitalized patient that contribute to the development of nosocomial pneumonia. The patients are often elderly with the associated age-related decline in immune system responsiveness (24). Administration of antibiotics is associated with the suppression of low virulence organisms that normally reside in the oropharynx and the development of Gram-negative colonization (25). Endotracheal intubation bypasses the upper airway defense mechanisms and provides direct access for oral secretions to enter the lung. This results in a high incidence of nosocomial pneumonias in intubated patients (26). Impaired mentation from drugs, anesthesia, and surgery predisposes the patient to aspiration (24). Surgery, especially thoracic and upper abdominal, is associated with an increased occurrence of pulmonary infection (24). Admission into an intensive care unit has been shown to increase the risk of acquiring nosocomial pulmonary infection (27).

The diagnosis of nosocomial pneumonia may be difficult (28). The signs and symptoms usually seen with pneumonia may not develop. When they do occur there may be underlying conditions that may produce similar findings. Because of this one must always consider the possibility of pulmonary infection in a hospitalized patient who undergoes deterioration in their clinical condition or who develops an infiltrate or pleural effusion on their chest radiograph.

RATE OF PROGRESSION

Pneumonias can be further classified into groups according to the acuteness of their clinical presentation. Acute pneumonias are those with an abrupt onset, developing in less than 24 hours. The patients typically have an abrupt onset of fever, sometimes with rigors. A productive cough is usually present, and they may complain of pleuritic chest pain. Radiographic changes are usually present at the time of presentation and without appropriate therapy will progress rapidly (Fig. 1). Acute pneumonias are usually due to bacterial infections by *S. pneumonia, H. influenzae, S. aureus,* and Gram-negative bacilli (15,25,29,30). Pneumonia due to *Legionella* may have a gradual onset, but the most common presentation is an acute illness that is clinically indistinguishable from pneumococcal infection (29). Anaerobic infections, which usually have a more gradual onset, may also present in an acute fashion (31). Anaerobic infections that produce necrotizing pneumonia typically have an acute

presentation (13). A biphasic illness characterized by respiratory symptoms, suggesting a viral infection followed by an acute respiratory infection, suggests that a *S. aureus* pneumonia has developed complicating an influenza infection (9).

Subacute infections are those in which the symptoms develop gradually over 1–7 days. The fever tends not to be as high as seen in cases with acute progression and is not associated with chills. The cough may be nonproductive. Systemic complaints such as myalgia, fatigue, headache, and sore throat may be present. The radiographic findings progress at a slower rate. *M. pneumoniae* and viruses frequently follow a subacute course (32). *Legionella* pneumonia may also progress in a subacute fashion (29) (Fig. 2). Anaerobic infections commonly have a subacute or chronic presentation. In one series of 147 anaerobic pulmonary infections, 57% had a subacute or chronic clinical course (13). Infections by the pathogenic fungi—*Histoplasma capsulatum, Coccidioides immitis, Cryptococcus neoformans,* and *Blastomyces dermatiditis*—are frequently asymptomatic or may have a subacute presentation (33–36).

Pulmonary infections that develop insidiously, with their symptoms being present weeks or months prior to presentation, can be termed chronic infections. Fever, if present, is usually low grade and may be intermittent. The cough may or may not be productive. The radiographic findings change slowly on serial radiographs, but may be advanced at the time of presentation (Fig. 3). Fungal infections due to *H. capsulatum, C. immitis, B.*

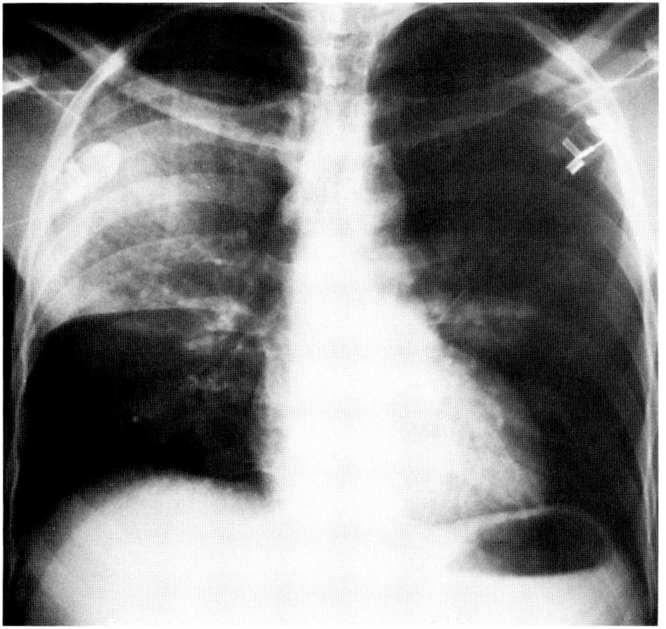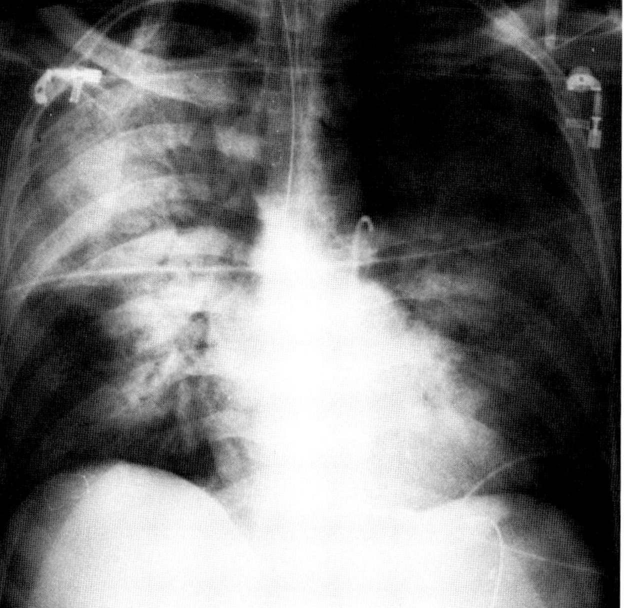

FIG. 1. Young man with *Streptococcus pneumoniae* pneumonia. **(A)** Initial radiograph demonstrates right upper lobe consolidation. **(B)** Patient's condition deteriorated rapidly with a chest radiograph obtained 36 hours later demonstrating increased right upper lobe infiltrate and new infiltrates in the right middle lobe, lingula, and left lower lobe. Patient died 2 days later.

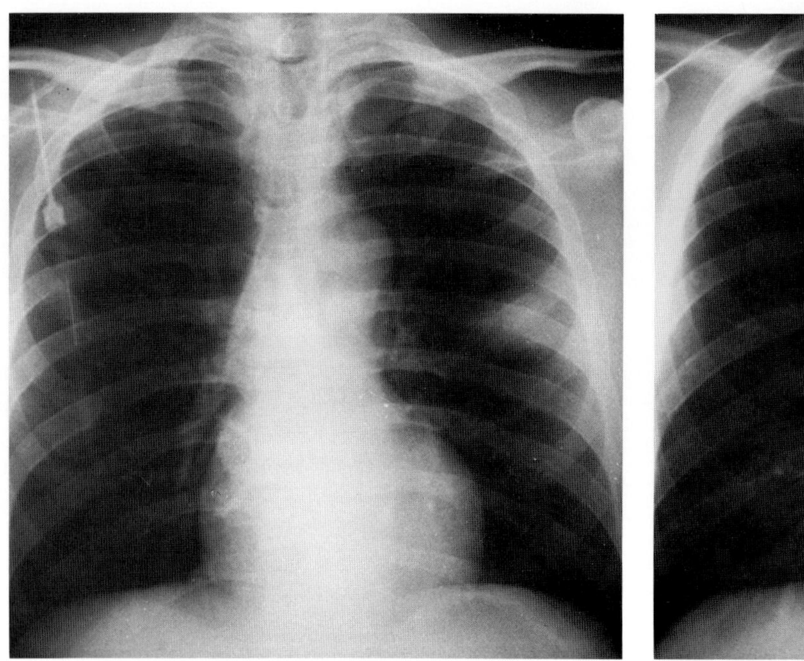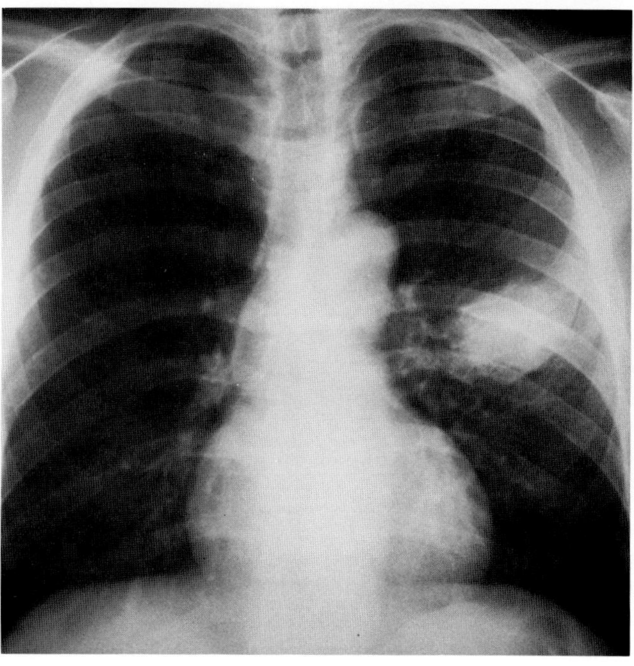

FIG. 2. Renal transplant patient who developed a fever and nonproductive cough. **(A)** Initial chest radiograph demonstrated a nodular infiltrate in the left midlung. Needle biopsy yielded *Legionella*. **(B)** Radiograph obtained 3 days later shows an interval increase in the size of the infiltrate.

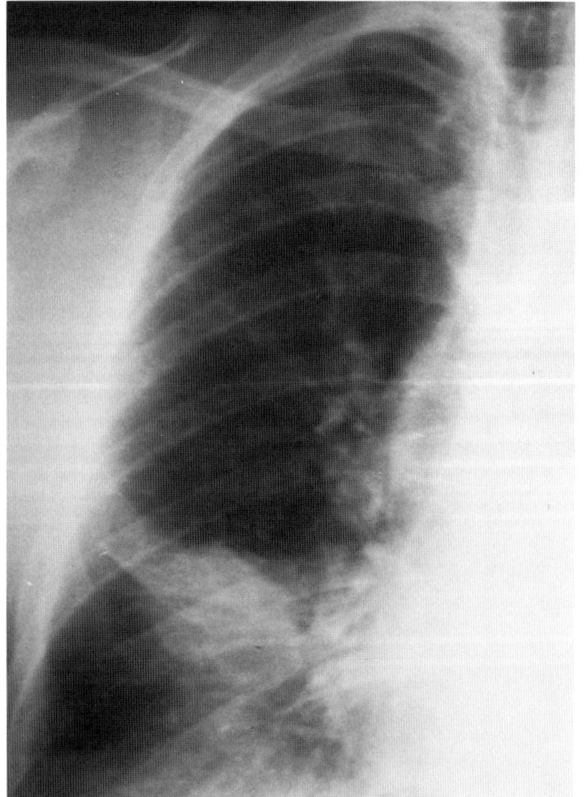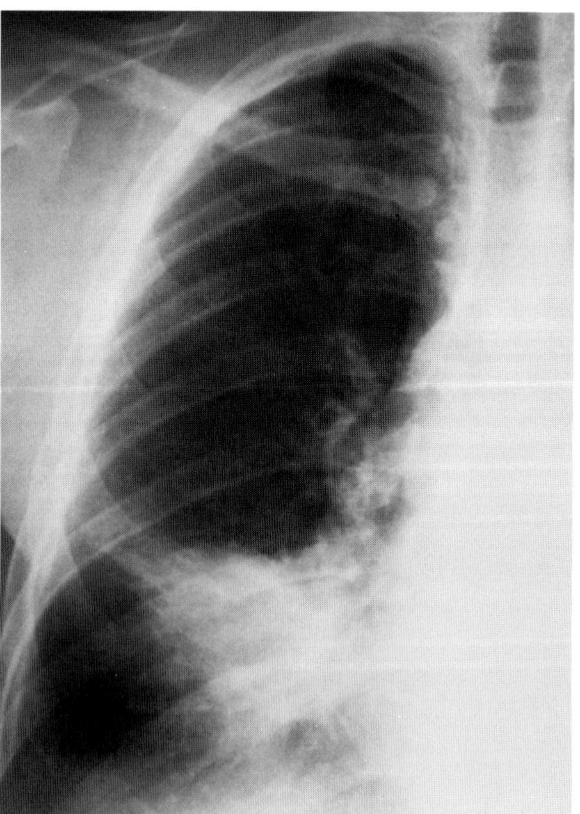

FIG. 3. Patient with a 1-month history of cough. **(A)** Initial chest radiograph shows a mass-like infiltrate in the right middle lobe. **(B)** Chest radiograph obtained 5 months later shows only a slight increase in the infiltrate. Needle biopsy of the mass yielded *Actinomyces israelii*.

dermatitidis, and *C. neoformans* may present in a chronic fashion (33–36). These fungal infections have several clinical presentations, which may be subacute or chronic in nature. Infections due to *Mycobacterium tuberculosis* and the atypical mycobacteria may also present in both a subacute or chronic fashion (37,38). Some anaerobic infections, including those that progress to the formation of a lung abscess, may be very indolent in their presentation (31). These infections may have very few symptoms, sometimes presently only with weight loss or unexplained anemia (13). Actinomycosis may have a chronic presentation that, in some cases, is so delayed that extension across the pleural space with chest wall involvement occurs (39) (Fig. 3).

ADDITIONAL HISTORICAL INFORMATION

Other historical facts may help identify the infecting organism. Travel history is important because the patient may acquire an infection endemic to an area already visited. A visit to the Ohio River Valley raises the possibility of *Histoplasma* infection and a trip to the Southwest suggests that *Coccidioides* is a potential agent (33,34). Occupational exposures should be considered when evaluating a patient with pneumonia. Bird handlers are at risk for psittacosis (40). Gardeners and florists may develop sporotrichosis (41). Chicken farmers may inhale chicken dropping particles that contain *Histoplasma* (33). Hunters may develop tularemia, whereas butchers and tanners may be exposed to anthrax or Q-fever (42–44).

Nonpulmonary signs and symptoms may provide a clue to the cause of a pneumonia. *Legionella* infections may be associated with gastrointestinal symptoms, such as jaundice, vomiting, and diarrhea (45). *Mycoplasma* pneumonia may be accompanied by myringitis (32). Halitosis or fetid sputum suggests an infection by anaerobic organisms (13).

RADIOLOGY

In most patients with pneumonia the initial chest radiograph will demonstrate changes in the lung parenchyma consistent with a pulmonary infection. These radiographic changes can be used to divide pneumonias into several general categories: lobar pneumonia, bronchopneumonia, nodular pneumonia, and interstitial pneumonia. The various radiographic patterns, although not specific, tend to be caused by certain groups of organisms. This list of potential organisms, when integrated with the clinical information, may significantly narrow the list of diagnostic possibilities. The narrowed diagnostic differential will allow for more rational evaluation and therapy of the patient.

It must be remembered, however, that there are no radiographic findings that are diagnostic of a specific organism. There is a wide range of radiographic findings that can be produced by a given organism, with overlap occurring between different organisms.

LOBAR PNEUMONIA

Lobar pneumonia is a term used to describe a pneumonia that primarily involves the alveolus and results in consolidation of involved lung. Inhaled microorganisms that reach the alveolus produce an inflammatory process that results in inflammatory exudate and edema filling the alveoli. Untreated, the process will spread through the pores of Kohn and the canals of Lambert to adjacent lung, involving first a segment and then given enough time the entire lobe. In the earliest stages a chest radiograph may only show a faint shadow. As the disease progresses a focal segmental area of consolidation will appear. The radiographs usually show involvement of only one or two segments. Without appropriate therapy the infiltrate will spread until the entire lobe is consolidated.

The bronchi are not primarily involved and remain air-filled. The air-filled bronchi, when surrounded by alveoli filled with inflammatory exudate, will produce air bronchograms. The presence of air bronchograms indicates that the density seen on the radiograph is due to consolidation of lung. Because the airways are not involved, there is little volume loss associated with the infiltrate.

Pneumonias that produce a lobar pattern of consolidation are frequently bacterial in etiology. Although *S. pneumoniae* is classically described as a lobar pneumonia, it frequently presents with segmental involvement (Fig. 4). Some series have found a patchy bronchopneumonic pattern to be more common than lobar consolidation (46). Pneumonia due to *K. pneumoniae* produces lobar consolidation. The initial radiograph may show nonsegmental consolidation that spreads to involve the entire lobe (11). Pneumonia caused by *Klebsiella* may be associated with enlargement of the lobe, with resultant bulging of the fissures (47). Infection due to *Legionella* initially presents with patchy peripheral infiltrates that progress to a consolidative pattern in 70 percent of the cases (48). Lobar consolidation may also develop in pneumonias due to *S. aureus, H. influenzae,* and *Nocardia* (49–52).

Fungal infections due to *Histoplasma, Coccidioides,* and *Blastomyces* may produce similar infiltrates (33,53–55). In the immunocompromised host, *Cryptococcus* may produce areas of consolidation (56). Parenchymal consolidation is commonly seen in patients with pri-

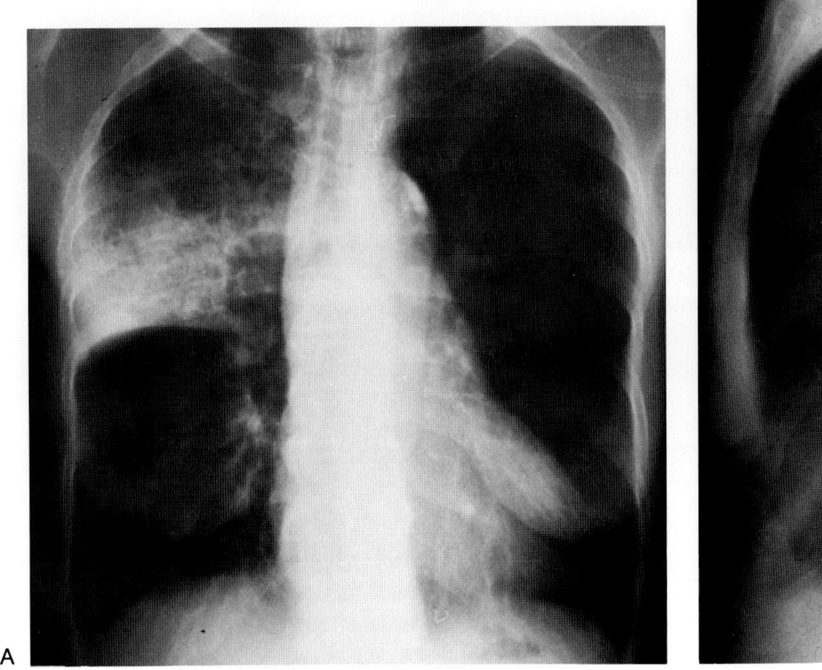 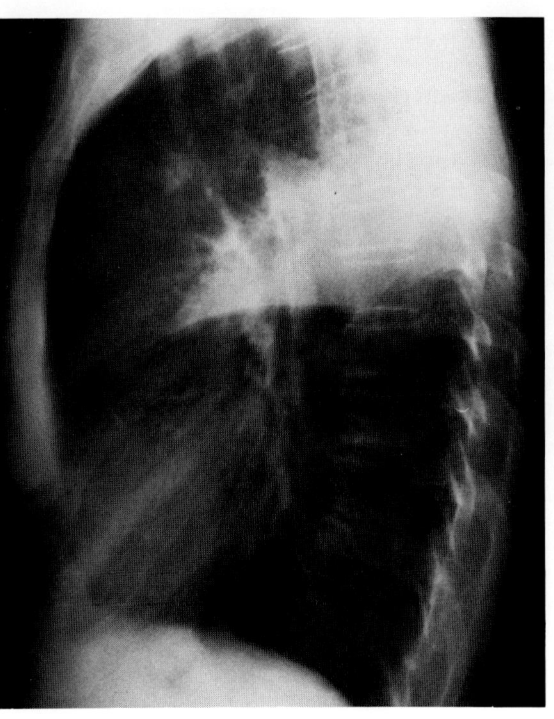

FIG. 4. Patient with pneumococccal pneumonia. Posteroanterior (**A**) and lateral (**B**) chest radiographs demonstrate consolidation involving the anterior and posterior segments of the right upper lobe.

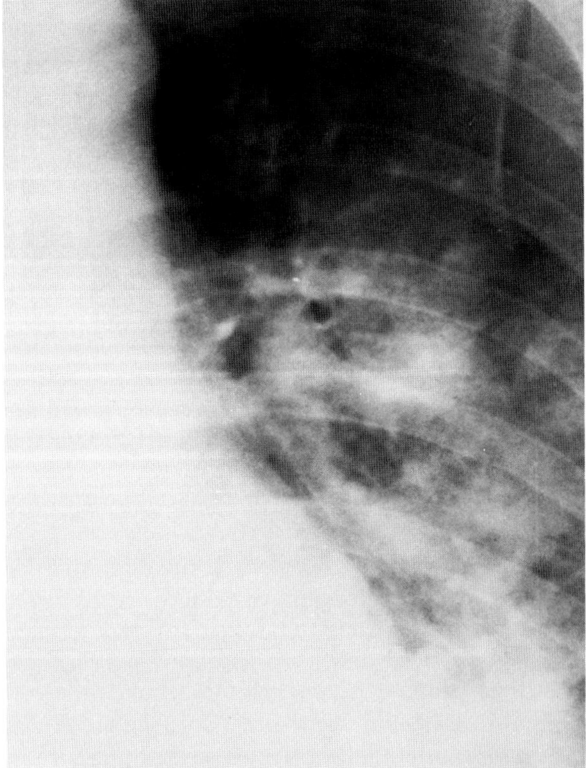 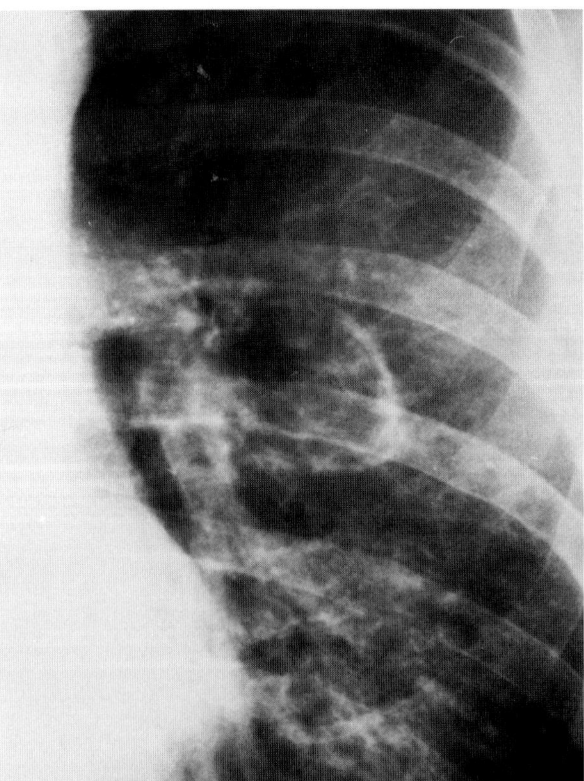

FIG. 5. Patient with glioblastoma multiforma who developed a nosocomial pneumonia due to *Staphylococcus aureus*. (**A**) Initial chest radiograph demonstrates a patchy left lower lobe infiltrate. (**B**) A radiograph obtained 9 days later shows partial clearing of the infiltrate and the development of pneumatoceles. (**C**) Computed tomography shows the thin wall of the pneumatocele.

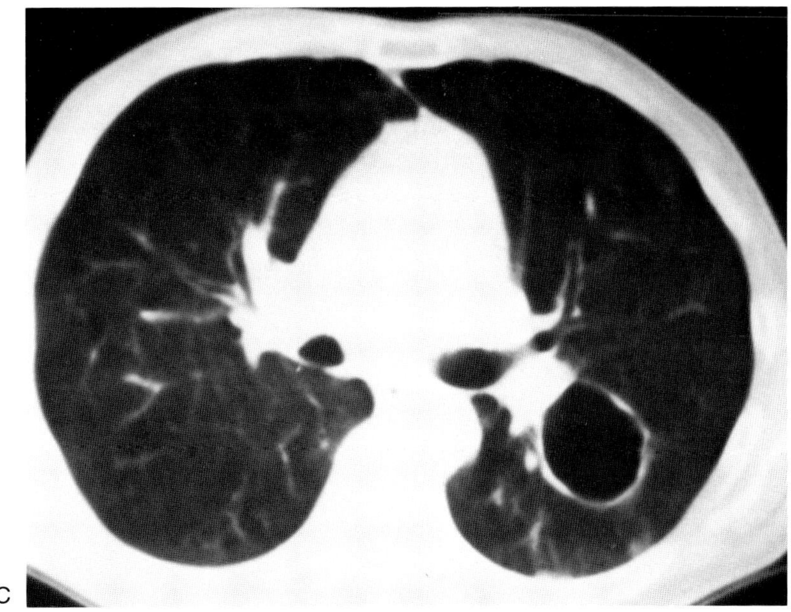

FIG. 5. *Continued.*

mary tuberculosis (57). The tuberculous and fungal pneumonias usually have a clinical presentation that allows their differentiation from bacterial infection.

BRONCHOPNEUMONIA

Bronchopneumonia results from an infection that primarily involves the bronchi. The infection may spread along the bronchi involving multiple parts of the lung. From the bronchus the infection may spread to involve adjacent alveoli. Progressive involvement of the alveoli results in the development of consolidation in a more lobar pattern.

Bronchopneumonia is characterized in its early stages by patchy infiltrates that may have a peribronchial distribution (Fig. 5). As the infection spreads to surrounding alveoli, the areas of consolidation may become more confluent, producing a pattern similar to that seen in lobar pneumonia. Atelectasis may be seen when bronchi are plugged with inflammatory exudate.

A bronchopneumonic pattern is frequently seen in pneumonia due to *S. aureus* (52) (Fig. 5). Gram-negative bacteria, including *Pseudomonas, Serratia, Escherichia,* and *Proteus,* cause pneumonias that frequently have a bronchopneumonic pattern (58–60). Community-acquired pneumonias due to *Hemophilus, Legionella,* and *Mycoplasma* may produce a bronchopneumonic type picture on the chest radiograph (32,48,51).

NODULES

Bacterial and fungal pneumonias may produce nodular or mass-like areas of consolidation. The densities vary in size from small nodules less than 1 cm to more mass-like areas of consolidation that are several centimeters in diameter. The margins of the lesions tend to be indistinct.

Nodular densities may be seen in fungal infections due to *Histoplasma, Cryptococcus, Coccidioides,* and *Blastomyces* (33,34,54–56) (Fig. 6). The nodules may be single or multiple. When multiple nodules are present they may be clustered together in one lobe. The nodular form of cryptococcosis is most frequently seen in patients with normal immune function (56). The nodules seen in coccidioidomycosis may represent either granulomas or a blocked cavity containing pus or caseous material (55). Blocked cavities may rupture into adjacent bronchi, with thin wall cysts remaining after the cavity has drained (Fig. 7). These cavities may resolve, refill with material, and again resemble nodules or persist as thin-walled cysts.

Immunocompromised patients may develop pulmonary infections due to opportunistic fungi, such as *Aspergillus* and *Phycomycetes,* and present with nodular infiltrates (61). Postprimary tuberculosis may also be associated with nodular areas of consolidation (57).

Bacterial infections by *Legionella, Nocardia,* and Gram-negative bacilli may produce nodular or mass-like areas of consolidation (49,50,60,62) (Fig. 2). Early in its course, pneumonia due to *S. pneumoniae* may appear as a round infiltrate. These infiltrates tend to progress more rapidly than those due to fungi or tuberculosis. Anaerobic pneumonia that results in abscess formation may produce a mass-like density that is typically basilar in location (63).

Hematogenous pneumonia results from septic emboli lodging in the pulmonary vasculature and producing fo-

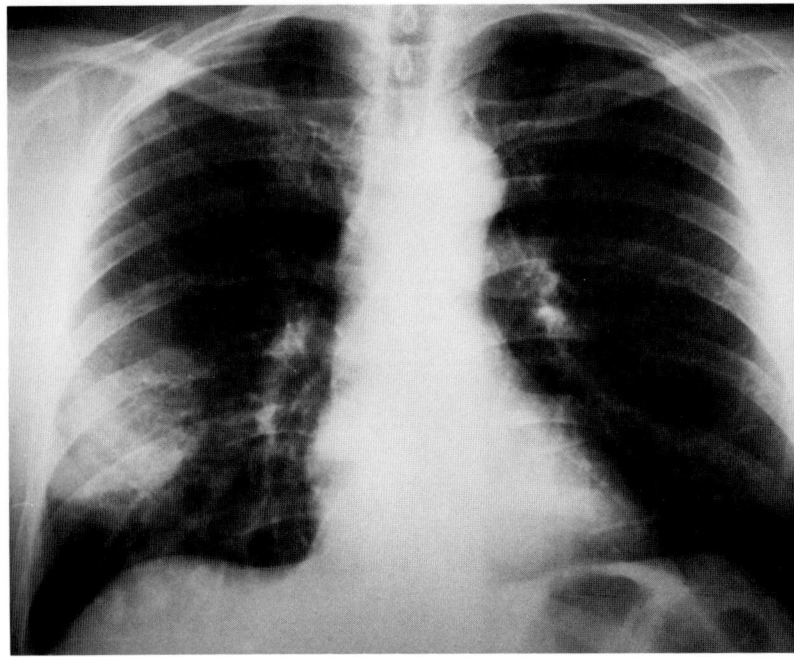

FIG. 6. Patient with a 1-month history of cough. Chest radiograph demonstrates a right lower lobe mass. Bronchoscopic biopsy yielded *Cryptococcus neoformans.*

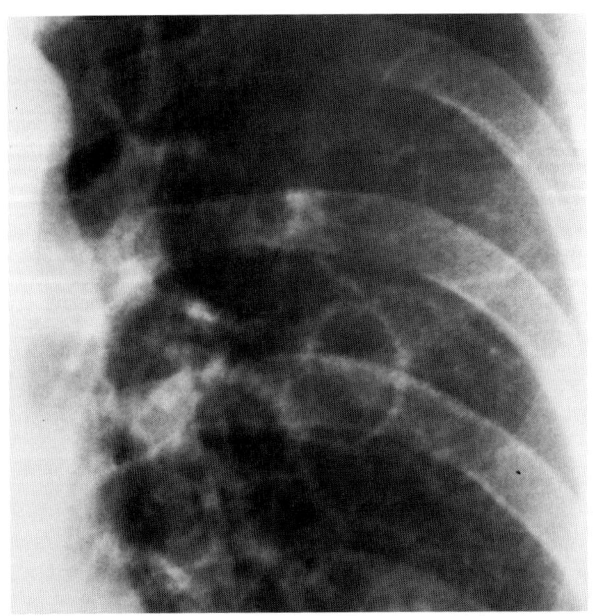

FIG. 7. Patient with pneumonia due to *Coccidioides immitis.* Chest radiograph shows a thin-walled cavity present in mid-left lung.

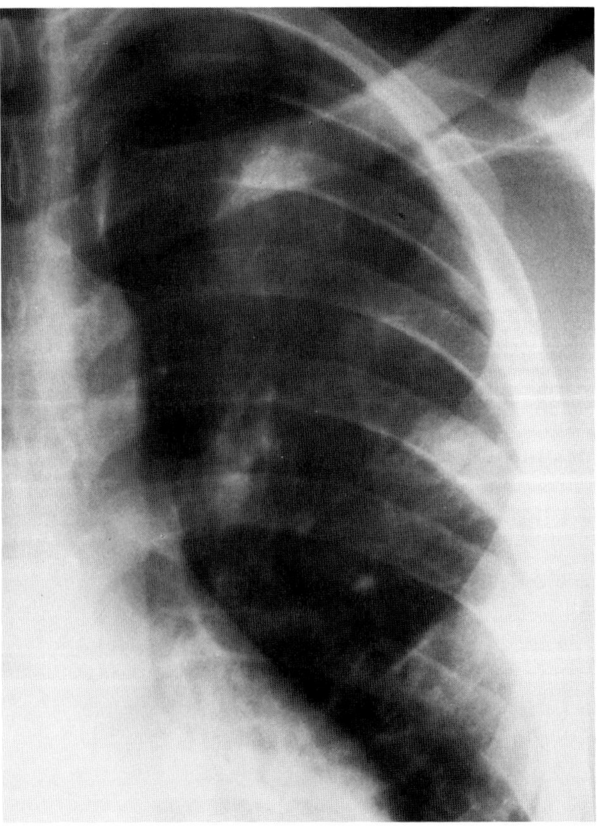

FIG. 8. Intravenous drug addict with *Staphylococcus aureus* endocarditis of the tricuspid valve. Chest radiograph shows multiple ill-defined nodular infiltrates due to septic emboli.

cal areas of pneumonitis. Septic emboli are associated with central venous lines, intravenous drug abuse, septic thrombophlebitis, and endocarditis. The chest radiograph typically demonstrates multiple ill-defined nodular infiltrates (Fig. 8). *Staphylococcus* is the most common cause of hematogenous pneumonia (64). Hospitalized patients with central venous lines, especially those who are immunocompromised, may also develop septic emboli due to *Candida* (65).

CAVITARY LESIONS

When the pulmonary infection produces necrosis of lung parenchyma, a lung abscess develops. Bronchi frequently communicate with the area of involved lung and allow drainage of the necrotic material. When air enters the abscess cavity, it becomes readily distinguishable from the surrounding consolidation (Fig. 9). If drainage is incomplete an air fluid level may be present. When the pneumonia is focal, a mass-like density with associated cavitation will be present on the chest radiograph. The walls of the cavity may vary in thickness. If the necrosis is more extensive, necrotizing pneumonia develops. In this form of pneumonia, multiple cavities develop

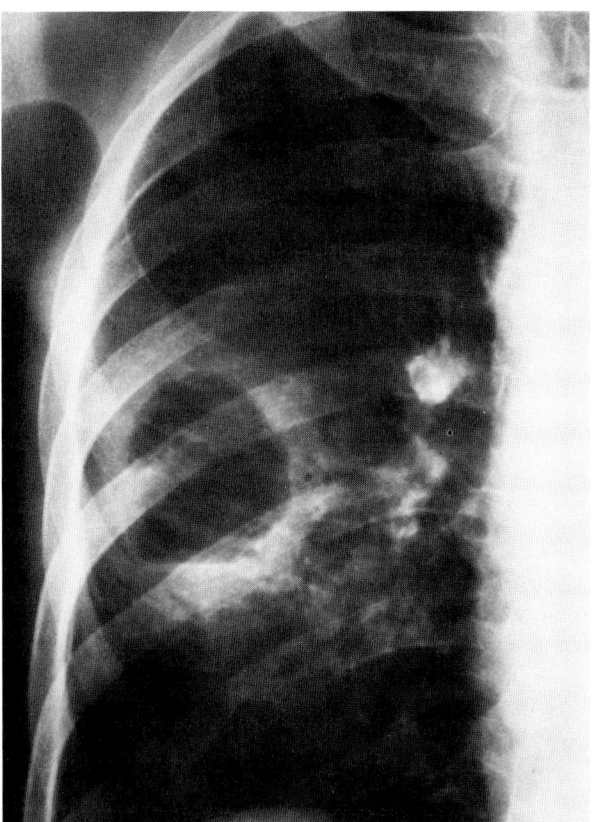

FIG. 9. Patient with anaerobic pneumonia of the right lung. Lung abscess developed that drained its contents into a bronchus resulting in an air-fluid level within the abscess cavity.

within the area of consolidation (Fig. 10). A rare complication of pneumonia occurs when the infection produces vascular occlusion resulting in the involved lung developing pulmonary gangrene.

Anaerobic infection following aspiration is commonly associated with lung abscess formation (13) (Fig. 9). Other bacterial infections that cause cavitation include: *S. aureus, Legionella, Nocardia, Actinomyces,* and Gram-negative bacilli (19,30,49,58,62) (Fig. 10). Cavitation occurs infrequently in pneumonia due to *S. pneumoniae* (29,46) (Fig. 11).

The granulomatous infections of the lung may produce cavitation. Primary tuberculosis typically presents with parenchymal consolidation, which is frequently associated with adenopathy. In up to 30 percent of these cases, cavitation will develop in the consolidated lung (57) (Fig. 12). Cavitation is seen very frequently in reactivation tuberculosis (Fig. 13). Atypical mycobacterial infections may also produce areas of cavitation within the involved lung (66,67). Pathogenic fungi, including *Histoplasma, Coccidioides,* and *Blastomyces,* have chronic forms of infection that result in the development of chronic cavitary lung disease (53–55,68). Sporotrichosis is a rare fungal disease that may produce thin-walled cavities within the lung (41).

Pneumatoceles are cavities in the lung that are not the result of parenchymal necrosis, but are thought to be due to injury to the bronchial and bronchiolar walls (69). Air leaks through the defect into the interstitium producing interstitial emphysema. If the defect acts as a ball-valve, air will accumulate distal to the point of obstruction producing a thin-walled, air-filled pneumatocele. These cavities are often multiple, appearing as areas of lucency within consolidated lung. They have a tendency to change in size and appearance. They frequently resolve spontaneously over weeks to months. They are seen in *S. aureus* pneumonia and are more common in children than adults (Fig. 5). In infants the pneumatocele may be confused with a pneumothorax.

Immunocompromised patients, especially those who are granulocytopenic, are at risk for developing invasive aspergillosis. In this infection the *Aspergillus* mycelia invade the blood vessels supplying the involved lung and thrombose them (61). This leads to the infarction of the involved lung and the development of cavitation. Radiographically this is characterized by the development of an air crescent sign (70). This sign is a curvilinear lucency that develops within the infiltrate. This lucency presents air within the cavity that is surrounding a mass of necrotic lung. The phycomycetes are a group of fungi that produce similar findings.

DIFFUSE INFILTRATES

Viral pneumonias typically present with diffuse reticular or reticulonodular infiltrates (Fig. 14). The nodular

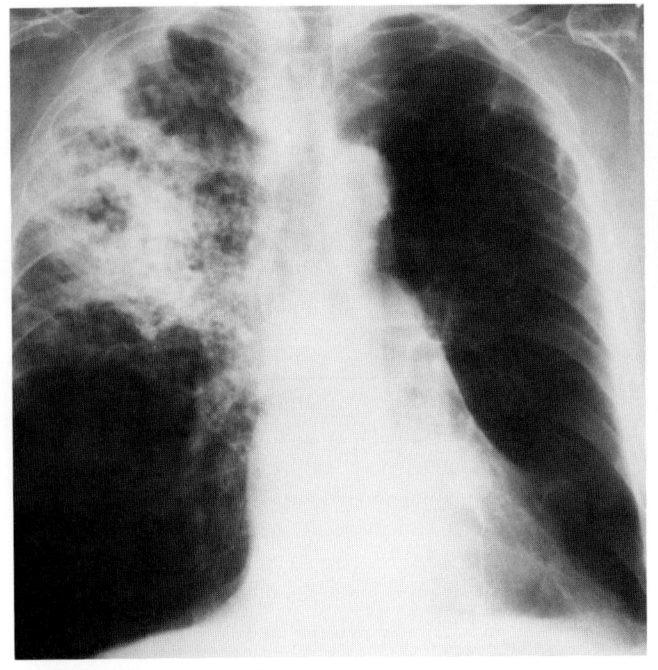

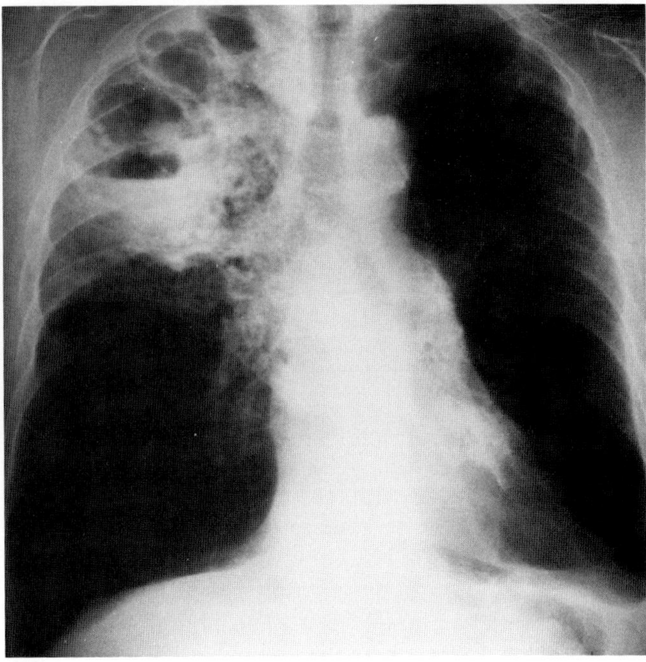

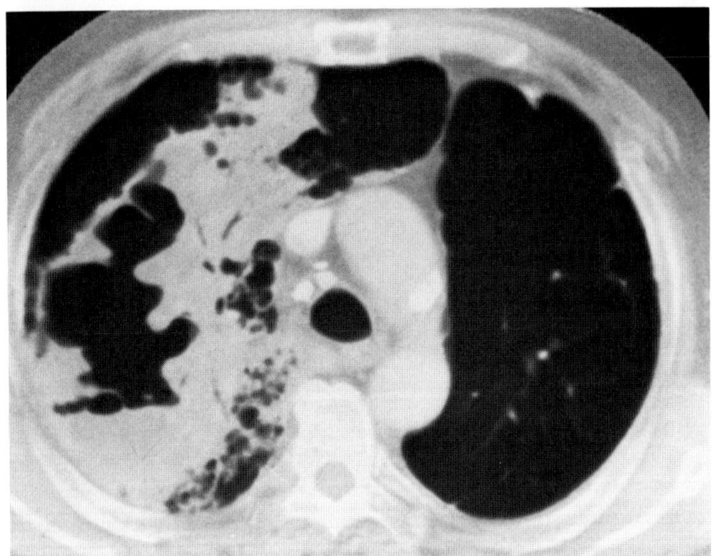

FIG. 10. Elderly nursing home resident admitted with pneumonia due to *Pseudomonas aeruginosa.* **(A)** Initial radiograph demonstrates a right upper lobe infiltrate. **(B)** One week later, a radiograph shows development of cavitation with air fluid levels being present. **(C)** Computed tomography shows the extent of parenchymal destruction by the Gram-negative pneumonia.

densities are small and ill-defined and represent peribronchial areas of inflammation (71). Viruses that produce pneumonia include influenza, adenovirus, cytomegalovirus, respiratory syncitial virus, herpes simplex, varicella zoster, and measles virus. Due to their small size, the nodular densities may be difficult to detect early in the infection. This is especially true on portable chest radiographs. They are not always diffuse in their distribution, especially early in the infection.

Pneumonia due to *M. pneumoniae* may present as either interstitial or air space disease (72). Interstitial infiltrates when present are reticulonodular in appearance and may be bilateral and diffuse in their distribu-

tion (Fig. 15). They tend to extend from the hila to the peripheral portions of the lung. In some cases the patients exhibit both interstitial infiltrates and areas of consolidation.

Infection due to *Pneumocystis carinii* also produces diffuse infiltrates (73). The inflammatory process in *Pneumocystis* infection is located in the alveoli and not the peribronchial regions. In spite of the alveolar location of the infection the infiltrates have an interstitial appearance early in the infection. Radiographs show a diffuse fine nodular or reticular infiltrate. As the infection progresses, the infiltrates become more confluent and take on the appearance of air space disease.

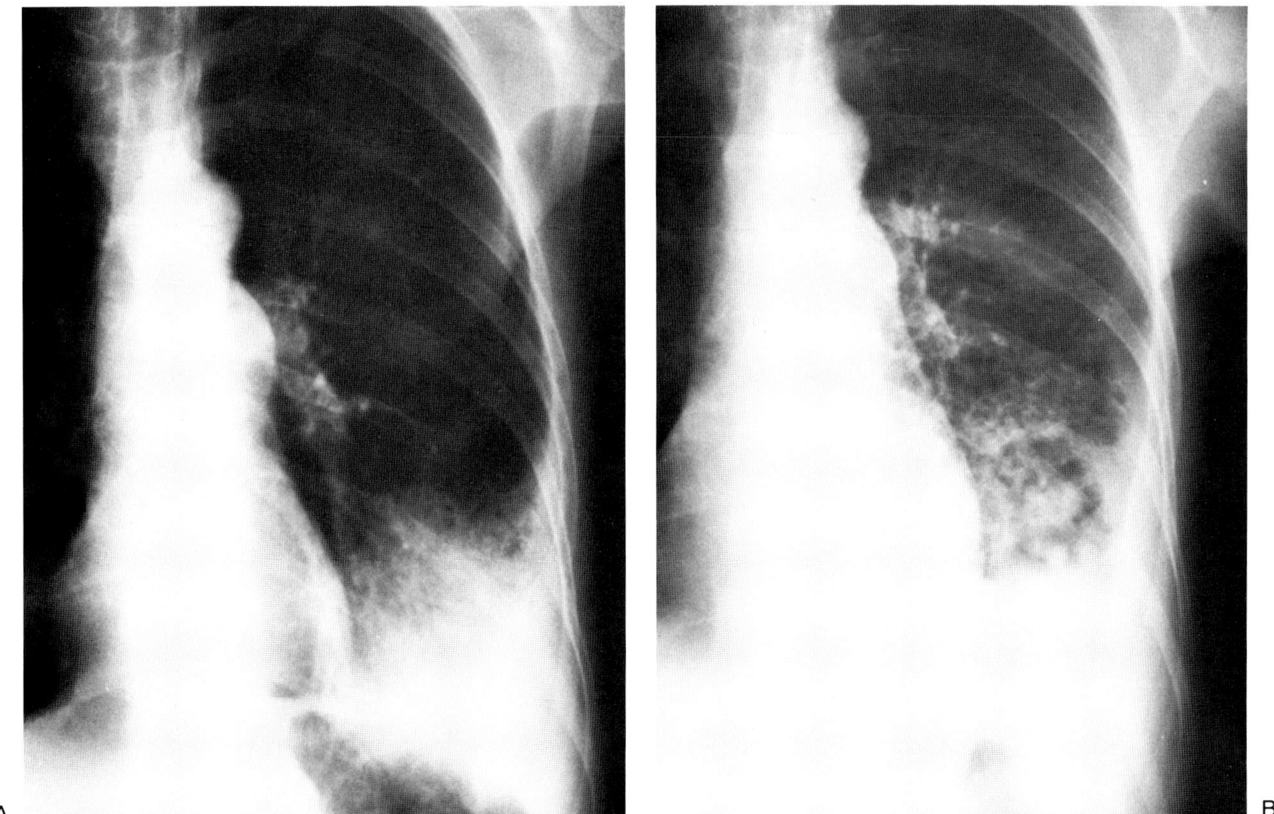

FIG. 11. Patient with cough, fever, and chills. Sputum culture grew *Streptococcus pneumoniae* (**A**). Initial radiograph shows a segmental area of consolidation in the left lower lobe. (**B**) Eight days later cavitation has developed. A small pleural effusion is also present.

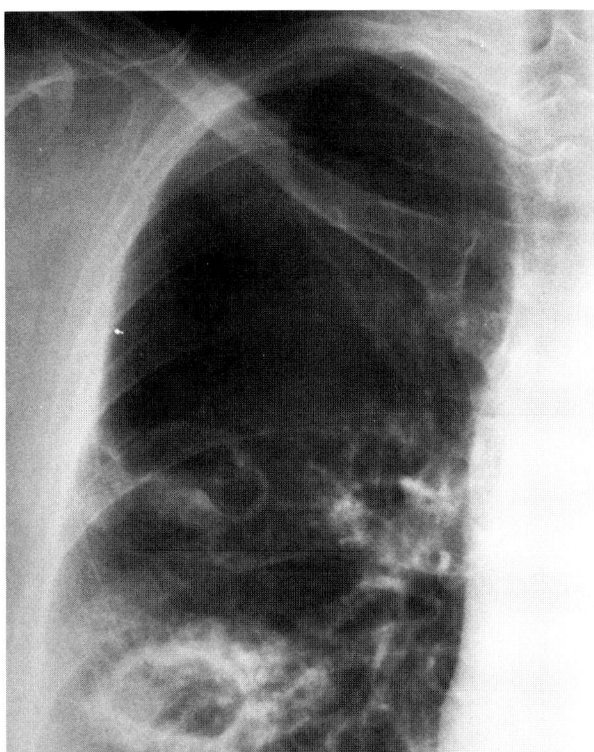

FIG. 12. Middle-aged man with a 3-week history of yellow sputum production. Sputum positive for *Mycobacterium tuberculosis.* Chest radiograph shows cavitary infiltrates in the mid- and lower right lung.

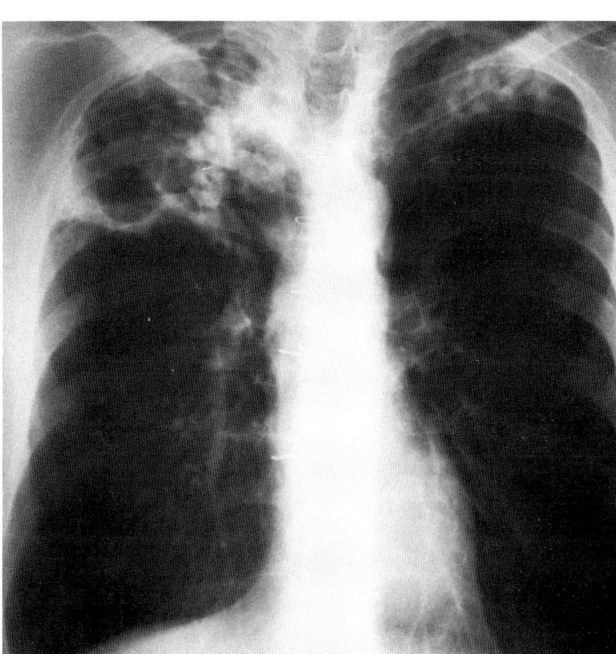

FIG. 13. Bilateral upper lobe infiltrates due to reactivation tuberculosis. Cavitation is clearly present in the right upper lobe.

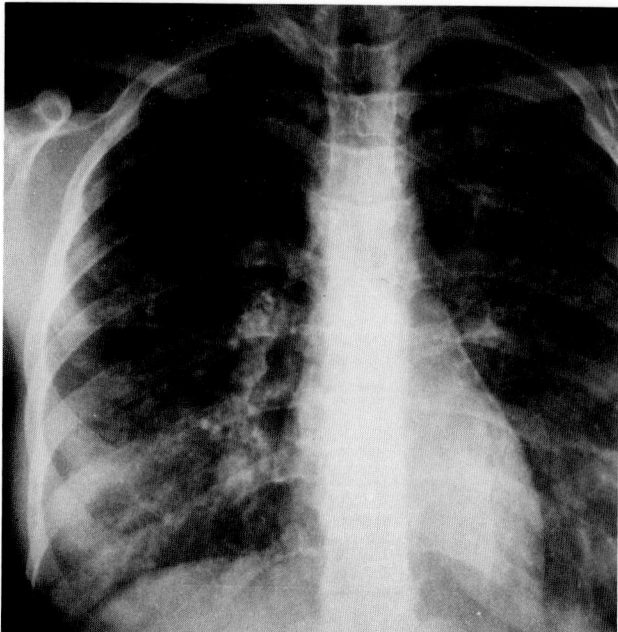

FIG. 14. Bilateral diffuse infiltrates in an adult with varicella pneumonia. The patient had been exposed to a child with chicken pox 10 days before and had developed skin lesions 2 days before the chest radiograph was obtained.

Disseminated tuberculosis, as well as disseminated fungal infections due to *Histoplasma, Coccidioides,* and *Blastomyces,* may produce a radiographic pattern described as miliary (74–76) (Fig. 16). The nodular densities are typically 2 to 4 mm in size. The lungs are diffusely involved because the infection is the result of

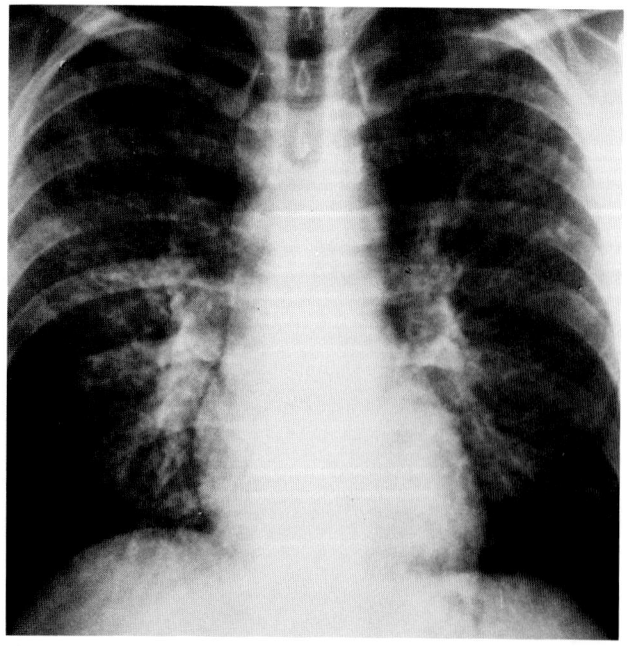

FIG. 15. Patient with a 2-week history of non-productive cough. Chest radiograph demonstrates diffuse interstitial infiltrates due to *Mycoplasma pneumoniae.*

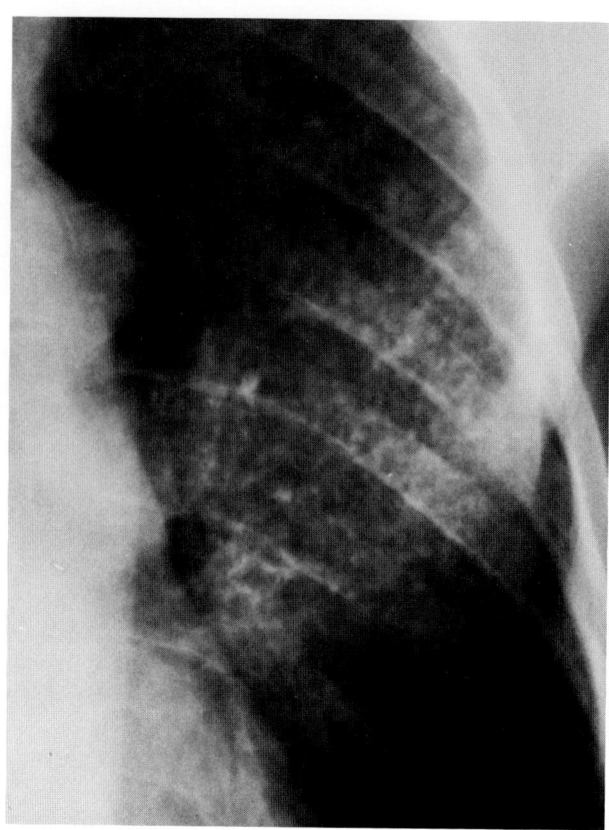

FIG. 16. Patient with miliary tuberculosis. Chest radiograph demonstrates diffuse infiltrates with innumerable small nodular densities.

hematogenous spread of the organism. Radiographically the various causes of this pattern can not be discerned from one another. Disseminated histoplasmosis may produce interstitial infiltrates that are composed of linear densities without nodular changes being seen (74).

Cryptococcal pulmonary infection in patients with acquired immune deficiency syndrome (AIDS) produces adenopathy and interstitial infiltrates (77). The infiltrates frequently have a nodular component to them. This pattern differs from that seen in individuals with normal immune function and those who are immunocompromised without AIDS.

PLEURAL EFFUSION

Pleural effusions may develop in response to a pulmonary infection. They are seen most commonly in bacterial pneumonia, occurring in approximately 40 percent of cases of acute bacterial pneumonia (78). These parapneumonic effusions are seen with pneumonia due to *S. aureus, S. pneumoniae, Legionella, H. influenzae, Nocardia,* Gram-negative bacilli, and anaerobic bacteria (29,48,49,51,52,59,63,79) (Fig. 11). Pleural effusions may be seen with infections by *Mycobacterium tubercu-*

losis, but are uncommon in pneumonia due to nontuberculous mycobacteria (80).

Parapneumonic pleural effusions evolve through three stages (81). The first stage is the exudate stage, which is characterized by sterile fluid that has a low white blood cell count and lactate dehydrogenase, and with a normal pH and glucose level. Radiographically these effusions move freely and are not loculated. In the second stage, the fibropurulent stage, the fluid contains bacteria, inflammatory cells, and cellular debris. Chest radiographs during this stage frequently show the fluid to be loculated. Loculated pleural fluid, however, may also occur with sterile parapneumonic effusions if preexisting pleural adhesions are present. Thoracentesis and pleural fluid analysis are the only certain way to separate the two types of fluid collections. Without therapy the effusion will progress to the organization stage. This final stage is characterized by the development of a thick pleural peel. The peel encases the lung and severely limits its function. The thick fluid that is present may erode through the chest wall or into the lung. Erosion through the visceral pleura results in the development of a bronchopleural fistula (Fig. 17).

Bronchopleural fistulas are the result of a fistula between a bronchus and the pleural space. Radiographically they are characterized by one or more air fluid col-

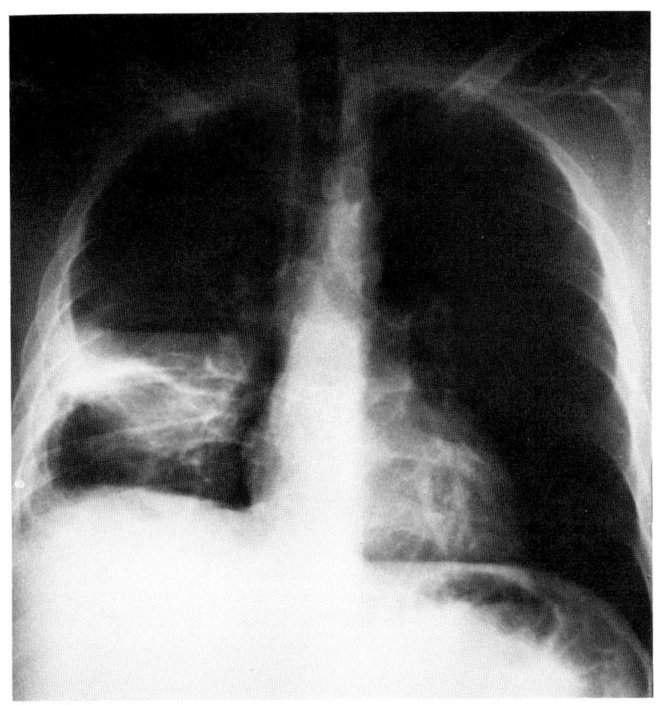

A

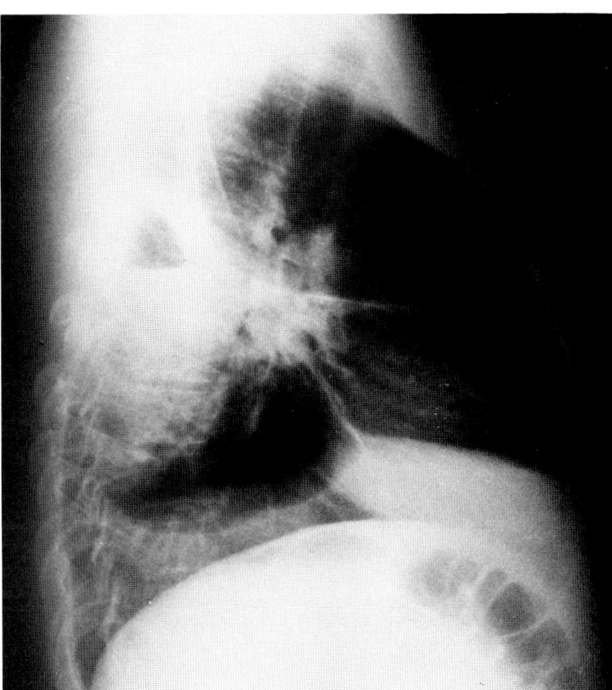

B

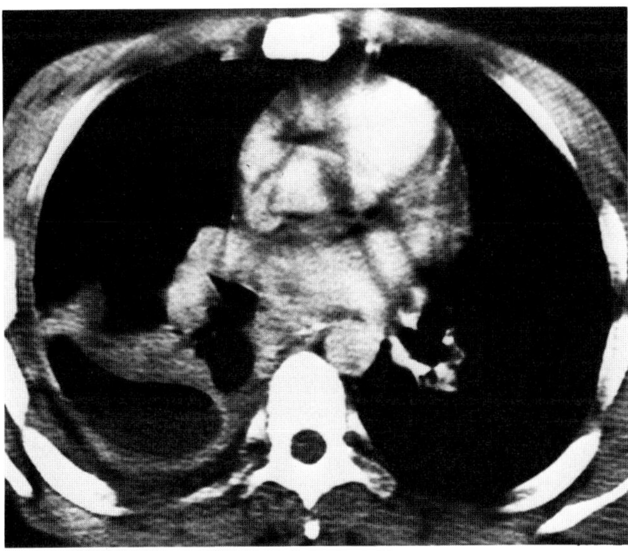

C

FIG. 17. Patient with anaerobic pneumonia involving the right lower lobe. **(A)** and **(B)** Chest radiograph shows a loculated pleural fluid collection in the posterior right chest. Air fluid level indicates the presence of a bronchopleural fistula. **(C)** Computed tomography shows loculated empyema with enhancing pleural rind and associated air fluid level. Consolidation is present in adjacent lung.

lections. These collections tend to be oblong, pleural-based fluid collections that form an obtuse angle with the lung. Because of their lenticular shape, the air fluid levels tend to have different lengths when viewed in different projections (82).

Bronchopleural fistulas sometimes need to be differentiated from lung abscesses. In most cases the radiographic appearance of the lung abscess will allow it to be distinguished from a bronchopleural fistula. The lung abscess tends to have a round appearance. The air fluid levels are approximately the same length when viewed in any projection. The abscess tends to have a thick wall that meets the chest wall at an acute angle.

ADENOPATHY

Hilar or mediastinal adenopathy is frequently encountered in cases of primary tuberculosis (57). Adenopathy, however, is rare in reactivation tuberculosis and with infections by atypical *Mycobacteria* (57,80). Another granulomatous infection, acute histoplasmosis, also frequently has adenopathy present at the time of initial presentation. Adenopathy, however, is uncommon with disseminated tuberculosis or fungal infection. Most acute bacterial infections are not associated with adenopathy. Adenopathy may, however, be seen in nocardiosis, tularemia, plague, and lung abscesses (49,83,84). Adenopathy

is not typically seen in viral infections or pneumonia due to *Mycoplasma* or *Pneumocystis*. In AIDS patients adenopathy is frequently seen with infections due to *Cryptococcus* and *Mycobacterium avium-intracellulare* (77).

Pulmonary neoplasm must always be considered in patients who present with hilar adenopathy and a peripheral infiltrate. The central adenopathy may represent neoplasm or reactive adenopathy. Infiltrates and adenopathy that do not clear following appropriate therapy for pneumonia should be evaluated for a possible underlying malignancy (Fig. 18). In fact many of the infiltrates distal to obstructing airway tumors are due to noninfectious processes and do not represent infection at all (85).

LOCATION

Location of the infiltrate may at times give a clue to the offending organism. The apical and posterior segments of the upper lobes are classically involved in reactivation tuberculosis (57) (Fig. 13). In spite of this characteristic distribution, tuberculosis is frequently not suspected at the time of initial evaluation (86). Fungal infections, such as chronic histoplasmosis, also tend to involve the upper lung fields (68). Dependent portions of the lung are typically involved in aspiration pneumonias (31). Lower lobe consolidation, especially if associated with volume loss, should raise the question of aspiration pneumonia. Aspiration pneumonia often involves more than one lobe and may be bilateral. *Mycoplasma* pneumonia more commonly involves the lower lobes than the upper lobes (32). A perihilar distribution of the infiltrates may be seen in pneumonia due to *Pneumocystis* (73).

Legionella usually presents with unilobar involvement, but frequently progresses to involve multiple lobes (48). The involved lobes may not be contiguous and may involve the contralateral lung. Multilobe involvement also is seen with *H. influenzae* and *S. aureus* (30,51).

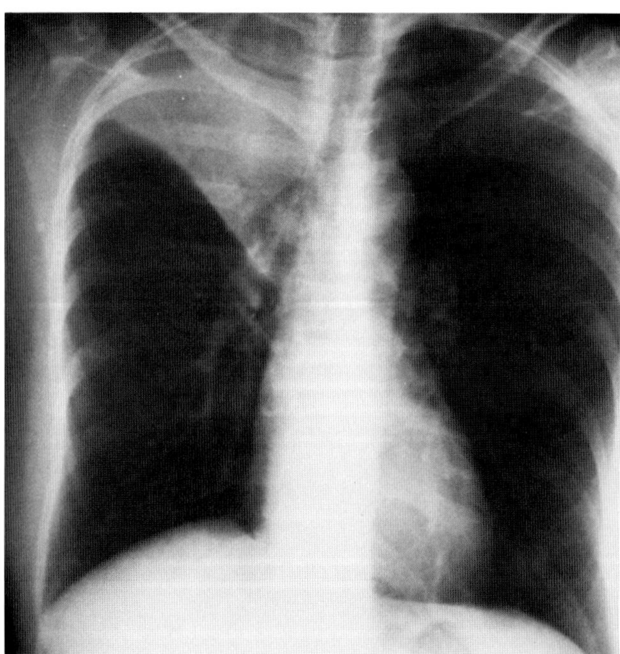

FIG. 18. Patient with cough and fever. Chest radiograph shows right upper lobe consolidation with associated volume loss. The symptoms resolved following a course of antibiotics, but the chest radiograph remained unchanged. Bronchoscopy demonstrated squamous cell carcinoma in the right upper lobe bronchus.

REFERENCES

1. Garibaldi RA. Epidemiology of community-acquired respiratory tract infections in adults. *Am J Med* 1985;78(suppl 6B):32–37.
2. Septimus EJ. Nosicomial bacterial pneumonias. *Sem Respir Infect* 1989;4:245–252.
3. Tew J, Calenoff L, Berlin BS. Bacterial or nonbacterial pneumonia: accuracy of radiographic diagnosis. *Radiology* 1977;124: 607–612.
4. Conces DJ. Opportunistic pneumonia: a systematic approach. *Postgrad Radiol* 1990;10:185–197.
5. Rosenow EC, Wilson WR, Cockerill FR. Pulmonary disease in the immunocompromised host (first of two parts). *Mayo Clin Proc* 1985;60:473–487.
6. Wilson WR, Cockerill FR, Rosenow EC. Pulmonary disease in the immunocompromised host (second of two parts). *Mayo Clin Proc* 1985;60:610–631.
7. Woodhead MA, Macfarlane JT. Comparative clinical and labora-

tory features of legionella with pneumococcal and mycoplasma pneumonias. *Br J Dis Chest* 1987;81:133–139.

8. Fang GD, Fine M, Orloff J, Arisumi D, et al. New and emerging etiologies for community-acquired pneumonia with implications for therapy. *Medicine* 1990;69:307–316.

9. Schwarzmann SW, Adler JL, Sullivan RJ, Marine WM. Bacterial pneumonia during the Hong Kong influenza epidemic of 1968–1969: experience in a city-county hospital. *Arch Intern Med* 1971;127:1037–1044.

10. Mackowiak PA, Martin RM, Jones SR, Smith JW. Pharyngeal colonization by gram-negative bacilli in aspiration-prone persons. *Arch Intern Med* 1978;138:1224–1227.

11. Holmes RB. Friedlander's pneumonia. *Am J Roentgenol* 1956;75:728–747.

12. Manfredi F, Daly WJ, Behnke RH. Clinical observations of acute Friedlander pneumonia. *Ann Intern Med* 1963;58:642–653.

13. Bartlett JG, Finegold SM. Anaerobic infections of the lung and pleural space. *Am Rev Respir Dis* 1974;110:56–77.

14. Chartard SA, Marks MI. Pulmonary infections in cystic fibrosis: pathogenesis and therapy. In Pennington JE, ed. *Respiratory infections: diagnosis and management*, 2nd ed. New York: Raven Press, 1988:276–297.

15. Keith TA, Schreiner AW. *Hemophilus influenzae* in adult broncho-pulmonary infection. *Ann Intern Med* 1962;56:27–38.

16. Lipsky BA, Boyko EJ, Inui TS, Koepsell TD. Risk factors for acquiring pneumococcal infections. *Arch Intern Med* 1986;146:2179–2185.

17. Ebright JR, Rytel MW. Bacterial pneumonia in the elderly. *J Am Geriat Soc* 1980;28:220–223.

18. Garb JL, Brown RB, Garb JR, Tuthill RW. Differences in etiology of pneumonias in nursing home and community patients. *JAMA* 1978;240:2169–2172.

19. Mufson MA. Pneumococcal infections. *JAMA* 1981;246:1942–1948.

20. Niederman MS. Gram-negative colonization of the respiratory tract: pathogenesis and clinical consequences. *Sem Respir Infect* 1990;5:173–184.

21. Craven DE, Barber TW, Steger KA, Montcalve MA. Nosocomial pneumonia in the 1990's: update on epidemiology and risk factors. *Sem Respir Infect* 1990;5:157–172.

22. Dondero TJ, Rendtorff RC, Mallison GF, et al. An outbreak of legionnaire's disease associated with a contaminated air-conditioning cooling tower. *N Engl J Med* 1980;302:365–370.

23. Bartlett JG, O'Keefe P, Tally FP, Louie TJ, Gorbach SL. Bacteriology of hospital-acquired pneumonia. *Arch Intern Med* 1986;146:868–871.

24. Celis R, Torres A, Gatell JM, Amela M, Rodriguez-Roisin R, Agusti-Vidal A. Nosocomial pneumonia: a multivariate analysis of risk and prognosis. *Chest* 1988;93:318–324.

25. Pierce AK, Sanford JP. Aerobic gram-negative bacillary pneumonias. *Am Rev Respir Dis* 1974;110:647–688.

26. Langer M, Mosconi P, Cigada M, Mandelli M. Long-term respiratory support and risk of pneumonia in critically ill patients. *Am Rev Respir Dis* 1990;140:302–305.

27. Dixon RE. Nosocomial respiratory infections. *Infect Control* 1983;4:376–381.

28. Karnad A, Alvarez S, Berk SL. Pneumonia caused by gram-negative bacilli. *Am J Med* 1985;79(suppl 1A):61–67.

29. Granados A, Podzamczer D, Gudiol F, Manresa F. Pneumonia due to *Legionella pneumophilia* and pneumococcal pneumonia: similarities and differences on presentation. *Eur Respir J* 1989;2:130–134.

30. Kaye MG, Fox MJ, Bartlett JG, Braman SS, Glassroth J. The clinical spectrum of *Staphylococcus aureus* pulmonary infection. *Chest* 1990;97:788–792.

31. Bartlett JG. Anaerobic bacterial infections of the lung. *Chest* 1987;91:901–909.

32. Mansel JK, Rosenow EC, Smith TF, Martin JW. *Mycoplasma pneumoniae* pneumonia. *Chest* 1989;95:639–646.

33. Goodwin RA, Loyd JE, Des Prez RM. Histoplasmosis in normal hosts. *Medicine* 1981;60:231–266.

34. Ampel NM, Wieden MA, Galgian JN. Coccidioidomycosis: clinical update. *Rev Infect Dis* 1989;11:897–911.

35. Littman ML, Walter JE. Cryptococcoses: current status. *Am J Med* 1968;45:922–932.

36. Witorsch P, Utz JP. North American blastomycosis: a study of 40 patients. *Medicine* 1968;47:169–200.

37. Contreras MA, Cheung OT, Sanders DE, Goldstein RS. Pulmonary infection with nontuberculous mycobacteria. *Am Rev Respir Dis* 1988;137:149–152.

38. Byram D, Hatton P, Williams S, Pearson SB. The form and presentation of tuberculosis over a 10-year interval in Leeds. *Br J Dis Chest* 1895;79:152–160.

39. Flynn MW, Felson B. The roentgen manifestations of thoracic actinomycosis. *Am J Roentgenol* 1970;110:707–716.

40. Schaffner W, Drutz DJ, Duncan GW, Koenig MG. The clinical spectrum of endemic psittacosis. *Arch Intern Med* 1967;119:433–443.

41. Pluss JL, Opal SM. Pulmonary sporotrichosis: review of treatment and outcome. *Medicine* 1986;65:143–153.

42. Brooks GF, Buchanan TM. Tularemia in the United States: epidemiologic aspects in the 1960's and follow-up of the outbreak of tularemia in Vermont. *J Infect Dis* 1970;21:357–359.

43. Laforce FM. Woolsorters' disease in England. *Bull NY Acad Med* 1978;54:956–963.

44. Clark WH, Lennette EH, Railsback OC, Romer MS. Q fever in California. Clinical features of one hundred eighty cases. *Arch Intern Med* 1951;88:155–167.

45. Kirby BD, Snyder KM, Meyer RD, Finegold SM. Legionnaires' disease: report of sixty-five nosocomially acquired cases and review of the literature. *Medicine* 1980;59:188–205.

46. Kantor HG. The many radiologic faces of pneumococcal pneumonia. *Am J Roentgenol* 1981;137:1213–1220.

47. Felson B, Rosenberg LS, Hamburger M. Roentgen findings in acute Friedlander's pneumonia. *Am J Roentgenol* 1949;53:559–563.

48. Kroboth FJ, Yu VL, Reddy SC, Yu AC. Clinicoradiographic correlation with the extent of legionnaire disease. *Am J Roentgenol* 1983;141:263–268.

49. Feigin DS. Nocardiosis of the lung: chest radiographic findings in 21 cases. *Radiology* 1986;159:9–14.

50. Raby N, Forbes G, Williams R. Nocardia infection in patients with liver transplants or chronic liver disease: radiologic findings. *Radiology* 1990;174:713–716.

51. Pearlberg J, Haggar AM, Saravolatz L, Beute GH, Popovich J. *Hemophilus influenzae* pneumonia in the adult. *Radiology* 1984;151:23–26.

52. Wiita RM, Cartwright RR, Davis JG. Staphylococcal pneumonia in adults: a review of 102 cases. *Am J Roentgenol* 1961;86:1083–1091.

53. Sheflin JR, Campbell JA, Thompson GP. Pulmonary blastomycosis: findings on chest radiographs in 63 patients. *Am J Roentgenol* 1990;154:1177–1180.

54. Halvorsen RA, Duncan JD, Merten DF, Gallis HA, Putman CE. Pulmonary blastomycosis: radiologic manifestations. *Radiology* 1984;150:1–5.

55. Bayer AS. Fungal pneumonias; pulmonary coccidioidal syndromes (part 1) primary and progressive coccidioidal pneumonias—diagnostic, therapeutic, and prognostic considerations. *Chest* 1981;79:575–583.

56. Khoury MB, Godwin JD, Ravin CE, Gallis HA, Halvorsen RA, Putman CE. Thoracic cryptococcoses: immunologic competence and radiologic appearance. *Am J Roentgenol* 1984;141:893–896.

57. Woodring JH, Vandiviere HM, Fried AM, Dillon ML, Williams TD, Melvin IG. Update: the radiographic features of pulmonary tuberculosis. *Am J Roentgenol* 1986;146:497–506.

58. Bailkian JP, Herman PG, Godleski JJ. *Serratia* pneumonia. *Radiology* 1980;137:309–311.

59. Unger JD, Rose HD, Unger GF. Gram-negative pneumonia. *Radiology* 1973;107:283–291.

60. Renner RR, Coccaro AP, Heitzmann ER, et al. *Pseudomonas* pneumonia: a prototype of hospital-based infection. *Radiology* 1972;105:555–562.

61. Libshitz HI, Pagani JJ. Aspergillosis and mucormycosis: two types of opportunistic fungal pneumonia. *Radiology* 1981;140:301–306.

62. Moore E, Webb WR, Gamsu G, Golden JA. Legionnaires' disease in the renal transplant patient: clinical presentation and radiographic progression. *Radiology* 1984;153:589–593.

63. Landay MJ, Christensen EE, Bynum LJ, Goodman C. Anaerobic

pleural and pulmonary infections. *Am J Roentgenol* 1980;134:233–240.

64. Press OW, Ramsey PG, Larson EB, Fefer A, Hickman RO. Hickman catheter infections in patients with malignancies. *Medicine* 1984;63:189–200.

65. Wey SB, Mori M, Pfaller MA, Woolson RF, Wenzel RP. Risk factors for hospital-acquired candidemia. *Arch Intern Med* 1989;149:2349–2353.

66. Christensen EE, Dietz GW, Ahn CH, et al. Radiographic manifestations of pulmonary *Mycobacterium kansasii* infections. *Am J Roentgenol* 1978;131:985–993.

67. Christensen EE, Dietz GW, Ahn CH, et al. Pulmonary manifestations of *Mycobacterium intracellularis*. *Am J Roentgenol* 1979;133:59–66.

68. Wheat LJ, Wass J, Norton J, Kohler RB, French MLV. Cavitary histoplasmosis occurring during two large urban outbreaks. *Medicine* 1984;63:201–209.

69. McGarry T, Giosa R, Rohman M, Huang CT. Pneumatocele formation in adult pneumonia. *Chest* 1987;92:717–720.

70. Gefter WB, Albelda SM, Talbot GH, Gerson SL, Cassileth PA, Miller WT. Invasive pulmonary aspergillosis and acute leukemia: limitations in the diagnostic utility of the air crescent sign. *Radiology* 1985;157:605–610.

71. Conte P, Heitzmann ER, Markarian B. Viral pneumonia: roentgen pathological correlations. *Radiology* 1970;95:267–272.

72. Putman CE, Curtis A, Simeone JF, Jensen P. *Mycoplasma* pneumonia: clinical and roentgenographic patterns. *Am J Roentgenol* 1975;124:417–422.

73. Forrest JV. Radiographic findings in *Pneumocystis carinii* pneumonia. *Radiology* 1972;103:539–544.

74. Wheat LJ, Connolly-Stringfield PA, Baker RL, et al. Disseminated histoplasmosis in the acquired immune deficiency syndrome: clinical findings, diagnosis and treatment, and review of the literature. *Medicine* 1990;69:361–374.

75. Goldstein E. Miliary and disseminated coccidioidomycosis. *Ann Intern Med* 1978;89:365–366.

76. Stelling CB, Woodring JH, Rehm SR, Hopper DW, Noble RC. Miliary pulmonary blastomycosis. *Radiology* 1984;150:7–13.

77. Miller WT, Edelman JM, Miller WT. Cryptococcal pulmonary infection in patients with AIDS: radiographic appearance. *Radiology* 1990;175:725–728.

78. Light RW, Girard WM, Jenkinson SG, George RB. Parapneumonic effusions. *Am J Med* 1980;69:507–512.

79. Fairbank JT, Mamourian AC, Dietrich PA, Girod JC. The chest radiograph in legionnaires' disease: further observations. *Radiology* 1983;147:33–34.

80. Albelda SM, Kern JA, Marinelli DL, Miller WT. Expanding spectrum of pulmonary disease caused by nontuberculous mycobacteria. *Radiology* 1985;157:289–296.

81. Light RW. Management of parapneumonic effusions. *Arch Intern Med* 1981;141:1339–1341.

82. Friedman PJ, Hellekant CAG. Radiologic recognition of bronchopleural fistula. *Radiology* 1977;124:289–295.

83. Rohfling BM, White EA, Webb WR, Goodman PC. Hilar and mediastinal adenopathy caused by bacterial abscess of the lung. *Radiology* 1978;128:289–293.

84. Dennis JM, Boudreau RP. Pleuropulmonary tularemia: its roentgen manifestations. *Am J Roentgenol* 1957;68:25–30.

85. Burke M, Fraser R. Obstructive pneumonitis: a pathologic and pathogenic reappraisal. *Radiology* 1988;166:699–704.

86. Counsell SR, Tan JS, Dittus RS. Unsuspected pulmonary tuberculosis in a community teaching hospital. *Arch Intern Med* 1989;149:1274–1278.

Thoracic Radiology, edited by
J.D. Newell, Jr., and R.D. Tarver,
Raven Press, Ltd., New York © 1993.

CHAPTER 3

Radiologic Evaluation of Bronchogenic Carcinoma

W. Richard Webb

In considering the radiologic evaluation of patients who are known or suspected of having lung cancer, two topics are of primary importance: (a) the assessment of a solitary pulmonary nodule and (b) the preoperative determination of tumor extent for the purposes of determining resectability.

EVALUATION OF THE SOLITARY PULMONARY NODULE

Although a large number of entities can result in the appearance of a solitary lung nodule on chest radiographs, the radiographic evaluation of such a lesion is primarily directed at distinguishing benign nodules that are usually inconsequential, from nodules that are malignant, or potentially malignant, and thus require treatment. The majority of solitary nodules detected radiographically are benign (1–4).

A variety of radiographic procedures can be used in the evaluation of patients with a solitary pulmonary nodule. Currently, plain chest radiographs and computed tomography (CT; specifically CT with thin collimation or high-resolution CT) are of the most value, sometimes followed by percutaneous lung biopsy. Simply stated, the goals of imaging in patients with an undiagnosed lung nodule are (a) to make a specific diagnosis, or (b) if a specific diagnosis cannot be made, to distinguish benign nodules from those that are potentially malignant, or (c) if benign and malignant nodules cannot be distinguished, to help determine what the subsequent evaluation should entail.

Plain Chest Radiographs

Some specific solitary nodules, such as pulmonary arteriovenous fistula, can be diagnosed on the basis of morphologic findings visible on plain films. However, in the large majority of such cases, it is advisable to obtain CT to confirm the diagnosis. The CT evaluation of solitary nodules is discussed in greater detail later.

A large number of plain film criteria have been reported to be of value in differentiating benign and malignant solitary pulmonary nodules. These include the size, shape, contour, edge definition, growth rate, and the presence or absence of satellite lesions and cavitation (Table 1). However, these plain film criteria rarely allow a specific diagnosis of benign or malignant to be made (4,5).

On the other hand, two specific radiographic findings provide very strong evidence that a solitary pulmonary nodule is benign: (a) the presence of a benign pattern of calcification within the nodule and (b) an absence of growth over 2 years. In patients with either finding, a solitary pulmonary nodule should be followed with sequential chest radiographs, but no other evaluation is usually necessary.

Calcification

Diffuse calcification of an entire nodule, dense calcification that is central (target calcification), laminated calcification, or irregular central popcorn calcification that is visible radiographically, virtually exclude malignancy (Fig. 1) (6). However, other patterns of calcification can sometimes be seen in patients with malignant tumors. For example, bronchogenic carcinomas (scar carcinomas) may incorporate an adjacent calcified granuloma, resulting in the radiographic appearance of a mass

W. R. Webb: Department of Radiology, University of California, San Francisco, San Francisco, California 94143–0628.

TABLE 1. *Plain radiographic findings of some value in distinguishing benign and malignant nodules*

	Benign	Malignant
Size	<3 cm	>3 cm
Shape	Round, elliptical	Irregular
Contour	Smooth	Spiculated
Edge	Well defined	Poorly defined
Doubling time	<1 month or >18 months	>1 month and <18 months
Satellite lesions	Yes	No
Cavitation	No	Yes

containing calcium; however, the calcification is often eccentric within the lesion rather than central (Fig. 2). In addition, bronchogenic carcinomas may themselves calcify; this calcification is often fine and stippled in appearance and may not be easily seen radiographically. In a study of 72 patients with malignant solitary pulmonary nodules, 10 had calcification visible on radiographs of the resected specimen, but only one had calcification detectable on standard chest radiographs (7). In the same study, 67 of 135 benign lesions (mostly granulomas and hamartomas) contained calcifications on specimen radiographs; in 46, these calcifications were also visible on standard chest radiographs (7).

Some malignant nodules can show patterns of calcification that appear benign. Metastatic malignant tumors (particularly osteogenic sarcoma, chondrosarcoma, and thyroid carcinoma) can show homogeneous calcification, but the nodules are usually multiple. Dense calcification in malignant primary carcinoid tumors has also been reported (8). Unless a nodule is diffusely and densely calcified, follow-up radiographs should generally be obtained in patients who are thought to have benign nodule calcification, to ensure that the nodule remains stable in size.

Growth Rate

The growth rate of a solitary pulmonary nodule (usually measured as doubling time) has been used to determine its likelihood of being malignant (9). A pulmonary nodule that doubles in volume in less than 1 month or more than 18 months is usually benign.

However, the overlapping growth rates of benign and malignant lesions, particularly among rapidly growing nodules, makes the use of doubling time hazardous as an absolute indicator of benignancy. Nevertheless, it is generally agreed that a solitary pulmonary nodule that does not grow over a 2-year period is benign and does not require resection. Only rare exceptions to this rule have been reported. Therefore, a vigorous search for old films must be the first step in the evaluation of a noncalcified solitary pulmonary nodule. If films 2 years or older show the pulmonary nodule to be unchanged, follow-up radiographs at intervals are all that are usually necessary.

If no old films are available, or if prior films are not old enough, the diagnostic approach may be based on the patient's age and the plain radiographic appearance of a lesion. If the patient is less than 30 years of age and the pulmonary nodule appears benign (small, round, and sharply defined), follow-up with standard chest radiographs is generally sufficient; lung cancers are rare in patients who are under the age of 30. However, if the patient is older than 30, has a history of an extrathoracic

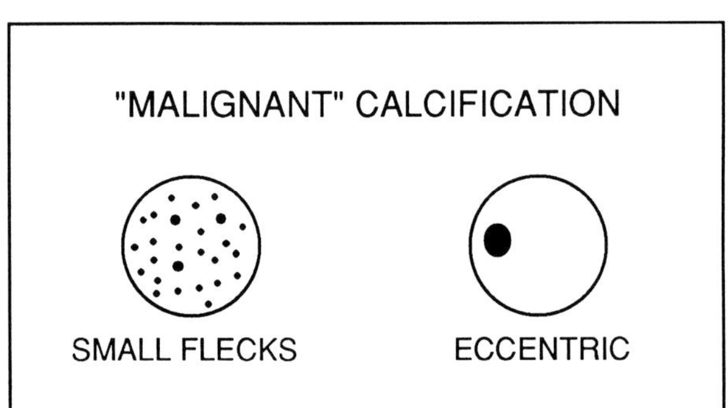

FIG. 1. Patterns of nodule calcification that suggest the presence of a benign or malignant nodule.

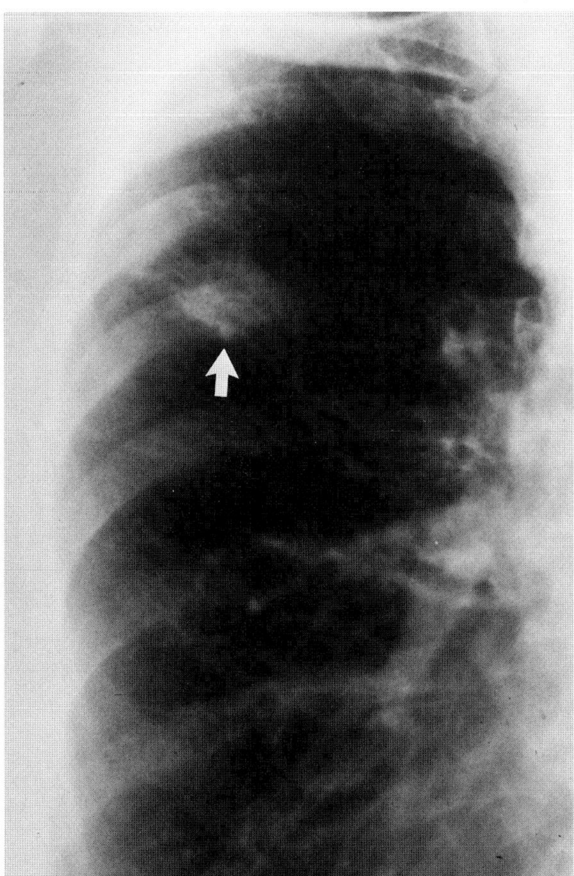
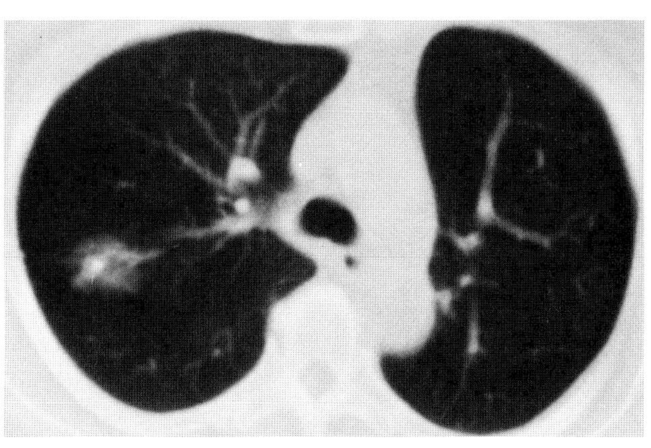

FIG. 2. Eccentric calcification in a carcinoma. (**A**) Plain radiograph shows an ill-defined right upper lobe nodule that contains an eccentric calcification (*arrow*). (**B**) A conventional CT scan confirms the presence of eccentric calcification within the nodule. In this patient, the calcification represents a preexisting granuloma that has been engulfed by the tumor. From Webb (4), with permission.

tumor (that raises the possibility of a solitary metastasis), or if the lesion does not appear benign (i.e., it is large, irregular, ill-defined, or spiculated), additional diagnostic procedures must be performed.

Also, occasionally a patient with an acute process, such as pulmonary embolism or focal pneumonia, can present with a nodular density on chest radiographs. In a patient with acute symptomatology, a follow-up radiograph in 1–2 weeks can sometimes show a decrease in size of a nodule, indicating its benign nature. In some patients without symptoms, repeat radiographs will show a similar decrease in size, indicating that the lesion is benign. Because of this, one or two follow-up films at 1- to 2-week intervals are often obtained in a patient with a solitary nodule, usually during their evaluation, to assess the stability of the lesion. However, it is not advisable in most subjects to obtain follow-up radiographs, *hoping* that a nodule will decrease in size. This can result in an unwarranted delay in treatment, and furthermore, in some patients with lung cancer, nodules become less well defined as they grow and can appear to decrease in size on chest radiographs.

Computed Tomography

CT is obtained in most patients with a solitary pulmonary nodule to define the morphology of the lesion, to detect calcification, and to help in biopsy planning. It has replaced conventional tomography for these purposes.

Delineation of Morphology

In patients with a solitary nodule suspected on plain radiographs, CT is often used to confirm that a nodule is present (e.g., to distinguish it from a pleural abnormality) and to define its morphologic characteristics. Specifically thin-section, high-resolution CT (HRCT) scans (10,11) are extremely valuable in demonstrating the morphology of focal pulmonary parenchymal lesions. We commonly obtain several contiguous HRCT scans through the nodule; such scans are also necessary for measuring nodule density.

A few types of nodular lung lesions have specific morphologic characteristics that are typical enough to allow a diagnosis to be made on CT. These include arteriovenous fistulas, rounded atelectasis, focal consolidation, pleural plaques, fungus balls, and mucous plugs (4).

In addition, the general morphologic characteristics of a nodule may suggest that it is benign or malignant. Pulmonary malignancies (particularly adenocarcinomas) are usually rounded, oval, or lobulated in shape and often appear irregular and spiculated on HRCT; this appearance strongly suggests malignancy (Fig. 3) (12–15). Also, air bronchograms are commonly seen on HRCT in adenocarcinomas (Fig. 3), whereas they are less common in benign nodules (14,15).

On the other hand, some nodules seen on chest radiographs appear benign on HRCT (i.e., their appearance would be atypical for carcinoma). Examples of focal lung lesions that can be classified as benign include nodules that appear linear or scar-like on HRCT (Fig. 4) and nodules that in reality consist of multiple small satellite nodules (Fig. 5).

The identification of multiple lung nodules using CT in a patient who has a single nodule visible on plain films suggests metastases as the likely diagnosis, but lung cancer in association with other causes of lung nodules (e.g., granulomas) must also be considered, particularly if one nodule is dominant. Furthermore, any patient with lung cancer has an increased risk (compared with the general population) of having a second lung cancer synchronous with the first. Thus, if two nodules are visible, both may be primary lung cancers, and both may be resectable. However, this is rare and occurs in less than 1 percent of patients (16,17).

CT Detection of Nodule Calcification

In addition to delineating the morphology of lung lesions, HRCT is ideally suited for the detection of nodule calcification. On HRCT, calcified lung nodules can often be recognized as calcified by simply viewing soft-tissue window scans (Fig. 6); a majority of calcified lung nodules can be detected in this manner (18,19). Nodules that are overtly calcified on HRCT usually have measured CT numbers in the range of 300–400 H. It is important to emphasize that the use of thin collimation (1–2 mm) is essential for detecting calcium; significant calcification can be missed on conventional CT scans with 1 cm collimation because of volume averaging.

Generally the use of HRCT to detect nodule calcification should be reserved for nodules that are smaller than

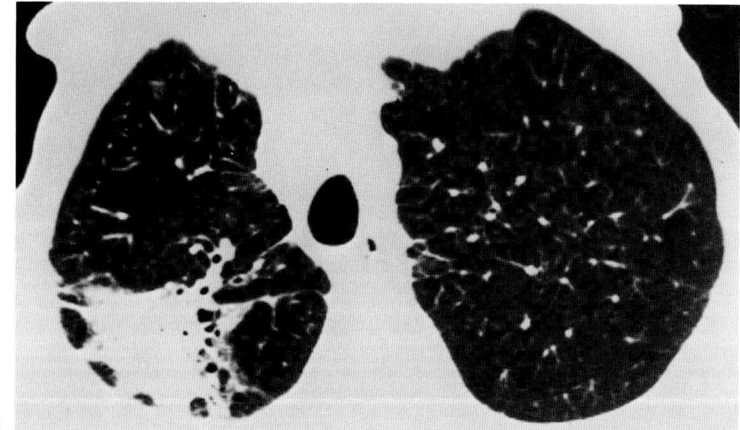

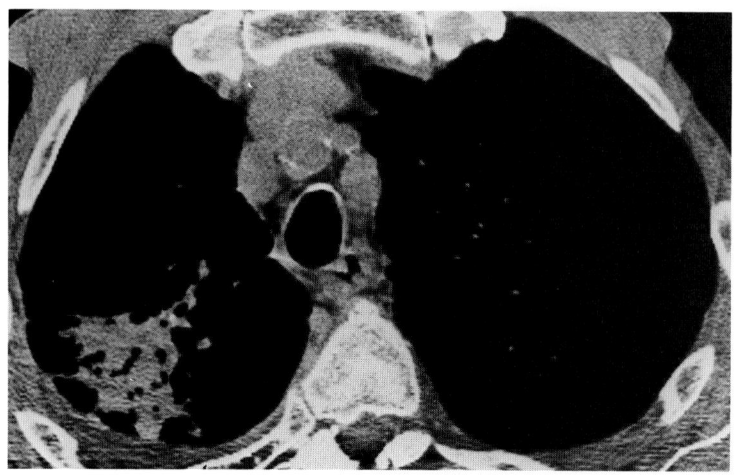

FIG. 3. HRCT of an adenocarcinoma. **(A)** Lung window scan shows a large ill-defined and spiculated nodule in the peripheral lung. This appearance is typical of adenocarcinoma. The tail-like extensions to the pleural surface usually represent fibrosis and do not imply tumor invasion of the pleura. **(B)** A soft-tissue window scan shows multiple air bronchograms within the nodule.

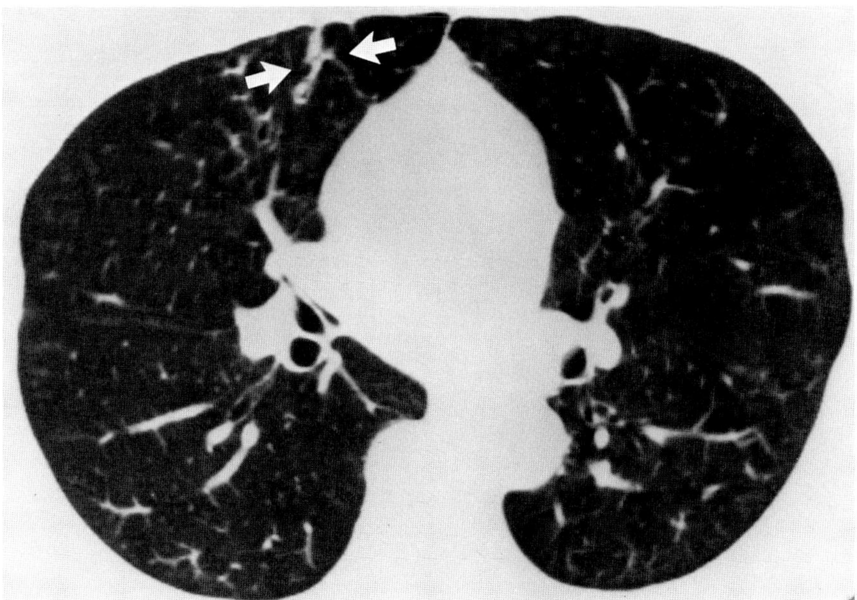

FIG. 4. HRCT of a small solitary nodule seen on plain radiograph. On HRCT, the nodule (*arrows*) consists of a linear area of scarring or atelectasis, and is associated with one or more ectatic bronchi. This lesion appears benign. Radiographic follow-up would be sufficient.

2.5 cm and appear relatively well defined on plain films or CT. Nodules that are larger than this, or appear spiculated or ill-defined, have a high likelihood of being malignant, and unless diffuse calcification was seen on HRCT, it would be hazardous to call such nodules benign (Fig. 6) (12,18).

CT using thin collimation can also be valuable in diagnosing pulmonary hamartomas. In one study (20), 30 of 47 patients with a hamartoma were correctly diagnosed using CT because of visible fat that was either focal or diffuse (18 patients) (Fig. 7), the combination of fat and calcification (10 patients), or diffuse calcification (2 patients). Visible fat within the nodules was more commonly seen than was calcification. CT numbers indicating the presence of fat ranged from −40 to −120 H.

CT Nodule Densitometry

In 1980, Siegelman et al. (21) suggested the use of quantitative CT densitometry for the detection of calcium in lung nodules, thus indicating their benignancy. He indicated that calcification invisible using plain radiographic or tomographic techniques could be detected by high CT numbers using CT with thin collimation. In his initial report (21), two-thirds of patients with benign nodules (and no patients with malignancies) had measured CT numbers within the nodule of greater than 164 H, and he regarded this number as the cutoff between benign (>164 H) and malignant (<164 H). Siegelman has subsequently confirmed his results in a larger series (12).

From 22 to 36 percent of lung nodules that cannot be shown to contain calcium using conventional tomograms are found to contain calcium using CT (12,22,23).

However, studies of individual scanners, scanner geometry, and reconstruction algorithms have emphasized the rather considerable variation in nodule density measurements that are obtained using different scanners, for nodules of different sizes, in different locations, and in patients of different size and chest wall thickness (24). These variables made the use of specific CT number criteria, which are applicable to one machine, difficult or impossible to use on another. Because of this, an anthropomorphic phantom for use in chest CT was developed (25). This phantom can simulate the shape, dimensions, and density of thoracic structures in most patients. Cylinders of various diameters, made of plastic to correspond to a density of 164–264 H on Siegelman's scanner, serve as the reference density for solitary pulmonary nodules (26). When using this phantom, after a patient with a solitary nodule is scanned using thin collimation, the phantom is assembled to simulate the same slice level, chest wall thickness, nodule location, and size, and then the phantom is scanned using the identical CT technique as was used in scanning the patient (Fig. 8). Then, the density of pixels in the patient's nodule and the phantom nodule are compared. If pixels in the lung nodule are denser than those in the phantom nodule, calcium is considered to be present (27). However, as stated previously, because lung carcinomas can contain some calcium, not all nodules shown to contain calcium should be called benign. It must be remembered that the calcifi-

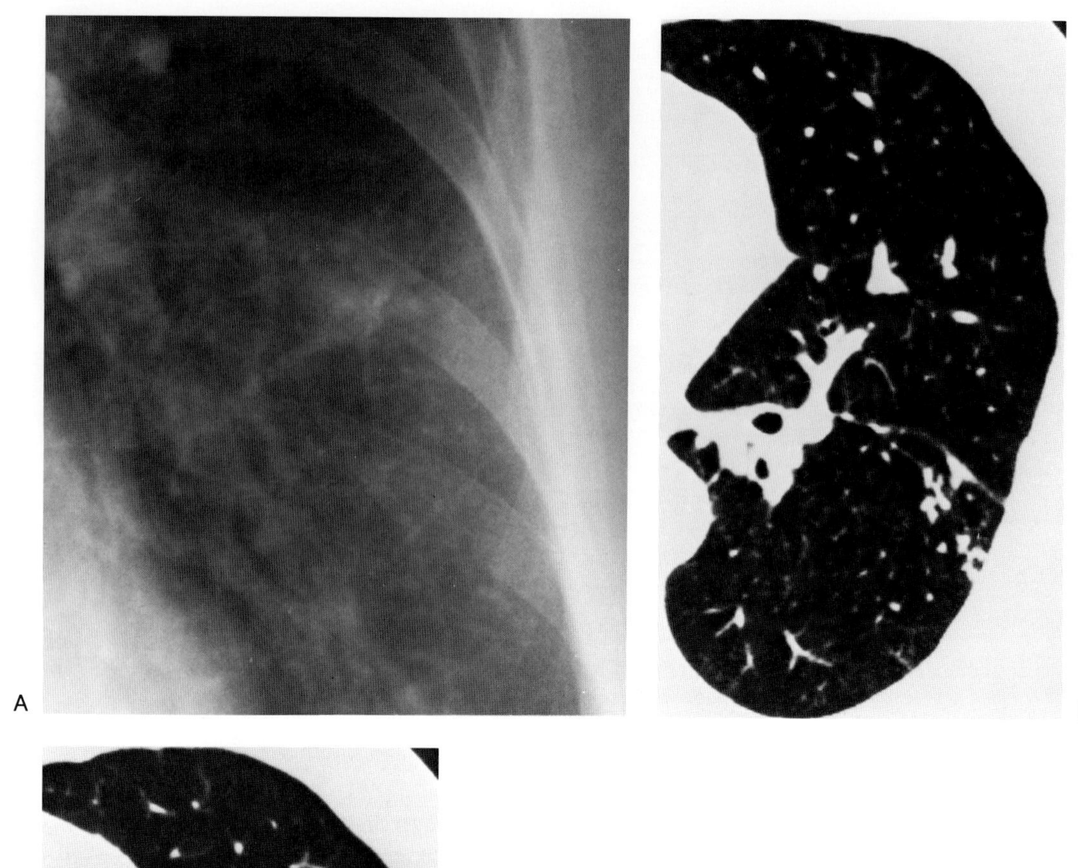

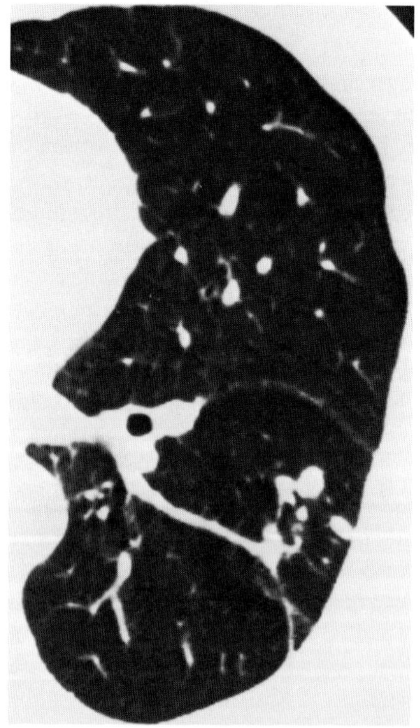

FIG. 5. (**A**) Plain chest radiograph shows an ill-defined left lung nodule. (**B** and **C**) HRCT at two levels shows that this nodule consists of multiple small satellites, rather than a single dominant mass as would be typical of carcinoma. This appearance is much more typical of a granulomatous disease. An atypical mycobacterium was found at needle biopsy. (B) and (C) from Webb (4), with permission.

cation must be benign in character (i.e., central and of significant size).

It has been shown in several studies that using a nodule densitometry phantom can increase the sensitivity of HRCT in detecting nodule calcification. In from one-third to one-half of cases in which a nodule can be called calcified using HRCT, the use of phantom nodule densitometry is necessary (18,19). At the same time, however, it is important to recognize that increasing the sensitivity of HRCT for detecting calcification can reduce its speci-

ficity to unacceptable levels. In one study that used phantom nodules having a density of 185 H, 10 of 85 nodules that were classified as calcified proved to be malignant (28).

Use of Imaging to Guide Biopsies

If plain radiographs and CT do not allow a specific diagnosis to be made, and no calcification is visible within the nodule, biopsy of the nodule may be neces-

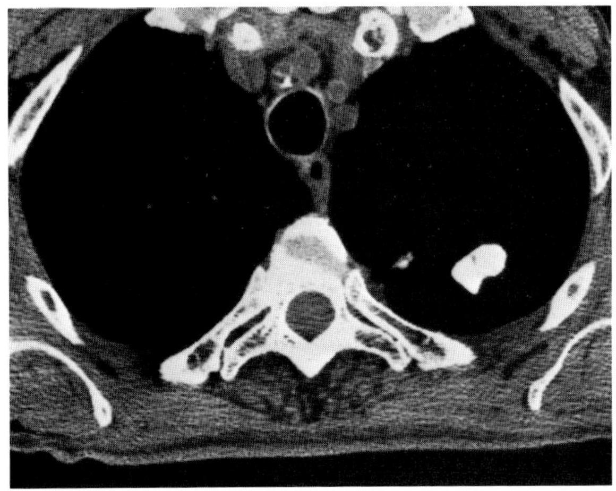

FIG. 6. HRCT through a left apical nodule seen on plain radiograph. On the plain radiograph, no definite calcification was visible. On HRCT, the nodule is densely and diffusely calcified. Despite its large size and irregular lobular shape, this nodule can be called benign with certainty.

sary. Depending on the clinical situation, and the beliefs of the patient's physician, several options are available. These may include needle lung biopsy, bronchoscopy, mediastinoscopy, or thoracotomy. To some degree, imaging studies can be valuable in making this choice.

Aspiration Lung Biopsy or Bronchoscopy?

Aspiration needle biopsy has become firmly established in the investigation of peripheral solitary pulmonary nodules that are suspected of being neoplastic (29). Lesions as small as 1 cm can be biopsied, although the minimum size varies with the skill of the radiologist. Confirmation of the tip of the needle within the lesion must be obtained. Biplane fluoroscopy, single plane fluoroscopy, and CT can be used.

Needle biopsy of the lung is a safe procedure. Although pneumothorax occurs in about 20 percent of patients, a chest tube is required in only a few percent. In

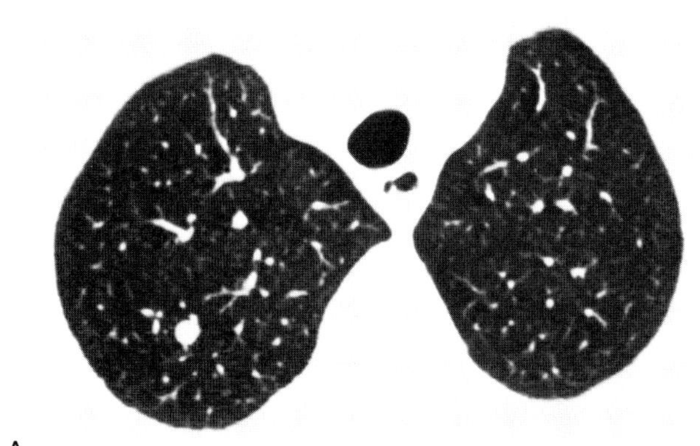

A

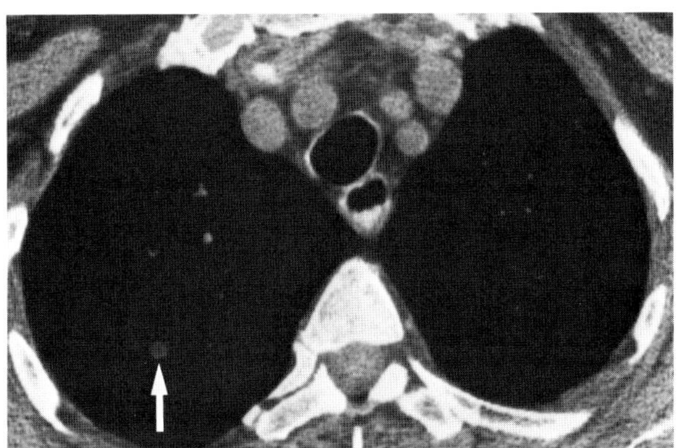

B

```
                    CT NUMBERS

        EXAM        390         STATION     1

    PRS     1        PROSPECTIVE      IMAGE      7
```

Y＼X	187	188	189	190	191	192	193	194	195
291	−804	−633	−265	−52	−62	−128	−200	−394	−436
292	−644	−270	−137	−97	−117	−101	−43	−158	−290
293	−364	−110	−60	−90	−83	−131	−102	−94	−217
294	−380	−119	−118	−145	−116	−137	15	−36	−14
295	−294	−101	−59	−107	−63	−167	−173	−177	−179
296	−404	−70	−86	−111	−88	−87	−64	85	−49
297	−637	−319	−22	−50	−20	−53	−32	−159	−520
298	−760	−464	−151	−83	−72	−169	−123	−272	−722
299	−889	−844	−632	−336	−142	−235	−396	−728	−950

C

FIG. 7. HRCT in a patient with a hamartoma. **(A)** A small, round, well-defined nodule is visible in the right upper lobe. **(B)** At a soft-tissue window setting, the nodule (*arrow*) is similar to subcutaneous fat in density and is difficult to see. **(C)** CT numbers measured from the nodule are in the range typically seen with fat-containing hamartomas. Follow-up has shown no change. From Webb (4), with permission.

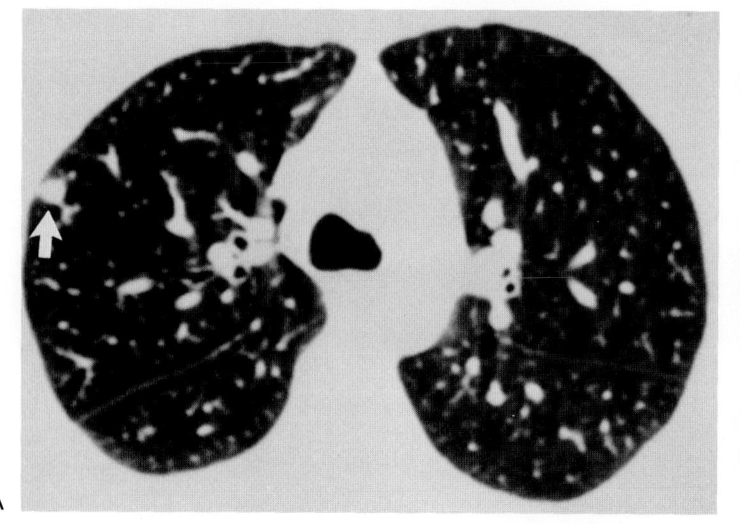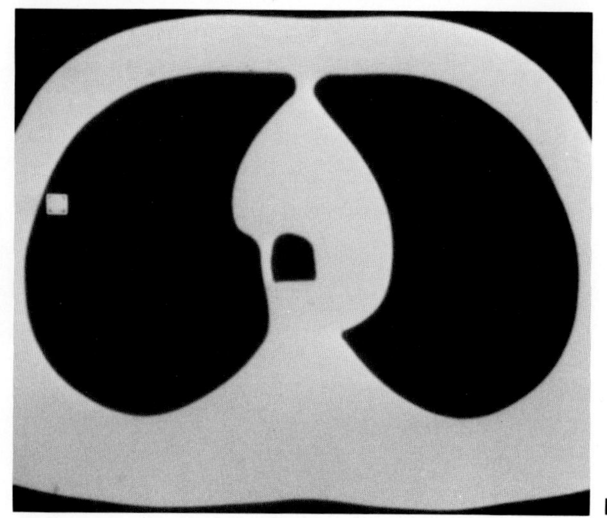

CT NUMBERS

EXAM   1799   STATION   1

PRS   1   PROSPECTIVE   IMAGE   12

Y \ X	117	118	119	120	121	122	123	124	125
202	-839	-618	-383	-241	-206	-283	-477	-742	-919
203	-627	-279	-61	12	30	-13	-146	-446	-782
204	-399	-64	32	36	38	27	-1	-196	-613
205	-265	13	35	33	31	19	23	-74	-482
206	-241	24	33	33	31	21	36	-52	-461
207	-339	-9	50	42	26	28	43	-113	-549
208	-533	-163	-2	34	37	26	-40	-316	-722
209	-765	-464	-226	-109	-86	-152	-323	-622	-890
210	-921	-799	-623	-499	-473	-562	-714	-880	-972

C

CT NUMBERS

EXAM   1799   STATION   1

PRS   1   PROSPECTIVE   IMAGE   5

Y \ X	126	127	128	129	130	131	132	133	134
283	-738	-640	-491	-401	-386	-347	-300	-370	-555
284	-648	-489	-294	-177	-126	-64	-24	-147	-430
285	-426	-269	-117	-35	18	82	94	-24	-319
286	-192	-81	5	38	87	141	118	2	-279
287	-118	-23	41	85	161	206	135	-25	-326
288	-187	-77	2	85	184	227	136	-88	-419
289	-354	-183	-55	52	146	186	72	-221	-554
290	-579	-396	-228	-103	3	42	-92	-405	-696
291	-737	-654	-538	-433	-337	-301	-375	-563	-751

D

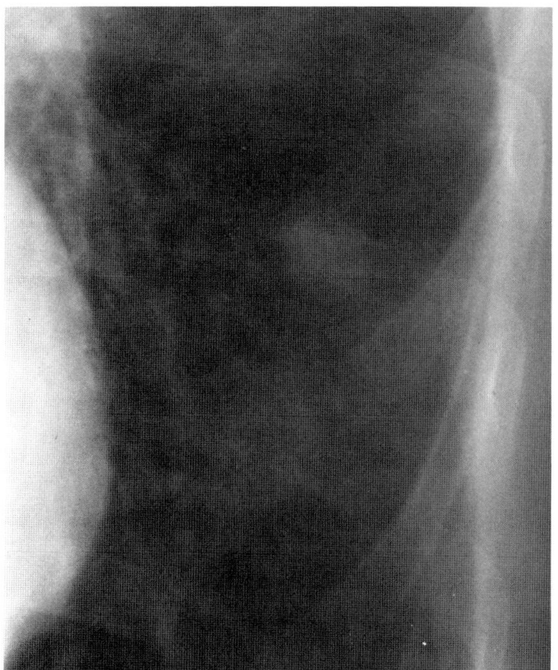

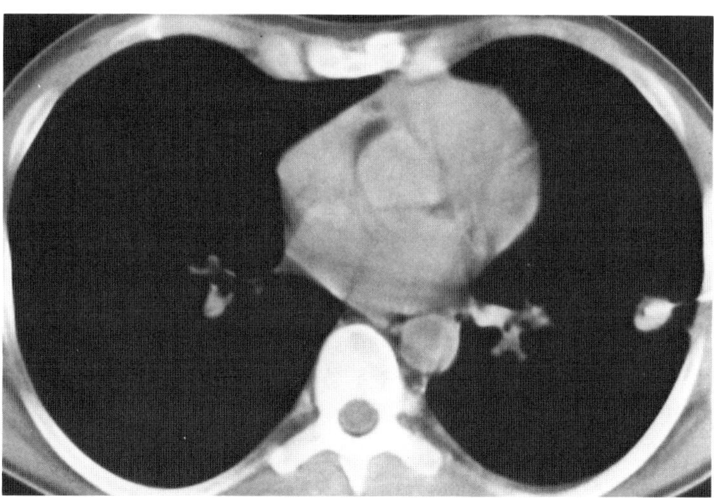

FIG. 9. (**A**) Chest radiograph shows a well-defined solitary nodule. (**B**) CT used for biopsy guidance shows the needle tip in the nodule. Biopsy showed fungal hyphae and necrotic debris, indicating the presence of a granuloma.

patients with carcinoma, hemorrhage and death are uncommon; dissemination of malignant cells from an aspiration biopsy may rarely occur.

Needle aspiration will yield malignant cells in more than 90 percent of neoplastic nodules (29). This percentage can be optimized by having a cytologist on hand at the time of the biopsy and repeating the biopsy if specimens are negative. Cytologic determination of cell type is good for squamous cell carcinomas and adenocarcinomas, but poor for undifferentiated tumors. The diagnosis of a benign nodule (e.g., hamartoma) can sometimes be made, although this usually requires a larger aspirate than for the diagnosis of malignancy.

The indications for needle aspiration biopsy of a lung nodule vary among institutions, often determined, at least in part, by the surgeon's preference. I think a case can be made for reserving needle biopsy for those patients with solitary pulmonary nodules who are not candidates for thoracotomy because of age, complicating ill-

ness, or because the lesion is suspected to be a metastatic deposit. Because of the relatively high false-negative rate (up to 10 percent) of needle biopsy in patients with carcinoma, a negative biopsy cannot be taken to mean that no tumor is present. If a patient can tolerate surgery, a solitary pulmonary nodule that could represent a malignancy is often resected without needle biopsy being performed. In patients suspected of having a benign nodule because of its appearance, growth rate, or the patient's age, needle biopsy can be used in an attempt to make a specific diagnosis of a benign lesion or to increase the likelihood of a benign process (i.e., if the biopsy is negative for cancer) prior to radiographic follow-up. It is important to note that the role of needle biopsy in patients with a solitary nodule can vary considerably from one institution to the next.

We commonly use CT guidance for needle aspiration lung biopsy, because of the precision with which the needle can be guided to the nodule in question (Fig. 9). Also,

FIG. 8. Use of a nodule phantom for nodule densitometry. (**A**) Thin-collimated CT in a patient with a small right upper lobe nodule (*arrow*). No calcification was visible on soft-tissue window scans. (**B**) The nodule phantom has been assembled to simulate the same level of the thorax (aortic arch), the same chest wall thickness, and the same nodule size and location. On this scan, the nodule appears square because it has been surrounded by a region of interest for measurement of CT numbers. (**C**) CT numbers measured from the region of interest indicated in the phantom show the phantom nodule to contain pixels that are primarily in the range of 30–40 H. (**D**) CT numbers measured from a region of interest surrounding the patient's nodule show many pixels exceeding 100 H and some exceeding 200. Low numbers (<50 H) are only seen at the edges of the nodule. Because the patient's nodule is denser than the phantom nodule, it can be said to be calcified. Because the calcification is diffuse, it can be considered benign. This nodule is unchanged on follow-up. From Webb (4), with permission.

CT can be helpful in planning a needle aspiration biopsy, even if CT is not used for the biopsy itself. First, CT can indicate the depth of the lesion, and the needle can be marked for the appropriate depth. Second, CT can help in planning the biopsy approach. If bullae lie in the path of the needle, or the needle must cross a fissure to reach the lesion, the risk of pneumothorax is increased, and a different approach might be used.

Bronchoscopy is most accurate in diagnosing central masses having an endobronchial component, whereas needle biopsy is best for peripheral lesions. Thus, the location of the lesion can be important in choosing the biopsy procedure. CT can be quite valuable in this regard. If an endobronchial lesion is detected with CT, or bronchial narrowing at the site of a hilar mass is visible, bronchoscopy directed to the proper level is most appropriate (30). In some patients, CT will show an endobronchial lesion beyond the visibility of the bronchoscope, and thus guide the biopsy attempt.

RADIOLOGIC STAGING OF LUNG CANCER

Plain radiographs and CT are the imaging techniques of most value in staging patients with lung cancer. Although each can provide significant anatomic information regarding the extent of intrathoracic tumor, it must be realized that these techniques have limited accuracy for diagnosing the presence of chest wall or mediastinal invasion by tumor, and the presence of mediastinal node metastases. However, the appropriate use of imaging studies, including magnetic resonance imaging, is valuable in determining whether invasive diagnostic procedures are necessary for staging, which invasive procedures should be performed, in guiding these procedures, and in planning eventual surgery (31).

The role of plain radiographs in lung cancer staging should not be underestimated. The presence of a bronchogenic carcinoma is often first suspected or confirmed on plain radiographs. Furthermore, the local extent of the tumor can sometimes be assessed quite accurately using plain films, allowing invasive diagnostic or staging procedures (i.e., bronchoscopy or mediastinoscopy) to be performed without further radiographic evaluation.

However, the ability of plain radiographs to define the extent of lung, hilar, or mediastinal masses is limited. CT is generally obtained in patients with lung cancer, because of its better definition of several areas important in lung cancer staging, particularly the mediastinum. Recently, magnetic resonance (MR) has been used in some specific situations to provide anatomic information not obtainable using CT. In certain instances it can be very helpful (32).

STAGING OF BRONCHOGENIC CARCINOMA

In patients with lung cancer, the anatomic extent of the tumor is usually most important in determining what therapeutic approach will be chosen. A TNM classification system is used in lung cancer staging (Table 2); this is based on the appearance and location of the primary tumor (T), the presence or absence of hilar or mediastinal lymphadenopathy (N), and the presence or absence of distant metastases (M) (33–35). Although this system is useful in radiologic lung cancer staging, it is not usually necessary in the clinical setting to classify the

TABLE 2. *Lung cancer staging system (35,38)*

T (primary tumor)

T0	No evidence of a primary tumor
T1	A tumor 3 cm or less in greatest diameter, limited to the lung, and without invasion proximal to a lobar bronchus
T2	A tumor larger than 3 cm; a tumor that invades the visceral pleura or produces collapse or consolidation of less than an entire lung; the tumor must be more than 2 cm distal to the carina
T3	A tumor invading parietal pleura, chest wall, diaphragm, or mediastinal pleura or pericardium; a tumor less than 2 cm from the carina, or producing collapse on consolidation of an entire lung
T4	A tumor of any size with invasion of the mediastinum or involving the heart, great vessels, trachea, esophagus, vertebral body, or carina, or producing malignant pleural effusion

N (nodal involvement)

N0	No node metastases
N1	Metastases to ipsilateral hilar nodes
N2	Metastases to ipsilateral mediastinal nodes or subcarinal nodes
N3	Metastases to contralateral hilar or mediastinal lymph nodes, or scalene or supraclavicular lymph nodes

M (distant metastases)

M0	Metastases absent
M1	Metastases present

Resectable stages

Stage I	T1	N0	M0
	T2	N0	M0
Stage II	T1	N1	M0
	T2	N1	M0
Stage IIIA	T3	N0	M0
	T3	N1	M0
	T1	N2	M0
	T2	N2	M0
	T3	N2	M0

Unresectable stages

Stage IIIB	N3, M0, any T
	T4, M0, any N
Stage IV	M1, any T, any N

tumor stage precisely using chest radiographs or CT (36,37). Rather, it is most important to determine, as accurately as possible, the anatomic extent of the tumor and its relationship to various intrathoracic structures. This can indicate whether or not the lesion is likely to be surgically resectable, what biopsies would be most appropriate, and, to some degree, what surgical procedure would be required. In this chapter, the critical determinates of lung cancer staging are emphasized as pertains to resectability.

Generally speaking, tumors are considered to be unresectable if they are classified as T4, N3, or M1 in the new staging classification (Table 2) (35,38,39). However, it is important to note that different surgeons have different anatomic criteria for considering a tumor unresectable, and a careful and detailed discussion of the radiographic findings with the involved surgeon is necessary in individual cases (40).

Invasive Primary Tumors

A primary tumor is classified T4 and is usually considered unresectable if it has invaded the mediastinum with involvement of the heart, great vessels, trachea, esophagus, vertebral body, carina, or produces a malignant pleural effusion (35,38,39). Tumors invading the chest wall, including the superior pulmonary sulcus, diaphragm, mediastinal pleural, pericardium, or proximal main bronchus, are not considered unresectable, and are classified as T3 (Table 2). CT can be quite helpful in determining tumor extent. In a recent survey of thoracic surgeons (40), 71 percent use CT to help decide if the primary tumor is resectable and to guide their surgery. Thus, using CT in an attempt to determine primary tumor extent seems quite appropriate.

Invasion of the Chest Wall or Mediastinum

Chest Wall Invasion

Direct invasion of the pleura and chest wall by a peripheral bronchogenic carcinoma may or may not indicate that the tumor is unresectable (41–44). Superior sulcus (Pancoast) tumors are a case in point (42,45). Although they were once considered unresectable in the presence of extrapulmonary invasion, local radiation followed by *en bloc* resection of the tumor and adjacent chest wall have resulted in 5-year survival rates of approximately 30 percent in some series (42,45).

Unless obvious rib destruction is present, the diagnosis of chest wall invasion on plain radiographs is difficult (46,47). Pleural thickening adjacent to a lung mass is nonspecific and need not indicate chest wall invasion. The CT diagnosis of chest wall invasion can also be prob-

lematic, although CT should be obtained if this diagnosis is suspected. A variety of CT findings that have been considered to indicate chest wall invasion have been investigated. These include the presence of (a) obtuse angles at the point of contact between tumor and pleura, (b) more than 3 cm of contact between tumor and the pleural surface, (c) pleural thickening adjacent to the mass, and (d) increased density of extrapleural fat (Fig. 10) (48). Surprisingly, none of these findings has proven to be of great value in making this diagnosis. Although the presence of a gross soft tissue mass or rib destruction indicates the presence of chest wall invasion (Fig. 10), obviously, these findings are not very sensitive. In one study (48), the overall accuracy of CT was only 39 percent in diagnosing chest wall invasion. In another study (49), where a combination of findings was used, sensitivity was 87 percent, specificity 59 percent, and accuracy 68 percent; in this study, the presence of local chest pain was more specific (94 percent) and accurate (85 percent) than CT in making this diagnosis. Recently, CT criteria for diagnosing chest wall invasion were evaluated in a series of 112 patients who had surgery (50). The findings assessed included (a) obliteration of the extrapleural fat plane, (b) the length of the tumor-pleura contact, (c) the ratio between the tumor-pleura contact and the tumor diameter, (d) the angle of the tumor with the pleura, (e) a mass involving the chest wall, and (f) rib destruction. Obliteration of the extrapleural fat plane (Fig. 11) (sensitivity 85 percent, specificity 87 percent) and a ratio of 0.9 between the length of tumor-pleura contact and the tumor diameter (Fig. 10) (sensitivity 83 percent, specificity 80 percent) were most accurate in making this diagnosis (50).

Care must be taken in diagnosing chest wall invasion when a tumor simply abuts the pleura. Tumors adjacent to the pleura—even when associated with local pleural thickening, pleural effusion, or other findings that seem to suggest chest wall invasion—may not be invasive (48,49). Thus, with a lesion that is otherwise resectable, surgery should not be denied the patient because of an appearance that suggests chest wall invasion. In patients with Pancoast tumors, vertebral body invasion, or invasion of the mediastinum or great vessels above the lung apex, prevent surgical resection (35,38). CT can sometimes be valuable in detecting such extensive invasion (47).

MR in the sagittal or coronal planes can be advantageous in imaging some tumors invading the chest wall, particularly those at the lung apex (51–54). In patients with a Pancoast tumor who are being considered for resection, the extent of chest wall invasion and involvement of the subclavian artery or brachial plexus is often better shown with coronal MR than on transaxial CT or MR images (Fig. 12). This anatomic information can be of great value in helping the surgeon decide if resection is possible and what approach to use.

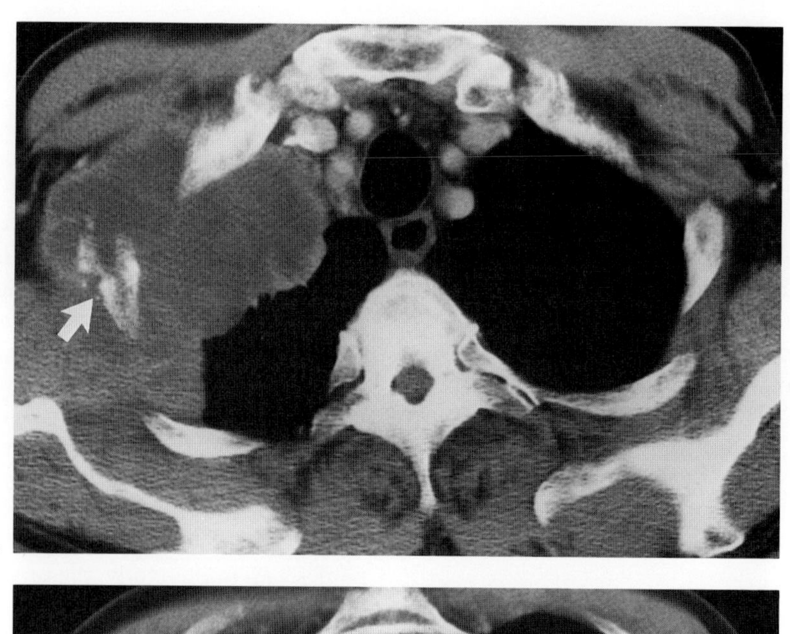

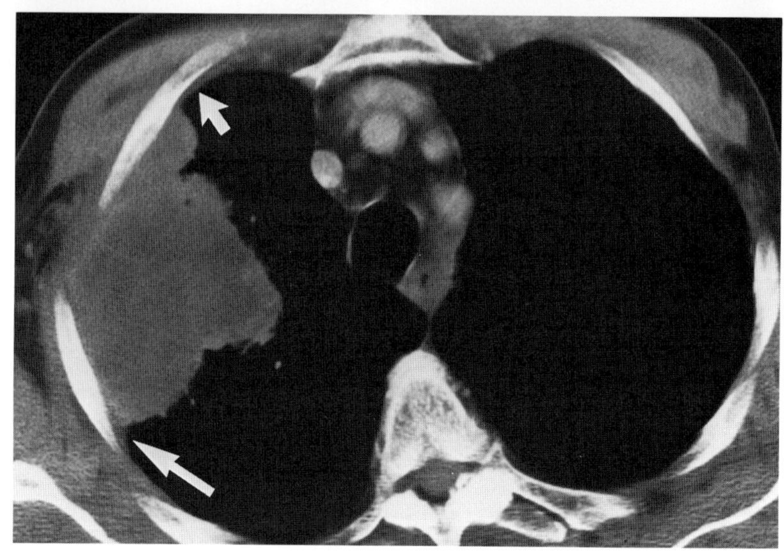

FIG. 10. Chest wall invasion by bronchogenic carcinoma. **(A)** In the upper thorax, a large inhomogeneous carcinoma within the peripheral lung has resulted in extensive chest wall invasion. Rib destruction (*arrow*) and a large chest wall mass are visible. **(B)** At a lower level, there is no gross chest wall invasion, but several CT findings associated with invasion are visible. Note the presence of obtuse angles at the point of contact between tumor and pleura (*large arrow*), pleural thickening adjacent to the mass (*small arrow*), more than 3 cm of contact between tumor and the pleural surface, and a ratio of more than 0.9 between the length of tumor-pleura contact and the tumor diameter.

Mediastinal Invasion

In patients with lung cancer, contiguous invasion of the mediastinum with involvement of the heart, great vessels, trachea, or esophagus precludes resection (35,39,44). Invasion of the mediastinal pleura or pericardium does not prevent resection, although significant invasion of mediastinal fat usually does.

On plain radiographs, findings that suggest mediastinal invasion include a mediastinal mass and diaphragmatic paralysis (which in turn implies involvement of the phrenic nerve), but radiographs are insensitive to the presence of invasion.

As with the CT diagnosis of chest wall invasion, tumor mass in contiguity with the mediastinal pleura or thickening of the mediastinal pleura does not necessarily indicate mediastinal extension or unresectability. However, a significant mediastinal mass contiguous with a lung tumor, which surrounds or compresses mediastinal vessels, the esophagus, or the central bronchi, and results in replacement of mediastinal fat by soft tissue density, strongly suggests this diagnosis (Fig. 13).

Other CT findings that are associated with mediastinal invasion include (a) obliteration of the fat plane that is normally seen adjacent to the descending aorta or other mediastinal vessels, (b) tumor contacting more than one-

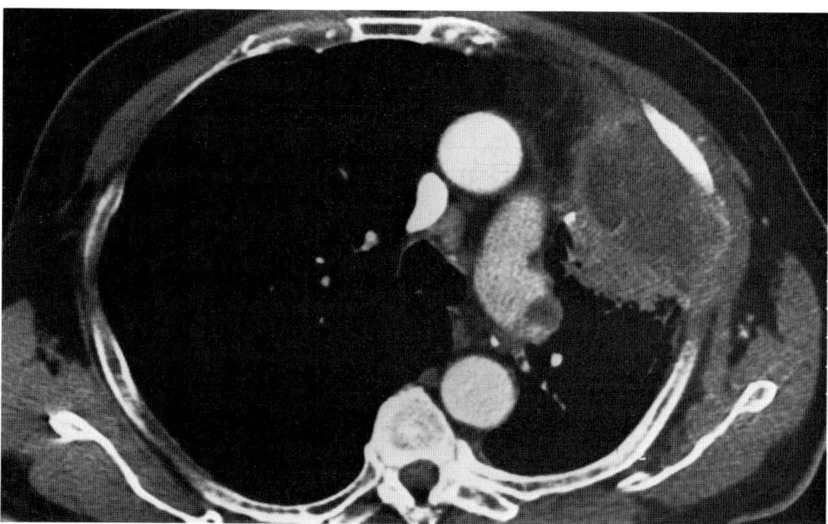

FIG. 11. In a patient with a necrotic carcinoma resulting in chest wall invasion, CT shows obliteration of fat planes normally seen in the intercostal spaces.

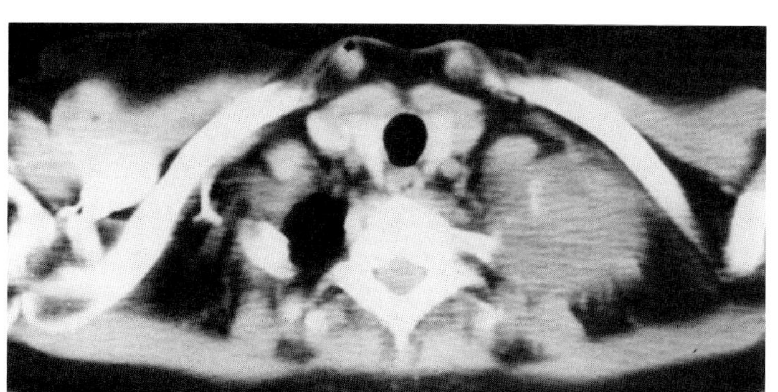

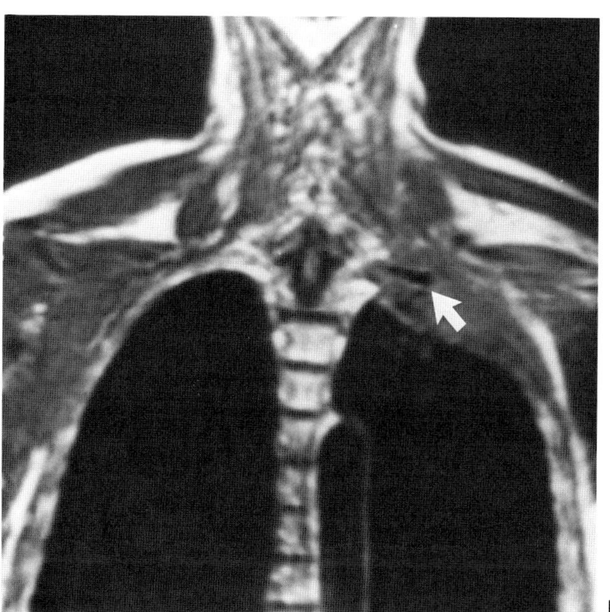

FIG. 12. Pancoast tumor with chest wall invasion. **(A)** CT shows soft-tissue invasion in the lung apex. **(B)** Coronal MR imaging shows the extent of chest wall invasion better than does CT. Tumor surrounds the subclavian artery (*arrow*), making this lesion unresectable. From Webb (37), with permission.

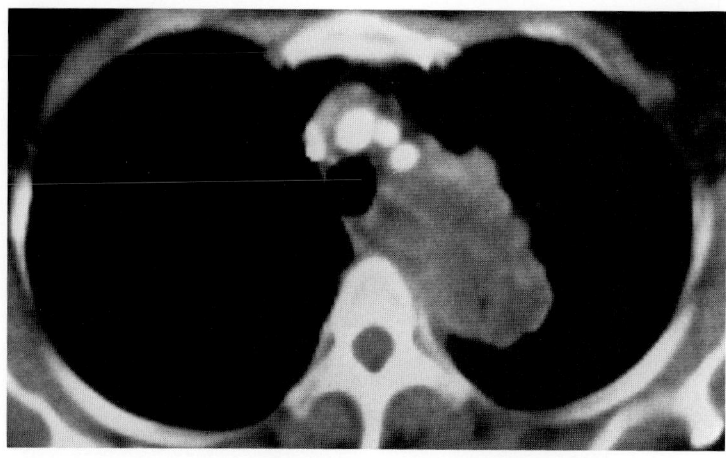

FIG. 13. Mediastinal invasion by tumor. Contrast-enhanced CT shows a tumor mass within the medial left lung, contacting and directly invading the mediastinum with replacement of mediastinal fat by soft tissue. Mediastinal tumor surrounds great vessels.

fourth of the circumference of the aortic wall, (c) tumor contacting more than 3 cm of the mediastinum, (d) mediastinal pleural thickening, and (e) a mediastinal mass effect (Fig. 14) (55). However, in patients who do not show obvious mediastinal invasion, these CT findings are only about 50 percent accurate in predicting invasion or unresectability, even in combination (55). On the other hand, if none of these findings is present, the tumor is likely to be resectable (55). In some patients, HRCT can aid in the diagnosis of mediastinal invasion (Fig. 15).

In patients who have findings that suggest mediastinal invasion, mediastinoscopy or transbronchoscopic or percutaneous needle aspiration biopsy should be performed prior to any attempt at surgical cure. Because of the limited accuracy of CT, unless CT findings are gross, confirmation of the diagnosis is necessary.

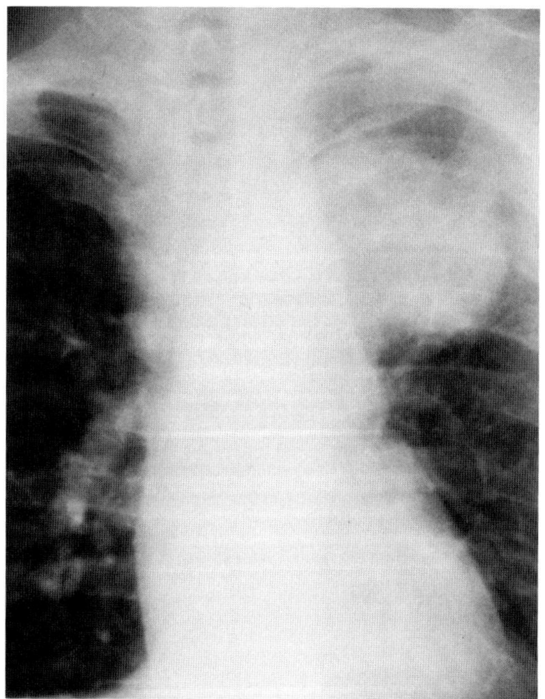

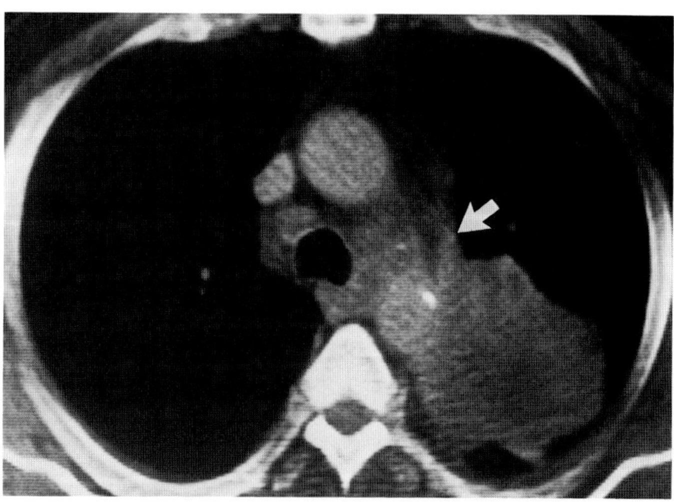

A

B

FIG. 14. CT in a patient with mediastinal node metastases and mediastinal invasion. **(A)** Chest radiograph shows a large left lung mass. There is widening of the right paratracheal mediastinum, suggesting the presence of right mediastinal lymph node enlargement. **(B)** CT shows a large mass in the left lung and a number of findings that can indicate the presence of mediastinal invasion. The mass contacts more than 3 cm of the mediastinum, obliterates the fat plane that is normally seen adjacent to the descending aorta, contacts more than one-fourth of the circumference of the aortic wall, and results in mediastinal pleural thickening (*arrow*). Aorticopulmonary window lymph node enlargement and enlargement of right paratracheal lymph nodes are present. Both mediastinal node metastases and mediastinal invasion were present. From Webb (36), with permission.

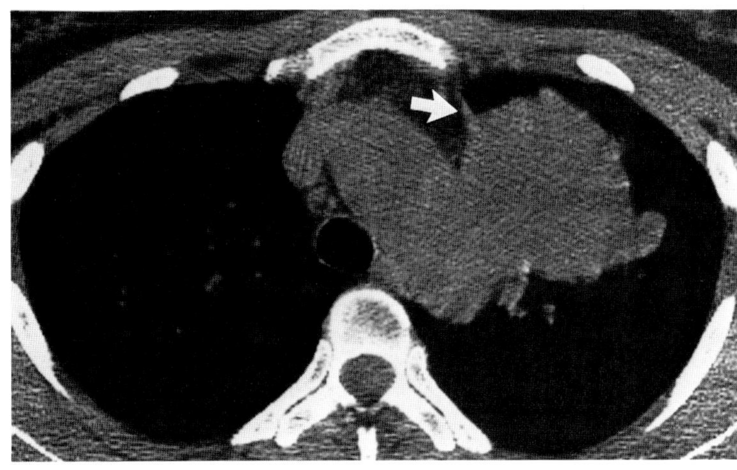

FIG. 15. Mediastinal invasion shown on HRCT. Tumor contacts the left aortic wall, and mediastinal fat lateral to the aorta is replaced by soft tissue. Mediastinal pleural thickening (*arrow*) is seen anteriorly.

As with CT, MR is incapable of accurately demonstrating mediastinal pleural invasion or minimal invasion of mediastinal fat. Only when there is significant obliteration of fat planes or compression or displacement of mediastinal vessels, can mediastinal invasion be diagnosed with a reasonable degree of accuracy using either technique. In one study, the accuracy of CT in diagnosing mediastinal invasion was 56 percent and that of MR was 50 percent (56); in a more recent study (57), the accuracies were higher, measuring 89 and 93 percent, respectively, for CT and MR. MR has been found to be significantly more accurate than CT in diagnosing mediastinal invasion (32), and it is occasionally performed in this setting, particularly when vascular invasion is suspected (58,59).

Pleural Effusion

In a patient with bronchogenic carcinoma, pleural effusion can occur for a variety of reasons, including pleural invasion, obstructive pneumonia, and lymphatic or pulmonary venous obstruction by tumor. Although the presence of effusion indicates a poor prognosis, only those patients with demonstration of tumor cells in the pleural fluid or on closed pleural biopsy samples are considered unresectable (35,38,39). Other patients with effusion are considered to have resectable lesions, despite their poor prognosis. Usually plain radiographs are sufficient for diagnosis of pleural effusion, leading to thoracentesis and/or pleural biopsy.

Central Bronchial Lesions

Although tumor masses that cause total lung collapse or consolidation, or involve the proximal bronchus may be difficult to treat surgically, they are not generally considered unresectable unless they involve the carina. In this situation, it is difficult to perform a pneumonec-

tomy, resect all the tumor, and surgically close the remaining airway (34,38).

In some cases, plain radiographs or CT (Fig. 16) can demonstrate the relationship of a proximal tumor mass to the main bronchus, carina, or trachea, but as a rule, bronchoscopy is more accurate in this regard. At bronchoscopy, minimal mucosal involvement by tumor can be diagnosed, whereas on CT or plain radiographs, only discrete masses are visible. Bronchoscopic confirmation of an apparent carinal or tracheal tumor is usually necessary, unless the findings are gross.

Mediastinal Node Metastases

Ipsilateral mediastinal or subcarinal node metastases are classified N2 in the current staging system, and are considered potentially resectable; contralateral hilar or mediastinal node metastases are considered N3 and unresectable (35,38,39,44). Despite this, there remains some controversy in the surgical community regarding the resectability of tumors associated with N2 mediastinal metastases. Some surgeons believe that surgery should be attempted only if node metastases are limited [e.g., if mediastinoscopy is negative (60) or if node metastases are present at only one level (61)]. The presence of gross or bulky node metastases and node metastases that have invaded through the node capsule are associated with a poor survival after surgery and are generally considered unresectable (39,62).

Radiological Evaluation of Mediastinal Nodes

Because large mediastinal masses in patients with lung cancer are considered unresectable by virtually all surgeons (38,39,63), a patient who has a mediastinal mass visible on plain radiographs (indicating its large size) usually does not require CT, but mediastinoscopy or biopsy should be performed to confirm the presence of

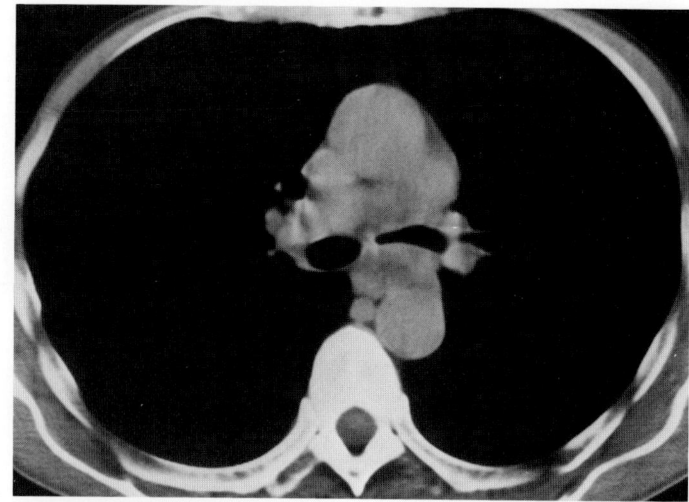

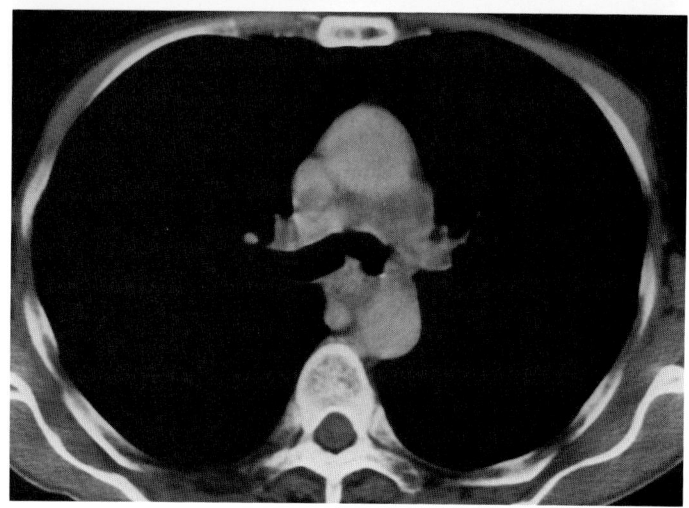

FIG. 16. Carinal invasion by carcinoma. **(A)** A carcinoma involves the left main bronchus with narrowing of the bronchial lumen. An extrinsic mass is present posterior to the bronchus. **(B)** Blunting of the posterior aspect of the carina suggests invasion by tumor. This was confirmed at bronchoscopy. From Webb (36), with permission.

mediastinal disease (Fig. 15) (62). On the other hand, plain radiographs are relatively insensitive for the detection of mediastinal adenopathy and, if normal, certainly do not exclude the presence of lymph node enlargement.

CT can be quite helpful in patients with bronchogenic carcinoma and no evidence of mediastinal mass on plain radiographs. However, although CT allows delineation of mediastinal lymph nodes and can detect lymph node enlargement, the accuracy of CT in predicting the presence or absence of mediastinal node metastases is limited. These limitations must be kept in mind.

A number of studies evaluating the accuracy of CT in diagnosing mediastinal node metastases from bronchogenic carcinoma have been performed (63–72). These studies cannot be easily compared because of the different criteria used in different studies for determining a mediastinal lymph node to be abnormal, different scanners and techniques, differences in the population of patients studied, and different methods for confirming or ruling out the presence of lymph node metastases (i.e., mediastinoscopy, palpation, and total nodal dissection). Not surprisingly, the results of these studies vary.

What conclusions can we draw from these studies? First, the larger the node diameter that is used to distinguish malignant nodes from benign, the more specific but less sensitive CT becomes in detecting metastases. On the other hand, using a small node diameter to distinguish malignant from benign increases sensitivity at the expense of specificity. A greatest node diameter of 1 cm is often used as the upper limits of normal; this value provides acceptable accuracy (approximately 80 percent) without sacrificing sensitivity. Currently, it has been suggested that the least or smallest node diameter, rather than greatest node diameter, more closely correlates with actual node size measured at resection, and therefore is the preferable measurement (73). Although this may be true, using least node diameter to measure mediastinal nodes may not significantly improve the accuracy of CT for diagnosing node metastases in lung cancer patients (63).

When the mediastinum is carefully explored surgically, and all nodes are submitted for histologic study (total nodal sampling), the sensitivity of CT found in experimental studies is lower than when the mediastinum is evaluated only by mediastinoscopy or palpation at surgery (71). With total nodal sampling, metastases in normal sized nodes will be detected. In some recent studies of CT, in which this technique has been used (32,63,68,69,71), the sensitivity (average 64 percent) and accuracy (average 72 percent) of CT in diagnosing mediastinal node metastases have been considerably lower than the sensitivity and accuracy rates (78 and 87 percent, respectively) reported in some earlier studies (65–67,70,72).

Despite these difficulties, however, most authors consider CT to be helpful in staging the mediastinal nodes. Although CT cannot be considered accurate enough to determine with certainty that mediastinal lymph nodes are or are not involved by tumor, it can provide information of value in guiding therapy and invasive diagnostic procedures.

Generally speaking, about 80–90 percent of patients who have no enlarged mediastinal nodes (nodes < 1 cm in greatest or least diameter) will be found to be free of node metastases at surgery. In such patients, thoracotomy without prior mediastinoscopy is probably appropriate, with a mediastinal node exploration conducted at surgery. Although some patients will be found to have microscopic or small intranodal metastases, their presence does not necessarily indicate that surgery should not have been performed. A growing body of literature (38,39,62) suggests that some patients with intranodal mediastinal metastases can be cured following surgical excision of nodes and radiation.

On the other hand, patients who have mediastinal lymph nodes measuring more than 1 cm in diameter have node metastases about 70 percent of the time (Fig. 17). It should be noted that patients with large nodes who have intranodal metastases may also be considered curable by some surgeons (38,39,62), as long as the nodes

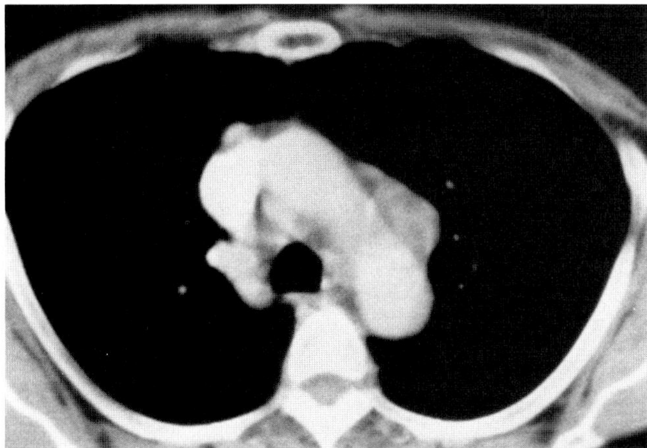

FIG. 17. Mediastinal lymph node metastases. Large mediastinal lymph nodes are clearly seen on CT. These nodes have a high likelihood of being involved by tumor. Mediastinoscopy should be performed prior to surgery.

are not contralateral, numerous, or bulky. Most surgeons will perform mediastinoscopy in patients who have enlarged mediastinal nodes seen on CT (40).

It must be emphasized that, in patients who have enlarged mediastinal nodes on CT, the node metastases found at surgery are not always in the nodes that appear large (63,69,74); large mediastinal lymph nodes in patients with bronchogenic carcinoma may be hyperplastic. Although the sensitivity of CT is about 70–80 percent in diagnosing mediastinal node metastases on a patient-by-patient basis, its sensitivity in detecting metastases in a specific node or node group is lower. For example, in one recent study (69), the sensitivity of CT in detecting mediastinal node metastases was 73 percent, but its sensitivity in diagnosing metastasis to a specific node was only 33 percent. In other studies the sensitivity of CT in diagnosing metastasis to a specific node group was found to be only 40 and 56 percent (63,74).

In general, MR is quite similar to CT in its ability to detect and define mediastinal lymph nodes (56,57, 68,75,76), and it has a similar accuracy in diagnosing mediastinal lymph node metastases (32,56,57,68,75,76). It has no real role to play in the diagnosis of mediastinal node metastases in patients with this disease.

Mediastinoscopy and CT

In addition to helping to determine which patients need mediastinoscopy prior to surgery, CT is also valuable as a guide for the invasive procedures performed before an attempt at a curative resection. Although mediastinoscopy is generally regarded as the gold standard of preoperative mediastinal evaluation, the mediastinoscope cannot evaluate all mediastinal compartments or lymph node groups, and a significant percentage (up to 33 percent) of patients with bronchogenic carcinoma who have a negative mediastinoscopy are proved to have mediastinal nodal metastases at surgery (61,63,77). Through a standard transcervical approach, the mediastinoscopist can evaluate pretracheal lymph nodes, nodes in the anterior subcarinal space, and lymph nodes extending anterior to the right main bronchus. Lymph nodes in the anterior mediastinum (prevascular space), aorticopulmonary window, and posterior portions of the mediastinum (posterior subcarinal space, azygoesophageal recess, etc.) are inaccessible using this technique, although some can be evaluated using a left parasternal mediastinoscopy. CT, on the other hand, allows evaluation of all these areas, shows where any enlarged nodes are, and can serve to guide needle aspiration biopsy, transbronchoscopic needle aspiration biopsy, or parasternal mediastinotomy if enlarged lymph nodes are visible in areas that cannot be evaluated using a standard approach.

In two recent reports, the accuracies of CT and mediastinoscopy were compared in large groups of patients with lung cancer (61,63). Simply stated, both studies found mediastinoscopy and CT to have the same, reasonably high, sensitivity for detecting mediastinal node metastases. However, as would be expected, mediastinoscopy was 100 percent specific (no normals were called abnormal), whereas CT had a specificity of only 50–65 percent. Thus, overall, mediastinoscopy was the more accurate study. In light of this, how should CT be used in evaluating and staging mediastinal nodes in lung cancer? Should mediastinoscopy be done instead of CT?

Some surgeons believe that positive lymph nodes found at mediastinoscopy rule out effective surgical treatment (60). In such patients, survival following surgical resection is poor compared with patients who have had a negative mediastinoscopy but have positive nodes found at surgery; this finding may relate the relative size of the abnormal nodes (abnormal nodes detected at mediastinoscopy are likely to be larger than those that are missed). Thus, in one study (60), the 5-year survival of patients with ipsilateral mediastinal metastases discovered at mediastinoscopy was 9 percent, whereas patients with a negative mediastinoscopy who had ipsilateral metastases discovered at surgery had a 5-year survival of 24 percent. However, despite this, and the fact that mediastinoscopy is more accurate than CT, it is usually recommended that CT should be performed and used to guide mediastinoscopy and biopsy (61,63).

In patients with small, peripheral lung nodules, mediastinal metastases are uncommon, and thoracotomy may be warranted without prior CT or mediastinoscopy, but this remains controversial (78,79). Among those surgeons who favor the use of mediastinoscopy because of its prognostic significance, CT and mediastinoscopy are recommended in all patients with lung cancer, even those with small nodules.

REFERENCES

1. Ray JF, Lawton BR, Magnin GE, et al. The coin lesion story: update 1976. Twenty years experience with early thoracotomy for 179 suspected malignant coin lesions. *Chest* 1976;70:332–336.
2. Bateson EM. An analysis of 155 solitary lung lesions illustrating the differential diagnosis of mixed tumors of the lung. *Clin Radiol* 1965;16:51–65.
3. Edwards WM, Cox RS, Garland LH. The solitary nodule (coin lesion) of the lung: an analysis of 52 consecutive cases treated by thoracotomy and a study of preoperative diagnostic accuracy. *Am J Roentgenol* 1962;88:1020–1042.
4. Webb WR. Radiologic evaluation of the solitary pulmonary nodule. *Am J Roentgenol* 1990;154:701–708.
5. Rotte KH, Meiske W. Results of computer-aided diagnosis of peripheral bronchial carcinoma. *Radiology* 1977;125:583–586.
6. Huston J, Muhm RR. Solitary pulmonary opacities: plain tomography. *Radiology* 1987;163:481–485.
7. O'Keefe MEJ, Good CA, McDonald JR. Calcification in solitary nodules of the lung. *Am J Roentgenol* 1957;77:1023–1033.
8. Zwiebel BR, Austin JHM, Grines MM. Bronchial carcinoid tumors: assessment with CT of location and intratumoral calcification in 31 patients. *Radiology* 1991;179:483–486.
9. Nathan MH. Management of solitary pulmonary nodules: an organized approach based on growth rate and statistics. *JAMA* 1974;227:1141–1144.
10. Mayo JR, Webb WR, Gould R, et al. High-resolution CT of the lungs: an optimal approach. *Radiology* 1987;163:507–510.
11. Webb WR. High-resolution CT of the lung parenchyma. *Radiol Clin North Am* 1989;27:1085–1097.
12. Siegelman SS, Khouri NF, Leo FP, Fishman EK, Braverman RM, Zerhouni EA. Solitary pulmonary nodules: CT assessment. *Radiology* 1986;160:307–312.
13. Kuriyama K, Tateishi R, Doi O, et al. CT-pathologic correlation in small peripheral lung cancers. *Am J Roentgenol* 1987;149:1139–1143.
14. Zwirewich CV, Vedal S, Miller RR, Müller NL. Solitary pulmonary nodule: high-resolution CT and radiologic-pathologic correlation. *Radiology* 1991;179:469–476.
15. Kuriyama K, Tateishi R, Doi O, et al. Prevalence of air bronchograms in small peripheral carcinomas of the lung on thin-section CT: comparison with benign tumors. *Am J Roentgenol* 1991;156:921–924.
16. Bower SL, Choplin RH, Muss HB. Multiple primary bronchogenic carcinomas of the lung. *Am J Roentgenol* 1983;140:253–258.
17. Stark P. Multiple independent bronchogenic carcinomas. *Radiology* 1982;145:599–601.
18. Zerhouni EA, Stitik FP, Siegelman SS, et al. CT of the pulmonary nodule: a cooperative study. *Radiology* 1986;160:319–327.
19. Khan A, Herman PG, Vorwerk P, Stevens P, Rojas KA, Graver M. Solitary pulmonary nodules: comparison of classification with standard, thin-section, and reference phantom CT. *Radiology* 1991;179:477–481.
20. Siegelman SS, Khouri NF, Scott WW, et al. Pulmonary hamartoma: CT findings. *Radiology* 1986;160:313–317.
21. Siegelman SS, Zerhouni EA, Leo FP, Khouri NF, Stitik FP. CT of the solitary pulmonary nodule. *Am J Roentgenol* 1980;135:1–13.
22. Proto AV, Thomas SR. Pulmonary nodules studied by computed tomography. *Radiology* 1985;156:149–153.
23. Huston J, Muhm JR. Solitary pulmonary nodules: evaluation with a CT reference phantom. *Radiology* 1989;170:653–656.
24. Zerhouni EA, Spivey JF, Morgan RH, Leo FP, Stitik FP, Siegelman SS. Factors influencing quantitative CT measurements of solitary pulmonary nodules. *J Comput Assist Tomogr* 1982;6:1075–1087.
25. Zerhouni EA, Boukadoum M, Siddiky MA, et al. A standard phantom for quantitative CT analysis of pulmonary nodules. *Radiology* 1983;149:767–773.
26. Khouri NF, Meziane MA, Zerhouni EA, Fishman EK, Siegelman SS. The solitary pulmonary nodule. Assessment, diagnosis, and management. *Chest* 1987;91:128–133.
27. Zerhouni EA, Stitik FP. Controversies in computed tomography of the thorax. The pulmonary nodule–lung cancer staging. *Radiol Clin North Am* 1985;23:407–426.
28. Swenson SJ, Harms GF, Morin RL, Myers JL. CT evaluation of solitary pulmonary nodules: value of 185-H reference phantom. *Am J Roentgenol* 1991;156:925–929.
29. Khouri NF, Stitik FP, Erozan YS, et al. Transthoracic needle aspiration biopsy of benign and malignant lung lesions. *Am J Roentgenol* 1985;144:281–288.
30. Naidich DP, Sussman R, Kutcher WL, Aranda CP, Garay SM, Ettenger NA. Solitary pulmonary nodules. CT-bronchoscopic correlation. *Chest* 1988;93:595–598.
31. Webb WR, Golden JA. Imaging strategies in the staging of lung cancer. *Clin Chest Med* 1991;12:133–150.
32. Webb WR, Gatsonis C, Zerhouni EA, et al. CT and MR imaging in staging non-small cell bronchogenic carcinoma: report of the Radiologic Diagnostic Oncology Group. *Radiology* 1991;178:705–713.
33. Mountain CF, Carr DT, Anderson WAD. A system for the clinical staging of lung cancer. *Am J Roentgenol* 1974;120:130–138.
34. Tisi GM, Friedman PJ, Peters RM, et al. Clinical staging of primary lung cancer. *Am Rev Respir Dis* 1983;127:659–664.
35. Friedman PJ. Lung cancer: update on staging classifications. *Am J Roentgenol* 1988;150:261–264.
36. Webb WR. Plain radiography and computed tomography in the staging of bronchogenic carcinoma: a practical approach. *J Thorac Imaging* 1987;2:57–65.

37. Webb WR. The role of magnetic resonance imaging in the assessment of patients with lung cancer: a comparison with computed tomography. *J Thorac Imaging* 1989;4:65–75.
38. Mountain CF. A new international staging system for lung cancer. *Chest* 1986;89:225S–233S.
39. Mountain CF. The biologic operability of stage III non-small cell lung cancer. *Ann Thorac Surg* 1985;40:60–64.
40. Epstein DM, Stephenson LW, Gefter WB, van der Voorde F, Aronchik JM, Miller WT. Value of CT in the preoperative assessment of lung cancer: a survey of thoracic surgeons. *Radiology* 1986;161:423–427.
41. Patterson GA, Ginsberg RJ, Poon PY, et al. A prospective evaluation of magnetic resonance imaging, computed tomography, and mediastinoscopy in the preoperative assessment of mediastinal node status in bronchogenic carcinoma. *J Thorac Cardiovasc Surg* 1987;94:679–684.
42. Paulson DL. Carcinoma in the superior pulmonary sulcus. *Ann Thorac Surg* 1979;28:3–4.
43. Piehler JM, Pairolero PC, Weiland LH, et al. Bronchogenic carcinoma with chest wall invasion: factors affecting survival following en bloc resection. *Ann Thorac Surg* 1982;34:684–690.
44. Scott IR, Müller NL, Miller RR, Evans KG, Nelems B. Resectable stage III lung cancer: CT, surgical, and pathologic correlation. *Radiology* 1988;166:75–79.
45. Miller JI, Mansour KA, Hatcher CR. Carcinoma of the superior pulmonary sulcus. *Ann Thorac Surg* 1979;28:44–47.
46. O'Connell RS, McLoud TC, Wilkins EW. Superior sulcus tumor: radiographic diagnosis and workup. *Am J Roentgenol* 1983;140:25–30.
47. Webb WR, Jeffrey RB, Godwin JD. Thoracic computed tomography in superior sulcus tumors. *J Comput Assist Tomogr* 1981;5:361–365.
48. Pennes DR, Glazer GM, Wimbish KJ, Gross BH, Long RW, Orringer MB. Chest wall invasion by lung cancer: limitations of CT evaluation. *Am J Roentgenol* 1985;144:507–511.
49. Glazer HS, Duncan MJ, Aronberg DJ, Moran JF, Levitt RG, Sagel SS. Pleural and chest wall invasion in bronchogenic carcinoma: CT evaluation. *Radiology* 1985;157:191–194.
50. Ratto GB, Piacenza G, Frola C, et al. Chest wall involvement by lung cancer: computed tomographic detection and results of operation. *Ann Thorac Surg* 1991;51:182–188.
51. Webb WR, Jensen BG, Gamsu G, Sollitto R, Moore EH. Coronal magnetic resonance imaging of the chest: normal and abnormal. *Radiology* 1984;153:729–735.
52. Heelan RT, Demas BE, Caravelli JF, et al. Superior sulcus tumors: CT and MR imaging. *Radiology* 1989;170:637–641.
53. Musset D, Grenier P, Carette MF, et al. Primary lung cancer staging: prospective comparative study of MR imaging with CT. *Radiology* 1986;160:607–611.
54. Haggar AM, Pearlberg JL, Froelich JW, et al. Chest-wall invasion by carcinoma of the lung: detection by MR imaging. *Am J Roentgenol* 1987;148:1075–1078.
55. Glazer HS, Kaiser LR, Anderson DJ, et al. Indeterminate mediastinal invasion in bronchogenic carcinoma: CT evaluation. *Radiology* 1989;173:37–42.
56. Martini N, Heelan R, Westcott J, et al. Comparative merits of conventional, computed tomographic, and magnetic resonance imaging in assessing mediastinal involvement in surgically confirmed lung cancer. *J Thorac Cardiovasc Surg* 1985;90:639–648.
57. Laurent F, Drouillard J, Dorcier F, et al. Bronchogenic carcinoma staging: CT vs MR imaging. Assessment with surgery. *Eur J Cardio-Thorac Surg* 1988;2:31–36.
58. Kameda K, Adachi S, Kono M. Detection of T-factor in lung cancer using magnetic resonance imaging and computed tomography. *J Thorac Imaging* 1988;3:73–80.
59. Kono M, Sako M, Adachi S, et al. MR imaging in the assessment of lung cancer patients: primary lung cancer staging, evaluation of therapeutic effect and diagnosis of recurrent tumor. *Nippon Igaku Hoshasen Gakkai Zasshi* 1989;49:831–840.
60. Pearson FG, DeLarue NC, Ilves R, et al. Significance of positive superior mediastinal nodes identified at mediastinoscopy in patients with resectable cancer of the lung. *J Thorac Cardiovasc Surg* 1982;83:1–11.
61. Ratto GB, Mereu C, Motta G. The prognostic significance of preoperative assessment of mediastinal lymph nodes in patients with lung cancer. *Chest* 1988;93:807–813.
62. Martini N, Flehinger BJ, Zaman MB, Beattie EJ. Results of resection in non-oat cell carcinoma of the lung with mediastinal lymph node metastases. *Ann Surg* 1983;198:386–397.
63. Staples CA, Müller NL, Miller RR, Evans KG, Nelems B. Mediastinal nodes in bronchogenic carcinoma: comparison between CT and mediastinoscopy. *Radiology* 1988;167:367–372.
64. Dales RE, Stark RM, Raman S. Computed tomography to stage lung cancer: approaching a controversy using meta-analysis. *Am Rev Respir Dis* 1990;141:1096–1101.
65. Baron RL, Levitt RG, Sagel SS, White MJ, Roper CL, Marbarger JP. Computed tomography in the preoperative evaluation of bronchogenic carcinoma. *Radiology* 1982;145:727–732.
66. Daly BDT, Faling LJ, Pugatch RD, et al. Computed tomography. An effective technique for mediastinal staging in lung cancer. *J Thorac Cardiovasc Surg* 1984;88:486–494.
67. Faling LJ, Pugatch RD, Jung-Legg Y, et al. Computed tomographic scanning of the mediastinum in the staging of bronchogenic carcinoma. *Am Rev Respir Dis* 1981;124:690–695.
68. Grenier P, Dubray B, Carette MF, Frija G, Musset D, Chastang C. Preoperative thoracic staging of lung cancer: CT and MR evaluation. *Diagn Inter Radiol* 1989;1:23–28.
69. Gross BH, Glazer GM, Orringer MB, Spizarny DL, Flint A. Bronchogenic carcinoma metastatic to normal-sized lymph nodes: frequency and significance. *Radiology* 1988;166:71–74.
70. Khan A, Gersten KC, Garvey J, Kahn FA, Steinberg H. Oblique hilar tomography, computed tomography, and mediastinoscopy for prethoracotomy staging of bronchogenic carcinoma. *Radiology* 1985;156:295–298.
71. McKenna RJ, Libshitz HI, Mountain CE, McMurtrey MJ. Roentgenographic evaluation of mediastinal nodes for preoperative assessment in lung cancer. *Chest* 1985;88:206–210.
72. Osborne DR, Korobkin M, Ravin CE, et al. Comparison of plain radiography, conventional tomography, and computed tomography in detecting intrathoracic lymph node metastases from lung carcinoma. *Radiology* 1982;142:157–161.
73. Glazer GM, Orringer MB, Gross BH, Quint LE. The mediastinum in non-small cell lung cancer: CT-surgical correlation. *Am J Roentgenol* 1984;142:1101–1105.
74. McLoud T, Kosiuk JP, Templeton PA, et al. CT in the staging of bronchogenic carcinoma: update of analysis by correlative lymph node mapping and sampling. *Radiology* 1989;173(P):69.
75. Poon PY, Bronskill MJ, Henkelman RM, et al. Mediastinal lymph node metastases from bronchogenic carcinoma: detection with MR imaging and CT. *Radiology* 1987;162:651–656.
76. Webb WR, Jensen BG, Sollitto R, et al. Bronchogenic carcinoma: staging with MR compared with staging with CT and surgery. *Radiology* 1985;156:117–124.
77. Graves WG, Martinez MJ, Carter PL, Barry MJ, Clarke JS. The value of computed tomography in staging bronchogenic carcinoma: a changing role for mediastinoscopy. *Ann Thorac Surg* 1985;40:57–59.
78. Pearlberg JL, Sandler MA, Beute GH, Madrazo BL. T1 N0 M0 bronchogenic carcinoma: assessment by CT. *Radiology* 1985;157:187–190.
79. Heavey LR, Glazer GM, Gross BH, Francis IR, Orringer MB. The role of CT in staging radiographic T1N0M0 lung cancer. *Am J Roentgenol* 1986;146:285–290.

Thoracic Radiology, edited by
J.D. Newell, Jr., and R.D. Tarver,
Raven Press, Ltd., New York © 1993.

CHAPTER 4

Emphysema and Bronchiectasis

John D. Newell, Jr.

Emphysema, asthma, and bronchitis are grouped together and labeled obstructive pulmonary disease. The diagnosis of mild to moderate asthma or bronchitis is made clinically, and there is usually no need for medical imaging at this point. Both asthma and bronchitis can present with bronchial wall thickening and increased lung volumes, but these findings can be absent in patients with known asthma or bronchitis. The computed tomography (CT) examination likewise may show some bronchial wall thickening and airtrapping, but is usually not obtained on patients with mild to moderate asthma or bronchitis without any other complicating factors. The radiologist is usually called on to assess the presence of bronchiectasis, allergic bronchopulmonary aspergillosis (ABPA), or emphysema in patients with clinical evidence of airflow obstruction and with a presumptive diagnosis of asthma, bronchitis, emphysema, or some combination of these three conditions. The radiologist may also discover other diseases coexisting or masquerading as simple asthma, bronchitis, or emphysema. Mitral stenosis, idiopathic pulmonary fibrosis, hypersensitivity pneumonitis, mycobacterial disease, and obstructive lesions of the trachea and central bronchi are just a few of the conditions that may be encountered in the workup of patients referred to radiology as obstructive lung disease. In this group of patients the presence of emphysema or bronchiectasis is useful information to formulate optimal medical management for these patients. It has been difficult to assess the pathologic changes in emphysema and bronchiectasis using conventional chest radiographic techniques. The development of CT and high-resolution CT (HRCT) has provided the radiologist with tools to visualize pulmonary pathology *in vivo,* and is particularly useful in assessing emphysema and bronchiectasis. A recent study illustrated the HRCT findings of diffuse lung disease, including emphysema and interstitial lung disease (1). This study nicely demonstrated the radiologic–pathologic correlation between HRCT scans of excised lungs and the corresponding thin, paper-mounted lung sections obtained at the same levels as the HRCT scans. It is hoped that, in the future, with three-dimensional image processing work stations becoming available, further qualitative and quantitative analyses of emphysema and bronchiectasis will be done to aid in the diagnosis and management of these conditions (2).

EMPHYSEMA

Emphysema is defined as abnormal enlargement of distal air spaces beyond the terminal bronchiole that is accompanied by destruction of the alveolar walls and without evidence of obvious fibrosis (3,4). In the more recent definitions of emphysema (4), simple airspace enlargement due to either congenital or acquired conditions has been excluded, and also airspace enlargement associated with fibrosis has been excluded.

In the early 1960s the discovery of homozygous α_1-protease inhibitor (α_1-PI) deficiency and its association with premature and familial emphysema brought insight into the possible pathophysiologic mechanisms that might produce emphysema (5). The current hypothesis is that emphysema is caused by an imbalance in proteases and antiproteases in the lungs. Studies of animal models of emphysema have lead to considerable support for this theory (6,7).

The clinical diagnosis of emphysema is usually made in a patient who has a clinical history of cigarette smoking, dyspnea, and abnormal pulmonary function tests. The physiologic testing shows chronic airflow obstruction and some abnormality in the central and peripheral airways secondary to bronchitis or bronchiolitis. There

J. D. Newell, Jr.: Department of Radiology, University of Colorado Health Sciences Center; and National Jewish Center for Immunology and Respiratory Medicine, Denver, Colorado 80206.

have been studies to show that the best structure–function correlation in individuals with moderate or severe chronic airflow obstruction associated with cigarette smoking is emphysema (4). Emphysema correlates well with indices of airflow obstruction such as decreased forced expiratory volume (FEV_1). The presence of inflammatory and structural changes in the peripheral airways are next in importance pathologically and generally speaking, the central airway changes, although often present, do not correlate well with the FEV_1. It should be pointed out, though, that emphysema may occur without any evidence of chronic airflow obstruction or any clinical symptoms. It is common to see mild degrees of emphysema at autopsy in patients who had a cigarette smoking history, although the patients may not have suffered any significant respiratory ailments during life (4).

In addition to abnormal FEV_1 measurements, the correlation of increased total lung capacity and a decrease in diffusing capacity from pulmonary function testing are physiologic measurements that correlate well with emphysema. If a patient is referred for HRCT evaluation, it is helpful to know ahead of time whether or not there are abnormalities in FEV_1, total lung capacity, or diffusing capacity.

The areas of involvement of the pulmonary acinus within the secondary pulmonary lobule provide the basis for classifying the different types of emphysema. In the following sections, the approach to diagnosing emphysema using conventional radiography (CR) and then CT will be discussed first. A discussion of centriacinar, panacinar, and distal acinar emphysema will follow this sec-

tion. This section on emphysema will conclude with a discussion of CT's ability to quantitate the amount of emphysema present using density mask software.

Diagnosing Emphysema Using CR

The CR findings for emphysema are not very sensitive (8), and it is difficult to distinguish the different forms of emphysema from each other on CR. It is relatively easy to diagnose moderate to severe emphysema using CT and to distinguish the different forms of emphysema by CT.

In order to assess emphysema using CR, it is important to obtain a good upright postero-anterior (PA) and lateral radiograph of the chest using 110–120 kVp. The examinations should be obtained at full inspiration. One of the newer film-screen systems that have been designed specifically for chest radiography, such as the Insight HC system that was described in Chapter 1, should be used for the examination.

Centrilobular emphysema produced by cigarette smoke involves the upper lobes more than the lower lobes, whereas panacinar emphysema involves the lower lobes more (Fig. 1). This difference in regional involvement of the lung can be helpful in distinguishing these two forms of emphysema on both CR and CT. A fairly recent study examining the ability of CR to diagnose emphysema used arterial deficiency and hyperlucent lungs as the most reliable criteria for diagnosing emphysema (8). The qualitative assessment of emphysema was

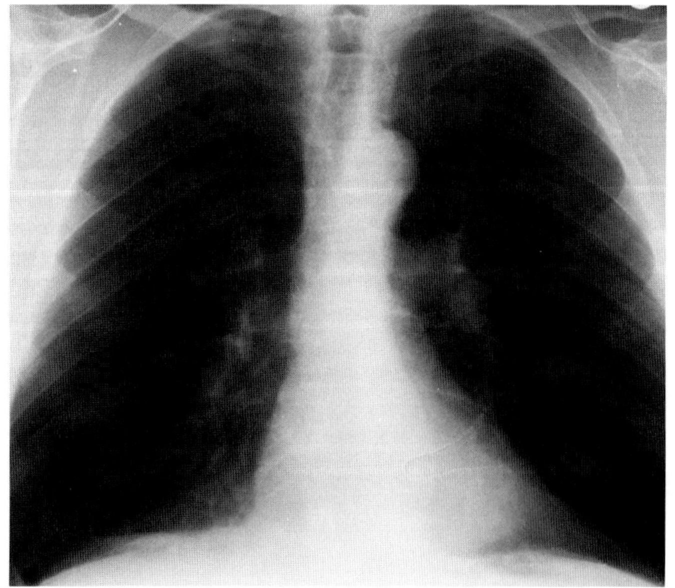
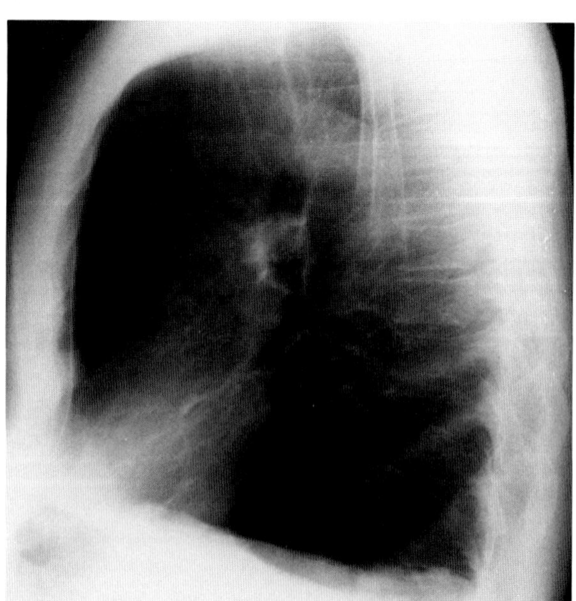

A   B

FIG. 1. (A) PA and **(B)** lateral chest radiographs taken from an elderly male with severe centrilobular emphysema. Note the increased lung volumes, with flattening of the contour of the diaphragm on both the frontal and lateral views of the chest. Focal areas of increased radiolucency with associated vascular attenuation can be seen in both lungs.

determined by hyperlucent lungs and the presence of arterial deficiency. The hyperlucency is quite discrete in distal acinar emphysema where subpleural bleb and bullae formation occur (Fig. 2). However, the hyperlucency is more diffuse and more difficult to appreciate in centriacinar emphysema and in panacinar emphysema. It was emphasized herein that three main abnormalities occurred in the pulmonary vascularity in emphysema.

The first abnormality is narrowing of the vessels that are present in the areas of abnormal lung. The second abnormality is that there are fewer arterial branches present than normal. The third vascular abnormality is that there may be complete absence of pulmonary vessels in some areas of emphysema. This is especially true in distal acinar emphysema where large subpleural bullae displace the adjacent pulmonary vessels.

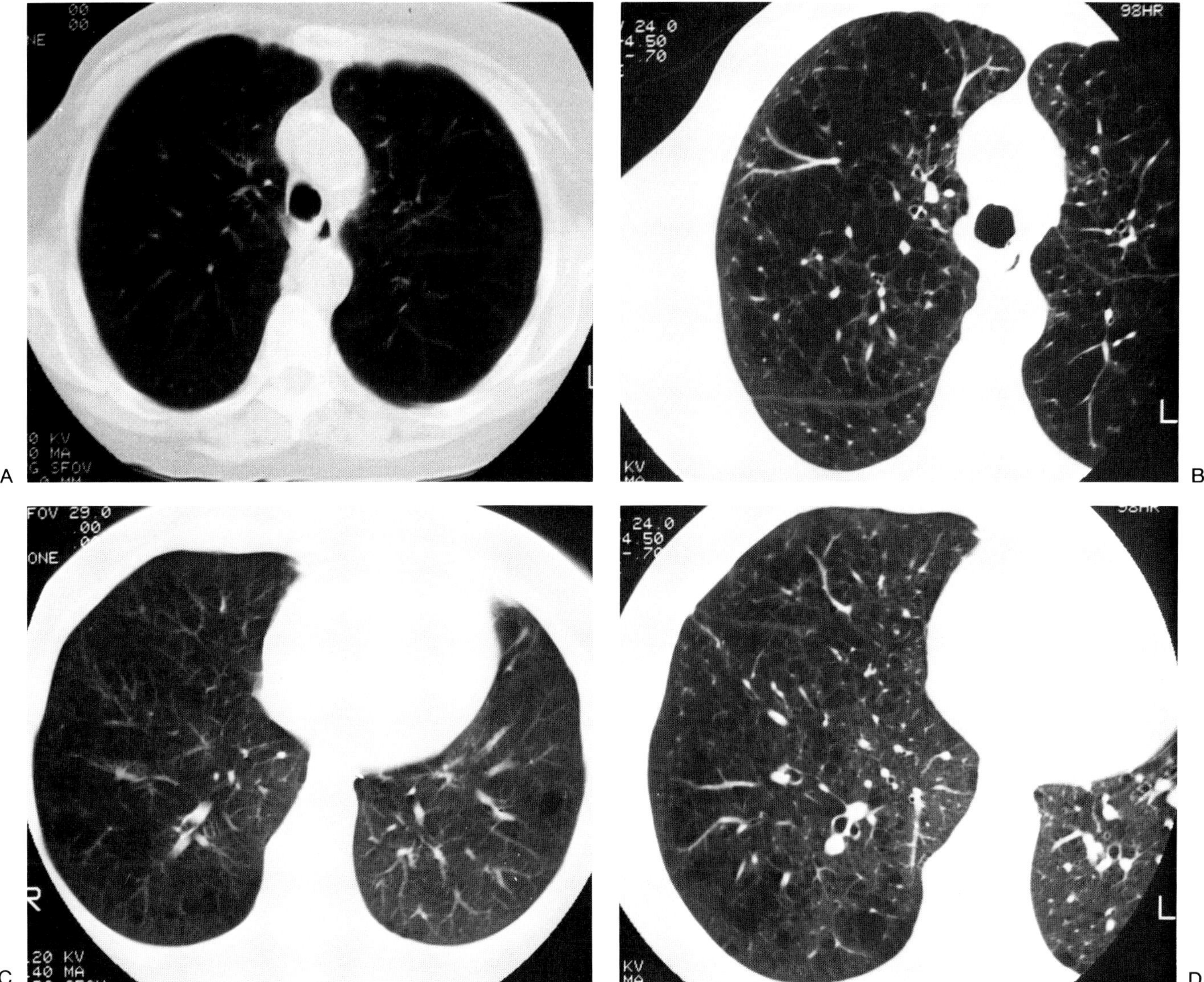

FIG. 2. Conventional and HRCT studies were obtained on an elderly male with a smoking history. (**A**) Conventional CT examination of the upper lungs demonstrates multiple discrete areas of decreased lung density with vascular attenuation. It is difficult to identify any normal areas of lung in this image. (**B**) HRCT examination on the same patient shows multiple areas of decreased attenuation and vascular attenuation. There is very little normal lung present in this image. This image demonstrates how difficult it may be to distinguish advanced centrilobular emphysema from panacinar emphysema on any given CT image of the lung. (**C**) Conventional CT image through the lower lungs in the same patient. This demonstrates milder changes than in (A) or (B). The more severe upper lung involvement is more typical of centrilobular emphysema. (**D**) HRCT examination through the right lower lobe. Multiple discrete areas of decreased attenuation can be seen interspersed with areas of normal lung attenuation. A small artery can be seen near the smaller areas of decreased attenuation in this image that helps to confirm the centrilobular origin of the emphysema. Areas of decreased attenuation do not have a demonstrable wall, which is also typical of centrilobular emphysema.

In this chapter several quantitative measurements were obtained in order to improve the ability to diagnose emphysema. These quantitative indices were also not very sensitive in detecting early emphysema. No combination of quantitative criteria resulted in better recognition of moderately severe or severe emphysema than a subjective diagnosis of emphysema that was determined using the qualitative criteria (8).

However, the three most useful quantitative variables in this study for the diagnosis of emphysema were first the lung length as measured from the tubercle of the first rib to the dome of the diaphragm on the PA radiograph. It was noted that the lung length was greater than 27 cm in 79 percent of patients with severe emphysema, and greater than 30 cm in length in 26 percent of patients with severe emphysema. The second useful measurement was the retrosternal airspace as measured horizontally from the posterior aspect of the sternum to the anterior margin of the ascending aorta. This last measurement was made 3 cm below the sternomanubrial junction. In patients with severe emphysema the retrosternal airspace was greater than 2.5 cm in 65 percent of the patients and greater than 3.5 cm in 30 percent of the patients. The third measurement that was thought to be useful was the diaphragm level. This was assessed by the relationship of the diaphragm to the anterior ribs on the frontal radiograph. The diaphragmatic level was at or below the sixth anterior rib in 95 percent of the patients, and at or below the seventh anterior rib in 55 percent of those patients with severe emphysema. The actual level of the diaphragm may not be as important as a flattened contour (9). The diaphragm contour is considered flattened when the top of the diaphragm is less than 1.5 cm above a straight line drawn between the costophrenic junction and the vertebrophrenic junction on the frontal radiograph (10). The frequency of radiologic diagnosis of emphysema is increased in those patients with emphysema and associated chronic airflow obstruction with ventricular hypertrophy or failure (8). The frequency of radiologic diagnosis of emphysema is also increased in those patients with chronic airflow obstructive disease determined by clinical symptoms and pulmonary function tests (8).

It has been pointed out that one of the older traditional signs of emphysema, a small vertical heart, is of limited value in distinguishing chronic bronchitis from emphysema (8). The reason for this is that right ventricular hypertrophy is common in patients with severe emphysema. The notion that patients with severe emphysema would have small hearts and that patients with chronic bronchitis would have larger hearts due to right ventricular hypertrophy is not true (8).

The presence of large central pulmonary arteries is usually secondary to cor pulmonale in patients with severe emphysema of any variety. When the right interlobar pulmonary artery is greater than 16 mm in diameter on the PA radiograph or when the left descending pulmonary artery is greater than 18 mm in diameter on the lateral radiograph, pulmonary arterial hypertension is usually present (11). Echocardiography, right heart catheterization, nuclear scintigraphy, and magnetic resonance imaging are more sensitive techniques than CR to diagnose cor pulmonale. It is important to recognize cor pulmonale, because this condition warrants long-term oxygen therapy to prevent a rapid deterioration in the patients' cardiopulmonary function.

In summary, the most useful three signs in the diagnosis of emphysema on the plain radiographs are focal areas of hyperlucency, vascular attenuation, and flattening of the hemidiaphragms.

Diagnosing Emphysema Using CT

The development of conventional CT and HRCT over the past 10 years has provided a powerful new imaging tool to assess the pulmonary parenchyma. In the past 5 years, numerous articles (7–16) have appeared that have shown CT to be of great value in diagnosing emphysema.

Conventional CT and HRCT should be used in the initial evaluation of patients for emphysema. The initial examination of these patients uses HRCT technique with 1–2 mm collimation, 20 mm slice gap, high spatial resolution algorithm, and 20–25 cm retargeted image field of view for each lung. The initial examination will also include conventional CT scan techniques using contiguous 5 mm collimation through the hilar structures and contiguous 10 mm collimated CT scans through the remainder of the thorax. A typical display field of view is 40 cm. The reason for performing the conventional CT exam is to evaluate the possibility of early bronchogenic carcinoma in patients with a smoking history. It would not be necessary to do the conventional CT study on someone with α_1-PI deficiency who is typically younger and may not have a smoking history. The initial study usually does not require intravenous contrast material unless a suspicious hilar or mediastinal mass is seen on the conventional chest radiograph. The easiest quantitative techniques to evaluate the extent of emphysema, besides qualitative scoring of the images, is to use a density mask technique that we use on selected patients. This technique is discussed more later in this chapter.

The two primary findings to look for on CT to diagnose emphysema are areas of decreased lung attenuation and areas of vascular attenuation (Fig. 2). The areas of decreased attenuation may be quite discrete with thin walls as seen in distal acinar emphysema or they may be more diffuse as seen in panacinar emphysema. Differentiating between the kinds of emphysema present will be examined herein.

A recent CT pathologic correlation study reviewing the diagnosis of emphysema using CT concluded that

CT is a useful adjunct in assessing the presence and severity of emphysema (12). In this study, 32 patients, prior to surgical removal of suspected tumors, had CT scans performed. The CT scans were performed using 10 mm collimation and conventional CT scanning parameters. A qualitative CT scoring system was used. Each CT slice was assessed individually, and the right and left lungs were graded separately. The criteria for abnormal lung indicating emphysema were areas of low attenuation and areas of vascular disruption. Grade 0 indicated there was no abnormality. If less than 25 percent of the pulmonary parenchyma was considered abnormal on a slice, the score was grade 1. If 25–50 percent of the lung was abnormal on a single scan this indicated grade 2 changes. Grade 3 indicated that 50–75 percent of the lung was abnormal on a single scan. Grade 4 indicated more than 75 percent of one lung on a single scan suggested emphysema. All slices above the level of the diaphragm were assessed in each patient, and the maximum possible score in a patient from whom 20 slices were obtained was $8 \times 20 = 160$. The final score of each patient was calculated as a percentage of the maximum. There was significant correlation between the pathology of resected lung tissue specimens and a preoperative CT score of both the resected lobe and the whole lung. Compared with pulmonary function tests, the CT examination was a better predictor of emphysema and distinguished patients with moderate emphysema from patients with normal lungs.

Another recent study examined 60 male patients who had concurrent chest films, CT scans, and pulmonary function tests and who were suspected of having emphysema (13). This study was performed to try to assess the sensitivity of CT and CR for detecting emphysema and comparing these with pulmonary function tests. Could CT diagnose emphysema with normal pulmonary function? A method of scoring the CT examinations was used that was similar to the previously described study. The severity of emphysema on the chest x-ray was estimated by grading the presence of arterial deficiency and bullae formation. In this study, there was a significant correlation between CT scores for emphysema and the percentage of predicted values of $DLCO/V_A$, FEV_1, and FVC. A smaller significant correlation was noted between the chest x-ray scores for emphysema and the percentage of predicted values of $DLCO/V_A$, FEV_1, and FVC. When the diffusion capacity was decreased and there was evidence of airflow obstruction, as determined by pulmonary function testing data, the CT examination was as sensitive as pulmonary function testing and more sensitive than the chest x-ray in detecting emphysema. It was also pointed out that CT may be more sensitive than pulmonary function testing in detecting mild emphysema.

Another recent study emphasized the importance in assessing the emphysematous changes in the lung in chronic asthma patients who are also cigarette smokers (14). The emphysema present on the CT scans in these patients was assessed using a visual scoring system. It was concluded in this study that the CT scans were useful for detecting emphysematous changes in this particular asthmatic patient population. In all the subjects with emphysema scoring obtained, there was significant correlation between the $DLCO/V_A$ and pack-years of cigarette consumption.

There are certainly limitations of CT in the assessment of emphysema (15). A recent study examined 38 patients undergoing lobectomy or pneumonectomy for carcinoma of the lung. Each patient received CT examinations of the thorax prior to surgery. Twenty-seven of the patients had HRCT scans with 1.5 mm collimation and conventional scans with 10 mm collimation. An additional 11 patients in the study had CT examinations using only 10 mm collimation. A grid technique was used to analyze the CT images for the presence of emphysema. The severity of emphysema was graded between 1 and 4. The CT images that were analyzed using the grid system were compared with a pathologic score using panels of standards for emphysema. There was a slight improvement in the 1.5 collimated slices versus the 10 mm collimated slices in detecting emphysema when compared with the pathologic changes that were seen. CT was sensitive in demonstrating early distal acinar and irregular emphysema, however, CT consistently underestimated the extent of centriacinar and panacinar emphysema because these lesions were usually less than 5 mm in diameter. As mentioned previously, HRCT studies correlated better with the degree of emphysema present pathologically than conventional CT, however, even in retrospect, HRCT did not see the small areas of parenchymal lung destruction from emphysema when the emphysematous holes were less than 5 mm in diameter. The results of this study indicate that both conventional and HRCT scanning can miss early emphysema of the lung.

In the following sections the different types of emphysema and their appearance on CT will be discussed.

Centriacinar Emphysema

The central portion of the acinus is involved in centriacinar emphysema (4). The emphysema begins in the respiratory bronchiole and adjacent alveoli. The scarring and dilation that occurs there results in enlarged air spaces in the center of the pulmonary acinus. These changes can be directly visualized on CT examinations, but are more difficult to see on CR. The most common form of centriacinar emphysema is produced by cigarette smoking and is known as centrilobular emphysema. This form of emphysema involves the upper lobes more than the lower lobes.

The CR findings of centrilobular emphysema include vague areas of hyperlucency, with associated vascular attenuation in the upper lung zones, and there may be associated flattening of the diaphragms in patients with significant airflow obstruction and increased lung volumes (Fig. 1). CT shows discrete areas of decreased attenuation that have imperceptible walls separating them from adjacent normal lung (Fig. 3). The areas of decreased attenuation predominate in the upper lung zones. There is significant vascular attenuation with elongation of arteries, a decrease in the number of arterial branches, and an increase in the arterial branching angle. As the disease progresses there is coalescence of many emphysematous lesions, making it increasingly difficult to distinguish this form of emphysema from panacinar emphysema. There may also be associated panacinar and distal acinar emphysema in these patients. The upper lungs are involved first in centrilobular emphysema, and this may help in distinguishing this form of emphysema from panacinar emphysema.

There is another form of centriacinar emphysema that is secondary to the dilatation of the respiratory bronchioles. This form of emphysema occurs with exposure to coal dust and other mineral dusts. This kind of cen-

triacinar emphysema produces relatively uniform changes throughout the lungs and has been called focal emphysema (4). Focal emphysema is a part of the pathologic picture of coal workers' pneumoconiosis. The CR and CT appearances are similar to those described for centrilobular emphysema, except the upper lungs are not preferentially involved. The presence of nodules within the lung and hilar and mediastinal lymphadenopathy are usually present to help distinguish this form of emphysema from centrilobular emphysema. It should be kept in mind that patients with coal dust exposure may also be cigarette smokers and have centrilobular emphysema as well as focal emphysema.

Panacinar Emphysema

Panacinar emphysema involves all components of the acinus uniformly (4). This process occurs more in the lower lungs and may accompany centrilobular emphysema in cigarette smokers. The focal form of this emphysema is seen more often in older patients and involves the lung bases more than the lung apices. It should be noted that, as the emphysema becomes more severe, it is difficult to distinguish between centrilobular and panacinar emphysema pathologically. There are some pathologists who feel that centrilobular emphysema will progress to panacinar emphysema (4). Diffuse panacinar emphysema is commonly observed with homozygous α_1-PI deficiency. This form of emphysema involves the lungs diffusely and usually is worse in the lung bases than in the lung apices, but this is not always the case.

The CR appearance of panacinar emphysema from α_1-PI deficiency shows a very diffuse pattern of hyperlucency that predominates in the lung bases (Fig. 4). There is vascular attenuation associated with the areas of hyperlucency. There is associated flattening of the hemidiaphragms as significant airflow obstruction develops along with increased lung volumes.

CT shows diffuse areas of decreased attenuation without discrete margins (Fig. 5). This CT appearance of panacinar emphysema differs considerably from centriacinar emphysema and distal acinar emphysema where discrete margins between the emphysematous lung and adjacent normal lung are visible. There is significant vascular attenuation with elongation of arteries, a decrease in the number of arterial branches, and an increase in the arterial branching angle.

The CT appearance of panacinar emphysema overlaps the appearance of severe airtrapping secondary to airway obstruction from asthma, bronchitis, and bronchiolitis.

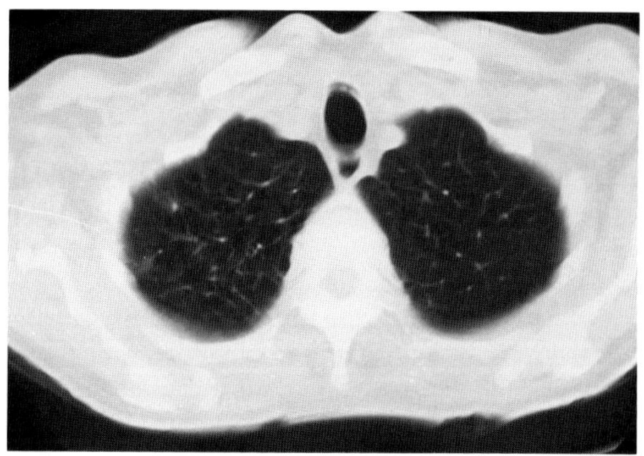

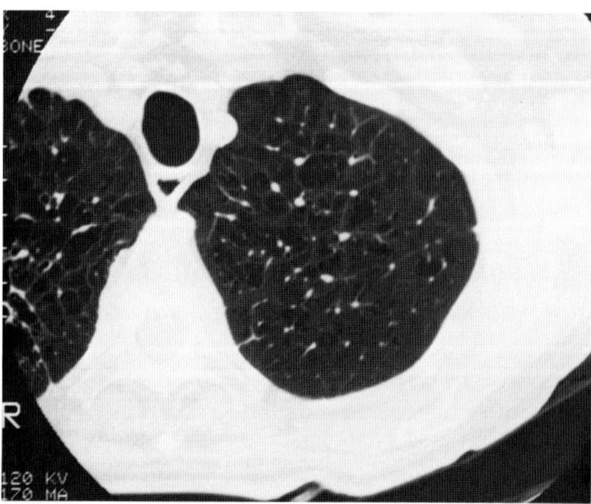

FIG. 3. **(A)** Conventional and **(B)** HRCT of the lung apices in a patient with early centrilobular emphysema. Findings are similar to those described in Fig. 2. HRCT image makes it easier to appreciate the early changes of centrilobular emphysema than the conventional CT image.

Distal Acinar Emphysema

Distal acinar emphysema involves the distal portion of the acinus, the alveolar ducts, and alveolar sacs (4).

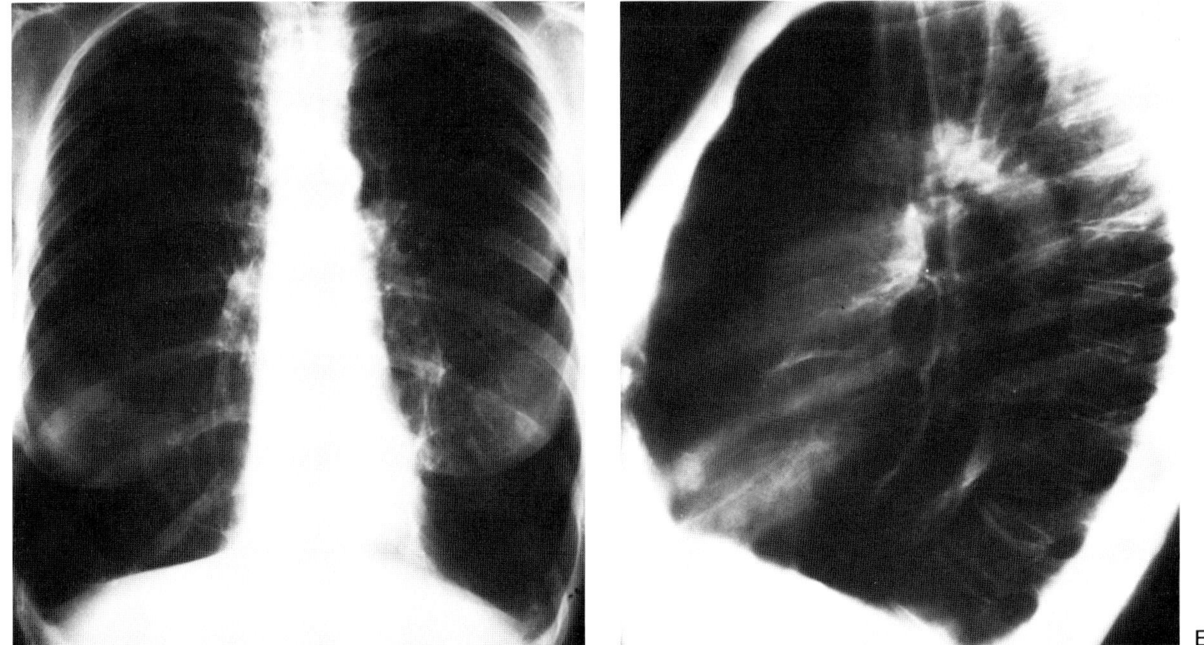

FIG. 4. (A) PA and **(B)** lateral radiographs of the chest of a young woman with α_1-PI deficiency and panacinar emphysema. These two views of the chest demonstrate increased lung volumes, marked flattening of the diaphragmatic contours, and marked decrease in the radiolucency of the lungs with associated vascular attenuation. The changes are more severe in the lower lobes, which helps to distinguish this form of emphysema from centrilobular emphysema secondary to cigarette smoking.

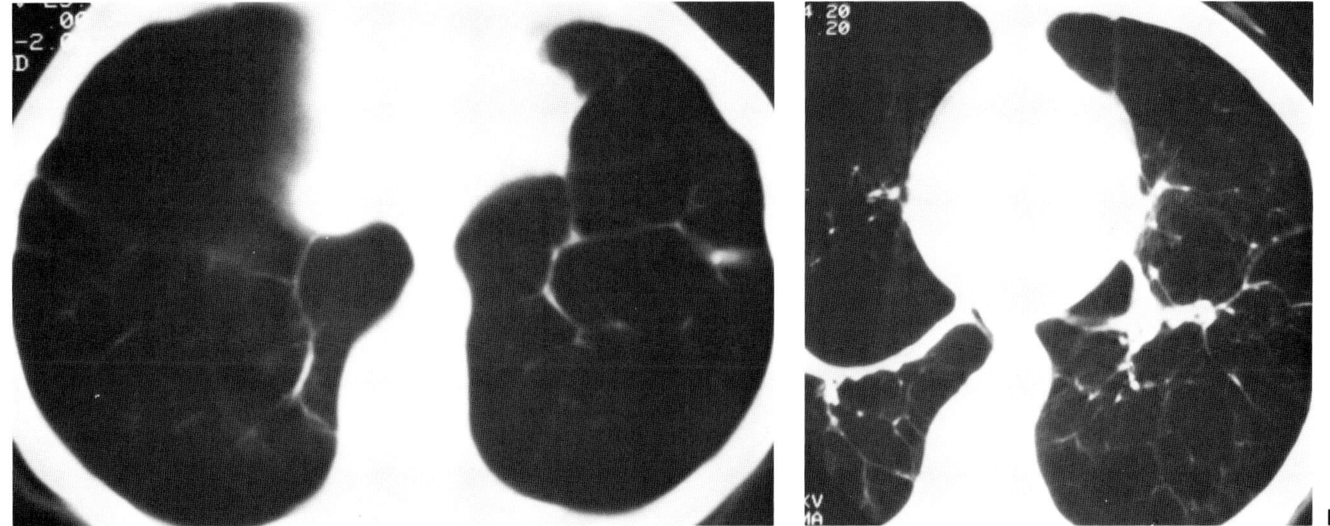

FIG. 5. (A) Conventional CT of the lower lung zones and **(B)** corresponding HRCT of the left lower lung. This study was obtained on the same patient with α_1-PI deficiency that was shown in Fig. 4. CT examinations show severe diffuse decrease in lung attenuation and marked vascular attenuation in both lungs. Pulmonary vessels are better seen in the high-resolution study. Lack of well-defined emphysematous lesions like those seen in centriacinar and distal acinar emphysema make the diagnosis of panacinar emphysema more challenging, even on HRCT scanning. Differentiating severe air trapping from early panacinar emphysema is difficult. It is also difficult to tell severe panacinar emphysema from severe centrilobular emphysema (see Fig. 2A,B).

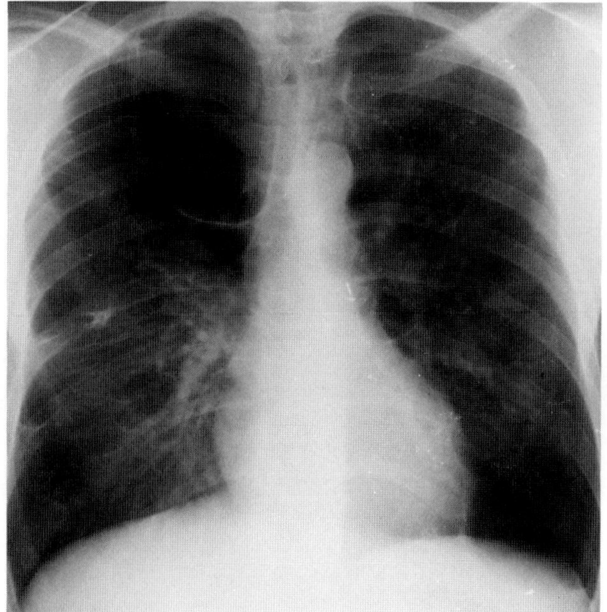

FIG. 6. PA chest radiograph from a middle-aged male with moderately severe distal acinar emphysema. A very large and discrete area of increased radiolucency with absent pulmonary vascularity is noted in the right upper lung. A similar lesion is seen in the left lower lung. Diaphragms also have a flattened contour. Bullae from distal acinar emphysema are the most clearly recognizable abnormality in patients with emphysema.

There is a close association of this form of emphysema with the interlobular septa and, for this reason, it is often referred to as paraseptal emphysema. This form of emphysema often demonstrates only mild airflow obstruction despite the presence of large bullae. The spontane- ous pneumothoraces seen in young adults are also associated with this form of emphysema. This form of emphysema may cause giant bullae that compress normal adjacent lung. If more than one-third of the hemithorax is occupied by one or more bullae, the patient may be a surgical candidate for bullae resection.

CR findings of distal acinar emphysema are discrete areas of hyperlucency with a thin wall, and without any pulmonary vasculature within the confines of the lesion (Fig. 6). CT of the lung is very useful for detecting distal acinar emphysema producing bullous lesions (16,17). The findings include focal areas of decreased attenuation with thin walls in a subpleural location without any vessels within the lesion (Fig. 7). In our experience, CT examination can identify small subpleural blebs, as well as large bullous lesions in patients with distal acinar emphysema. CT can separate operative patients with large subpleural bullae that occupy more than one-third of a hemithorax from the nonsurgical group whose CT demonstrates predominantly centrilobular emphysema and/ or panacinar emphysema.

Emphysema Associated with Pulmonary Fibrosis

It should be noted that there is a spectrum of airspace enlargement associated with pulmonary fibrosis (4). These conditions include fibrosing alveolitis and the fibrosis associated with granulomatous disease, such as silicosis, tuberculosis, sarcoidosis, or eosinophilic granuloma. This form of emphysema has been called both localized emphysema and irregular emphysema. Recent work has indicated that the mild scarring associated with

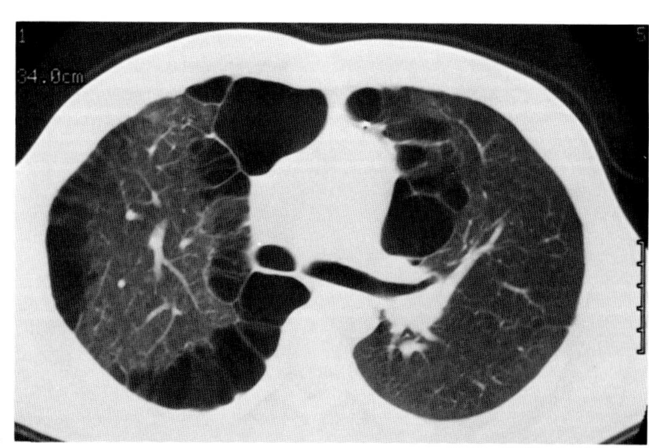

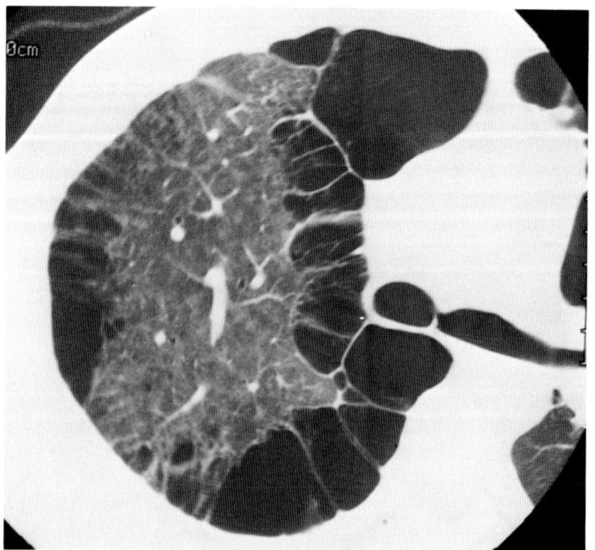

FIG. 7. (A) Conventional CT and **(B)** HRCT, of the same patient seen in Fig. 6 with distal acinar emphysema. CT examinations demonstrate multiple discrete areas of decreased attenuation with thin walls and absent pulmonary vascularity. Areas of decreased attenuation are in subpleural locations. These are true emphysematous lesions and not pulmonary cysts. The subpleural location should help distinguish these lesions from the cysts encountered in lymphangiomyomatosis (LAM) and esosinophilic granuloma.

irregular emphysema may overlap the occasional mild fibrosis seen in more classic emphysema. Irregular emphysema can be identified on conventional CT and HRCT examinations of the thorax, but is usually not seen on conventional chest radiographs. Irregular emphysema usually involves discrete lesions that closely resemble centriacinar emphysema on CT.

Quantitative CT Assessment of Emphysema

The density mask technique that was described in 1988 is the most useful readily available technique to assess quantitatively the amount of emphysema present both on conventional and HRCT examinations of the thorax (18,19). The density mask computer program is provided with the General Electric 9800 CT/T scanner. This program can be used to highlight the voxels within each slice obtained through the patient's lungs within a given density range to quantitate the amount of emphysema present. First, this program is used to determine the total amount of lung tissue present on each slice obtained through the lungs, typically 20–30 slices. The density mask technique, then, is applied to determine those pixel values less than −900 H. This range of densities represents abnormal areas of decreased attenuation within the lung parenchyma. The total percentage of abnormal lung is determined by dividing the volume of emphysematous lung by the total lung volume.

A recent study suggests that it may be possible to determine a quantitative index to assess patients with emphysema by obtaining only two conventional CT scans of the thorax with the patient at full expiration (20). A technique similar to the density mask technique was used to determine the amount of lung that was less than −900 H on two expiratory CT images of the thorax. One image was obtained at the level of the aorta, and the other one was obtained 6 cm below this level. The measurements from the two levels were averaged for the inspiration study and, similarly, a second average measurement was determined for the expiratory study. The amount of lung that was abnormal was expressed as a percentage of total lung present on the images and was termed pixel index. A pixel index greater than 15 percent correlated well with significant decreases in the pulmonary function test data that indicated the presence of obstructive lung disease, including percent of predicted values of DLCO, DLCO/V_A, and FEV_1, and the FEV_1/ FVC ratio.

It has been pointed out that using CT measurements of lung density has limitations. There is variation in these values depending on the type of CT scanner used, the kilovoltage used, and the reconstruction algorithm (18). However, CT measurements of lung parenchyma using the density mask technique seem to be the most readily available technique to obtain quantitative measurements of emphysema today.

BRONCHIECTASIS

The term bronchiectasis refers to abnormal dilation of the proximal and medium-sized bronchi, greater than 2 mm in diameter (21). The bronchi are dilated due to destruction of the muscular and elastic components of their walls (21). Bronchiectasis is thought of as a persistent and usually permanent pathologic process, although the cylindrical bronchial dilation seen in acute pneumonia may reverse completely.

The term process is used because bronchiectasis is not a discrete disease entity unless it is secondary to bronchial obstruction or untreated pulmonary infection (21). Bronchiectasis is more commonly a manifestation of a systemic disorder. These disorders include immotile cilia syndrome, cystic fibrosis, ABPA, immunodeficiency, α_1-PI deficiency, pulmonary sequestration, unilateral hyperlucent lung (Swyer–James–MacLeod syndrome), congenital cartilage deficiency (Williams–Campbell syndrome), Marfans syndrome, tracheobronchomegaly (Mounier–Kuhn syndrome), yellow nail syndrome, and ulcerative colitis (21).

The patient with bronchiectasis often presents with chronic cough, purulent expectoration, fever, weakness, weight loss, and hemoptysis. Dyspnea is reported in some patients with bronchiectasis, but this is not a universal finding. The most common complications are recurrent pneumonia, empyema, pneumothorax, and lung abscess. Cor pulmonale occurs in a minority of patients, but it is a serious complication that can be seen in patients with bronchiectasis.

The pathologic classification of bronchiectasis was divided into three groups by Reid (22): cylindrical, varicose, and cystic bronchiectasis. Mild bronchiectasis is described as cylindrical, with regular outlines of the bronchi; however, there is loss of the normal tapering of the distal bronchi and, usually, they end abruptly and squarely. More severe bronchiectasis is described as varicose bronchiectasis with irregular dilation of the bronchi and a bulbous termination. Cystic bronchiectasis is the most severe form of bronchiectasis and is characterized by bronchial dilation that increases progressively toward the periphery, with a ballooning of the distal abnormal bronchi with (fewer than normal) bronchial subdivisions.

Conventional Radiography

Bronchiectasis is defined on CR and CT as irreversible dilation of the airways. The conventional radiograph is insensitive to detecting early bronchiectasis. It is helpful in detecting advanced disease. CR is helpful in identifying people with recurrent pneumonia. These patients can then undergo CT to evaluate early bronchiectasis. As mentioned previously, there are groups of patients who are at higher risk to develop bronchiectasis than others. These patients should undergo CT even if the plain film does not indicate any evidence of bronchiectasis.

Upright PA and lateral chest radiographs obtained at full inspiration should be done on patients suspected of having bronchiectasis. A modern film-screen system that is specifically designed for thoracic imaging, such as the Insight HC system described in Chapter 1, should be used if at all possible.

The radiographic findings of bronchiectasis are well documented in the radiology literature (23). The findings on CR of bronchiectasis include atelectasis, thickening of bronchial walls (best appreciated when seen end on), and indistinctness of the central vessels due to inflammation involving the bronchovascular or axial intersitium. This early appearance of bronchiectasis overlaps the findings seen in asthma and bronchitis without bronchiectasis. The bronchial wall thickening will progress to dilated thick wall bronchi, which can be visualized as tramlines or parallel lines separated by a lucent bronchial lumen on CR. The tramlines may be associated with peribronchial opacification, atelectasis, and superimposed airspace pneumonia. If the tramlines are straight, the bronchiectasis is classified as cylindrical. As the disease progresses the tramlines will become tortuous in appearance, indicating that more severe varicose bronchiectasis has developed. The presence of large cystic structures with or without air fluid levels indicates that bronchiectasis has progressed to the most severe form, cystic bronchiectasis. These thick-walled structures may be in a line, resembling a string of beads, or clustered together like a bunch of grapes.

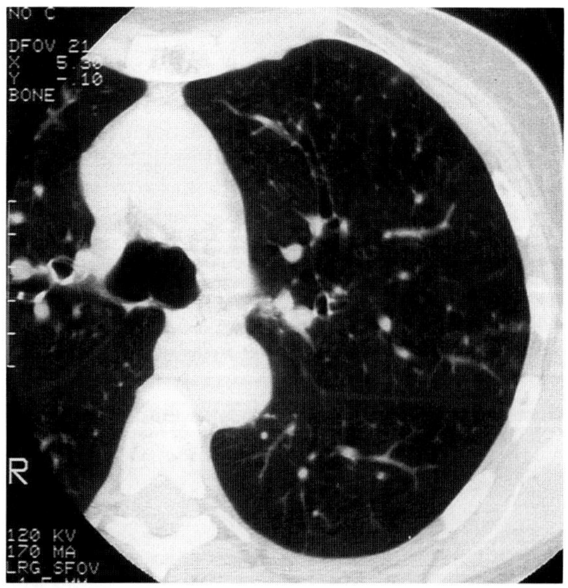

FIG. 8. HRCT of a patient with cylindrical bronchiectasis in the anterior segment of the left upper lobe. The abnormal bronchus coursed horizontally through a significant portion of the scan plane. This shows the thickened wall, dilated lumen, and nontapering nature of the abnormal bronchus. The bronchus is bigger than the adjacent artery. The smooth bronchial wall distinguishes cylindrical from varicose bronchiectasis.

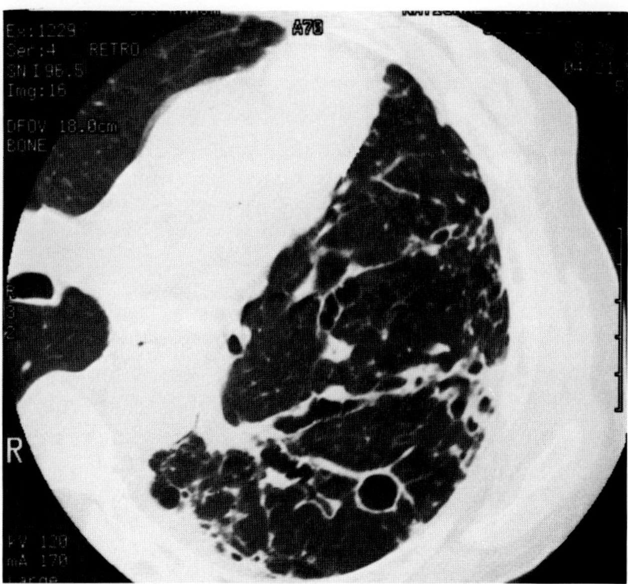

FIG. 9. HRCT of varicose bronchiectasis in a patient with chronic mycobacterial disease. Note the dilated and irregular bronchial lumen caused by irregular thickening of the bronchial wall in two centrally located bronchi in the dorsal aspect of the remaining left upper lung. This patient had previously undergone a partial left pneumonectomy prior to this study. In order to tell varicose from cylindrical bronchiectasis, the bronchus must be imaged along its long axis.

Computed Tomography

CT has dramatically improved the radiologist's ability to noninvasively diagnose bronchiectasis (24–26). Conventional chest radiographic examination is very insensitive in diagnosing bronchiectasis. In the past, prior to the advent of CT, it had been necessary to perform bronchography on patients suspected of having bronchiectasis. This is an invasive and unpleasant examination for the patient, and a demanding examination to be performed by the radiologist. This procedure has been almost completely eradicated following the advent of HRCT.

Conventional CT was first used to examine patients with suspected bronchiectasis. Conventional CT using 10 mm collimation was far better than CR but not good enough to displace bronchography. CT examinations (10 mm collimation) were insensitive in detecting cylindrical bronchiectasis.

The development of HRCT using 1–2 mm collimation and a 10 mm gap between images has pushed the resolution of CT to the point that bronchography is not necessary in the vast majority of patients who are being studied to determine if there is bronchiectasis present (25). Grenier et al. (25) reported an HRCT sensitivity of 97 percent and a specificity of 93 percent in the diagnosis of bronchiectasis. The HRCT examinations were compared with bronchograms that were also obtained on the patients in the study. It has been my experience that

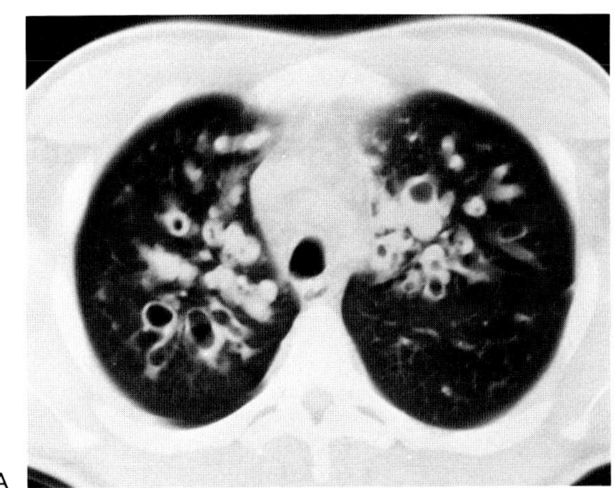
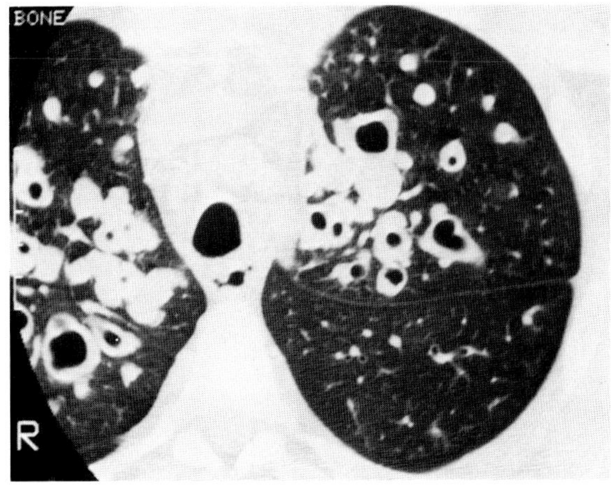

FIG. 10. Conventional CT and HRCT obtained from a 28-year-old male with cystic fibrosis and cystic bronchiectasis. Multiple cystic-shaped dilated bronchi are seen in both the left upper and right upper lobes. Multiple bronchiectatic lumen are either partially or completely obliterated by mucous plugging.

HRCT can replace bronchography in almost all patients with suspected bronchiectasis. If the HRCT examination demonstrates diffuse disease the patient is inoperable. If there is only one area of abnormality confined to a lobe or segment, then it may be necessary to do bronchography prior to thoracotomy.

It is important to use proper technique in assessing bronchiectasis. Collimation (1–2 mm) should be used, and the HRCT examinations should be obtained at 10 mm intervals. It is essential to use a high-spatial resolution algorithm, and it is preferable to retarget the images to a display field of view between 20 and 25 cm. A conventional contrast-enhanced CT examination using 5 and 10 mm collimation is recommended if there is a suspicion of an endobronchial lesion or atriovenous malformation (AVM).

Bronchi are normally not visible in the outer third of the lung on HRCT examinations. The bronchi are usually smaller than the accompanying artery and are thin-walled. In cylindrical bronchiectasis the bronchi will enlarge and when viewed in cross-section on HRCT will exceed the diameter of the adjacent vessel (Fig. 8). The walls of the bronchi will also thicken. The dilated bronchi, when seen in cross-section with their adjacent vessels, will have a signet-ring appearance. If the bronchi are viewed horizontally or in the same plane as the HRCT section, a tram track-like structure will be seen. The bronchus does not taper normally, and this produces the tram track or pipe-like appearance of the bronchus in cylindrical bronchiectasis.

As the bronchiectatic process continues varicose bronchiectasis will develop. The bronchus has all the features of cylindrical bronchiectasis, but also has an irregular beaded wall. This is difficult to appreciate when viewing the bronchus in cross-section, but can be seen when the abnormal bronchus is seen horizontally (Fig. 9).

The most severe form of bronchiectasis is cystic bronchiectasis. The features of varicose bronchiectasis will be seen along with additional large rounded structures replacing the normal bronchi, and air fluid levels may be seen within the dependent portion of the dilated bronchial lumen. Cystic bronchiectasis may demonstrate a line of cysts or a cluster of cysts on HRCT, similar to what was described for CR (Fig. 10). Volume loss within the affected segment may be especially noticeable in cystic bronchiectasis.

Central bronchiectasis is characteristic of allergic bronchopulmonary aspergillosis (27) (Fig. 11). The patients with ABPA have central bronchiectasis, along with upper lobe involvement and bronchial wall thickening.

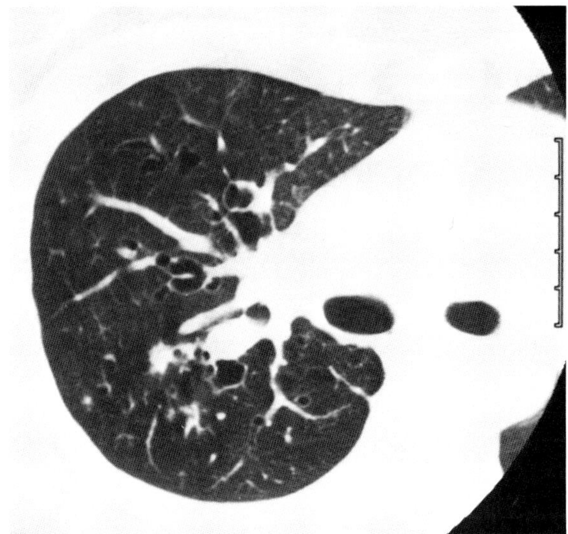

FIG. 11. HRCT of a woman with ABPA. Both cylindrical and varicose bronchiectatic changes are involving multiple central bronchi of the right middle lobe and the superior segment of the right lower lobe.

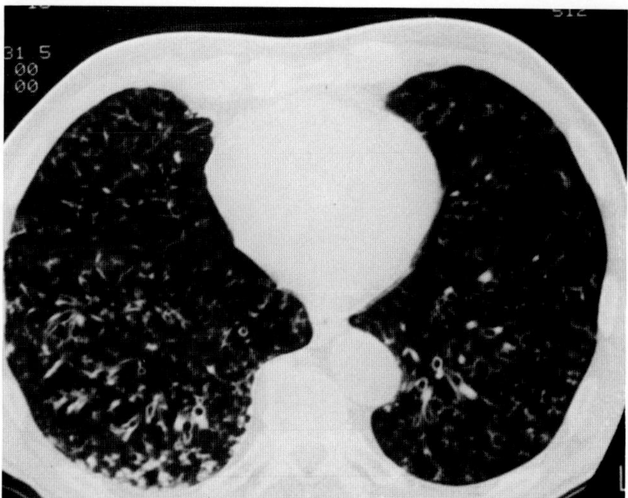

FIG. 12. HRCT of the lower lungs in a patient with panbronchiolitis. There is marked diffuse peribronchial thickening and small nodule formation. Numerous small bronchi are dilated in the mid and peripheral third of the right lower lung on this scan. Changes in the smaller airways are termed cylindrical bronchiolectasis.

Non-ABPA asthmatics also demonstrated bronchial wall thickening and upper lobe central bronchiectasis (27). Thus, there is considerable overlap in these two groups based on HRCT findings alone. It should be pointed out that, in this study, only the ABPA patients had evidence of varicoid or cystic bronchiectasis on HRCT.

Panbronchiolitis is a disease that affects the smaller airways and has a characteristic appearance on HRCT (28). There are numerous small dilated peripheral airways that can be seen in the outer third of the lung with bronchial wall thickening, and peripheral small nodule formation (Fig. 12).

HRCT studies for the evaluation of bronchiectasis have some limitations. Cardiac motion transmitted to the left lower lung and small amounts of breathing during image acquisition may both mimic bronchiectasis (29). Mucous plugs may simulate large vessels in patients with bronchiectasis, and this may be a bigger problem in patients with bronchial atresia and large peripheral mucous plugs. It should also be remembered that bronchial dilation accompanies most acute bacterial pneumonias. As the acute pneumonia resolves, the cylindrical bronchiectasis will usually resolve.

REFERENCES

1. Webb WR, Stein MG, Finkbeiner WE, et al. Normal and diseased isolated lungs: high-resolution CT. *Radiology* 1988;166:81–87.
2. Ney DR, Kuhlman JE, Hruban RH, et al. Three-dimensional CT—volumetric reconstruction and display of the bronchial tree. *Invest Radiol* 1990;25:736–742.
3. Terminology, definitions, and classification of chronic pulmonary emphysema and related conditions: a report of the conclusions of a CIBA guest symposium. *Thorax* 1959;14:286–299.
4. Snider GL, Kleinerman J, Thurlbeck WM, Bengali ZH. The definition of emphysema: report of a national heart, lung blood institute, division of lung diseases workshop. *Am Rev Respir Dis* 1985;132:182–185.
5. Laurell CB, Eriksson S. The electrophorectic alpha-1-globulin pattern of serum in alpha-1 antitrypsin deficiency. *Scand J Clin Lab Invest* 1963;15:132–140.
6. Gross P, Babjak M, Tolker E, Kaschak M. Enzymatically produced pulmonary emphysema: a preliminary report. *J Occup Med* 1964;6:481–484.
7. Snider GL, Lucey EC, Stone PJ. State of the art: animal models of emphysema. *Am Rev Respir Dis* 1986;133:149–169.
8. Thurlbeck WM, Simon G. Radiographic appearance of the chest in emphysema. *Am J Roentgenol* 1978;130:429–440.
9. Pratt PC. Role of conventional chest radiography in diagnosis and exclusion of emphysema. *Am J Med* 1987;88:998–1006.
10. Müller NI. Obstructive lung disease. In Freundlich IM, Bragg DG, eds. *A radiologic approach to diseases of the chest.* Baltimore: Williams & Wilkins, 1992;455–465.
11. Matthay RA, Schwarz MI, Ellis JH, Steele PP, Siebert PE, Durrance JR, Levin DC. Pulmonary artery hypertension in chronic obstructive pulmonary disease: determination by chest radiography. *Invest Radiol* 1981;16:95–100.
12. Bergin C, Muller N, Nichols DM, et al. The diagnosis of emphysema: a computed tomographic-pathologic correlation. *Am Rev Respir Dis* 1986;133:541–546.
13. Sanders C, Nath PH, Bailey WC. Detection of emphysema with computed tomography: correlation with pulmonary function tests and chest radiography. *Invest Radiol* 1988;23:262–266.
14. Kondoh Y, Taniguchi H, Yokoyama S, et al. Emphysematous change in chronic asthma in relation to cigarette smoking: assessment by computed tomography. *Chest* 1990;97:845–849.
15. Miller RR, Müller NL, Vedal S, et al. Limitations of computed tomography in the assessment of emphysema. *Am Rev Respir Dis* 1989;139:980–983.
16. Lesur O, Delorme N, Fromaget JM, et al. Computed tomography in the etiologic assessment of idiopathic spontaneous pneumothorax. *Chest* 1990;98:341–347.
17. Watanabe K, Kakitsubata Y, Kusumoto S, et al. Bullous lesions detected by computed tomography. *Radiat Med* 1986;4:119–123.
18. Muller NL, Staples CA, Miller RR, Abboud RT. "Density mask": an objective method to quantitate emphysema using computed tomography. *Chest* 1988;94:782–787.
19. Kinsella M, Muller NL, Abboud RT, et al. Quantitation of emphysema by computed tomography using a "density mask" program and correlation with pulmonary function tests. *Chest* 1990;97:315–321.
20. Knudson RJ, Standen JR, Kaltenborn WT, Knudson DE, Rehm K, Habib MP, Newell JD. Expiratory computed tomography for assessment of suspected pulmonary emphysema. *Chest* 1991;99:1357–1366.
21. Luce JM. Bronchiectasis. In Murray JF, Nadel JA, eds. *Textbook of respiratory medicine.* Philadelphia: WB Saunders Co., 1988;1107–1125.
22. Reid I. Reduction in bronchial subdivision in bronchiectasis. *Thorax* 1950;5:233–247.
23. Gudbjerg CE. Roentgenologic diagnosis of bronchiectasis. An analysis of 112 cases. *Acta Radiol* 1955;43:210–226.
24. Naidich DP, McCauley DI, Khouri NF, Stitik FP, Siegelman SS. Computed tomography of bronchiectasis. *J Comput Assist Tomogr* 1982;6:437–444.
25. Grenier P, Maurice F, Musset D, Menu Y, Nahum H. Bronchiectasis: assessment by thin-section CT. *Radiology* 1986;161:95–99.
26. Phillips MS, Williams MP, Flower CDR. How useful is computed tomography in the diagnosis and assessment of bronchiectasis? *Clin Radiol* 1986;37:321–325.
27. Neeld DA, Goodman LR, Gurney JW, Greenberger PA, Fink JN. Computerized tomography in the evaluation of allergic bronchopulmonary aspergillosis. *Am Rev Respir Dis* 1990;142:1200–1205.
28. Akira M, Kitatani F, Yong-Sik L, Kita N, Yamamoto S, Higashihara T, Morimoto S, Ikezoe J, Kozuka T. Diffuse panbronchiolitis: evaluation with high-resolution CT. *Radiology* 1988;168:433–438.
29. Tarver RD, Conces JD, Godwin JD. Motion artifacts on CT simulate bronchiectasis. *Am J Roentgenol* 1988;151:1117–1119.

Thoracic Radiology, edited by
J.D. Newell, Jr., and R.D. Tarver,
Raven Press, Ltd., New York © 1993.

CHAPTER 5

Radiology of Interstitial Lung Disease

David A. Lynch

Interstitial lung diseases are characterized by inflammation of the alveolar interstitium of the lung, often leading to pulmonary fibrosis. Although there are at least two hundred recognized causes of interstitial disease, the etiology of the two most common interstitial diseases—sarcoidosis and idiopathic pulmonary fibrosis (IPF)—remains unknown. Radiology plays a central role in the diagnosis, differential diagnosis, and staging of these disorders.

Inflammation in the alveolar interstitium, or alveolitis, which characterizes interstitial lung disease, is associated with accumulation of neutrophils, macrophages, or lymphocytes (1). These inflammatory cells, by releasing various mediators, give rise to pulmonary fibrosis. The intensity of the alveolitis probably governs the severity of the subsequent fibrosis. Alveolitis may also involve the air-containing spaces of the lung, altering the radiographic appearances. The inflammation may also affect the peribronchovascular interstitium supporting the main blood vessels and bronchi, or the subpleural and interlobular interstitium that are predominant peripheral. Granuloma formation is a prominent feature in some disorders, such as sarcoidosis and hypersensitivity pneumonitis.

The role of the radiologist in the management of interstitial lung diseases is fourfold:

1. Recognize the type of interstitial abnormality (nodules, lines, and cysts) and distinguish it from disorders that predominantly involve the airways or airspaces of the lung.
2. Develop a differential diagnosis, based on clinical information, the pattern of interstitial abnormality present, and associated abnormalities, such as adenopathy or pleural disease.

3. Evaluate the extent of disease and the severity of the alveolitis.
4. Determine the rapidity of change by comparing with previous studies.

IMAGING MODALITIES IN INTERSTITIAL LUNG DISEASE

Chest Radiographs: Value and Limitations

The chest radiograph remains the primary imaging modality for evaluation of pulmonary interstitial disease. An abnormal chest radiograph is often the first indicator of the presence of interstitial lung disease. Analysis of the radiographic pattern can have considerable value in the differential diagnosis of interstitial lung disease (Table 1). Associated radiographic clues may sometimes indicate the specific cause of the interstitial lung disease (Fig. 1) (Table 2).

Limitations of the chest radiograph in the interstitial lung diseases include the fact that a normal chest radiograph will occur in at least 10 percent of subjects with interstitial lung disease (2) (Fig. 2). With refinement of diagnostic criteria for interstitial lung disease, the true prevalence of a normal chest radiograph may be much higher. The occurrence of a normal chest radiograph with interstitial lung disease is most common in stage 1 sarcoidosis, hypersensitivity pneumonitis, and desquamative interstitial pneumonitis. Another limitation of the chest radiograph is the frequent lack of specificity of the findings. Whereas pattern recognition helps to narrow the differential diagnosis, it is rare to make a specific diagnosis of interstitial lung disease on the basis of the radiographic pattern alone. A further limitation of the chest radiograph is that it is difficult to quantify objectively improvement or deterioration. Although various methods for quantitation of chest radiographic abnor-

D. A. Lynch: Department of Radiology, University of Colorado Health Sciences Center, Denver, Colorado 80262.

TABLE 1. *Patterns of interstitial disease*

Nodules	Sarcoidosis
	Berylliosis
	PHX[a]
	Hypersensitivity pneumonitis
	Pneumoconiosis (silicosis, coal dust)
	Metastatic carcinoma
Miliary (fine nodules)	Tuberculosis
	Fungal infection
	Sarcoidosis
	Metastatic carcinoma
Linear/reticular	IPF
	Asbestosis
	Collagen vascular disease
Septal lines	Lymphangitis carcinomatosa
	Interstitial edema
	Drug hypersensitivity
	Lymphangiomyomatosis
Cysts	Lymphangiomyomatosis
	PHX
	Endstage honeycombing
	IPF
	Collagen vascular
	Asbestosis
	Hypersensitivity pneumonitis
	Sarcoidosis

[a] Pulmonary histocytosis X.

malities have been described, most of them correlate poorly with measures of physiologic change and are too complex or too insensitive to be used in clinical practice. Finally, it is rarely possible for the radiologist to determine the intensity of alveolitis on the basis of the chest radiographic appearance.

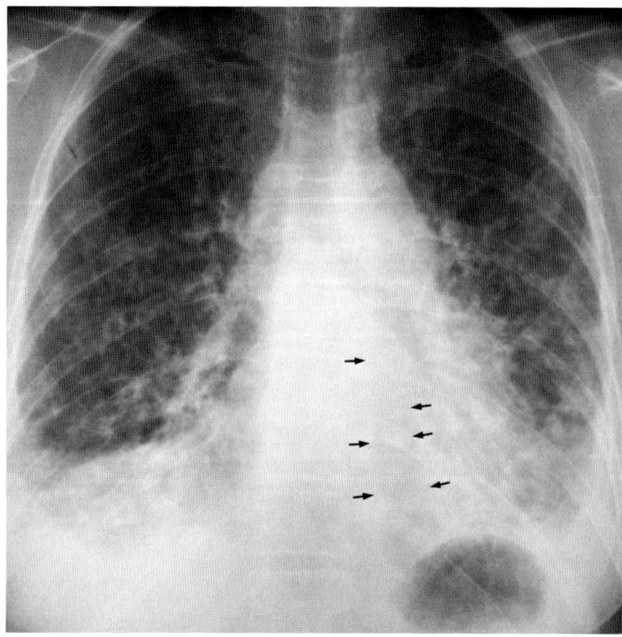

FIG. 1. Progressive systemic sclerosis (PSS). Chest radiograph shows bilateral basal reticulonodular interstitial densities, bilateral pleural effusions, and a dilated esophagus (*arrows*).

Gallium Scanning

The uptake of [67]gallium in the lungs is normally less than or the same as that in the surrounding soft tissues, and considerably less than the uptake in bone marrow or spine. In interstitial lung diseases an abnormal proportion of gallium accumulates in the lungs, mainly in the alveolar macrophages. Imaging of the lung is performed at 6, 24, and 48 hours after intravenous injection of gallium (3). Several indices for quantitation of abnormal gallium uptake have been proposed. The simplest index compares gallium uptake in the lung with the uptake in soft tissues and in the liver.

It is important to note that abnormal gallium uptake in the lung is entirely nonspecific. It may occur in drug toxicity, lymphangiography, pneumoconiosis, pulmonary alveolar proteinosis, sarcoidosis, IPF, and in infectious disorders such as *Pneumocystis carinii* pneumonia or miliary tuberculosis. In both IPF and sarcoidosis, the intensity of uptake within the lung correlates with evidence of active alveolitis on biopsy or bronchoalveolar lavage (4,5). However, the gallium scan may be normal in the presence of active lung disease. In addition gallium scans may remain abnormal in the presence of clinically inactive disease. Therefore, the significance of persistent abnormal pulmonary uptake of gallium is difficult to evaluate. Because of its lack of specificity, gallium scanning is not widely used for evaluation of interstitial lung disease.

Computed Tomography (CT) Scanning

From the early days of CT scanning it was recognized that this technique could be helpful in identifying and characterizing interstitial lung disease. However, the value of CT has increased dramatically with the introduction of specific high-resolution techniques (6). These techniques involve the use of narrow collimation (1–3 mm) and high-resolution, edge-enhancing reconstruction algorithms. Retargeting of reconstruction, with a field of view that includes one lung only, also increases resolution. Utilization of the correct technique is critical for accurate demonstration of early interstitial disease.

This technique of high-resolution CT (HRCT) scanning of the lung parenchyma has been shown to be more sensitive than chest radiographs for detection of early interstitial changes (7) (Fig. 2). However, CT scanning may sometimes be normal in cases of biopsy-proven interstitial lung disease. The accuracy of characterization of interstitial disease by HRCT is 76 percent, compared with an accuracy of 57 percent for the chest radiograph (8). The identification of hazy increase of lung density on HRCT correlates with evidence of active alveolitis on biopsy. CT offers considerable potential for quantification of the extent and severity of interstitial lung diseases. Semiquantitative scores of disease severity ob-

TABLE 2. *Radiographic clues in differential diagnosis of interstitial lung diseases*

Radiographic feature associated with interstitial lung disease	Diagnoses[a]
Mediastinum	
Dilated esophagus	PSS, CREST
Cardiomegaly	SLE, rheumatoid disease, amiodarone therapy, amyloid
Hilar/mediastinal adenopathy	Sarcoidosis, silicosis, lymphangitis carcinomatosa
Pleura	
Pneumothorax	PHX, lymphangiomyomatosis, any other interstitial disease
Pleural effusions	SLE, rheumatoid disease, lymphangitic carcinoma, lymphangiomyomatosis, amiodarone toxicity
Pleural plaques	Asbestosis
Chest wall	
Rib lesion	PHX
Soft tissue calcification	Dermatomyositis, PSS
Eroded or penciled clavicles	Rheumatoid disease, PSS
Distribution of lung disease	
Dominant upper lobe disease	Sarcoidosis, pneumoconiosis, PHX, chronic hypersensitivity pneumonitis
Dominant lower lobe disease	IPF, collagen vascular disease (rheumatoid disease or scleroderma), or asbestosis

[a] SLE, systemic lupus erythematosus.

tained from CT scans correlate moderately well with pulmonary function abnormalities in asbestosis (9), IPF (10), and sarcoidosis (11). However, appropriate techniques for objective or automated quantification of these diseases have not yet been developed.

Magnetic Resonance Imaging (MRI)

The lung is probably the most difficult organ in the body to image using MRI. The primary reasons for this difficulty are magnetic susceptibility artifacts due to numerable soft tissue-air interfaces, and the effect of respira-tory motion-induced phase artifact. If these difficulties could be overcome, MRI might be of value for distinction between active pulmonary inflammation (alveolitis) and established fibrosis (12).

RADIOGRAPHIC PATTERN RECOGNITION IN LUNG DISEASE

The primary chest radiographic signs of interstitial lung disease are decreased lung volumes, nodules, lines, honeycombing, and hazy increase in lung density. The

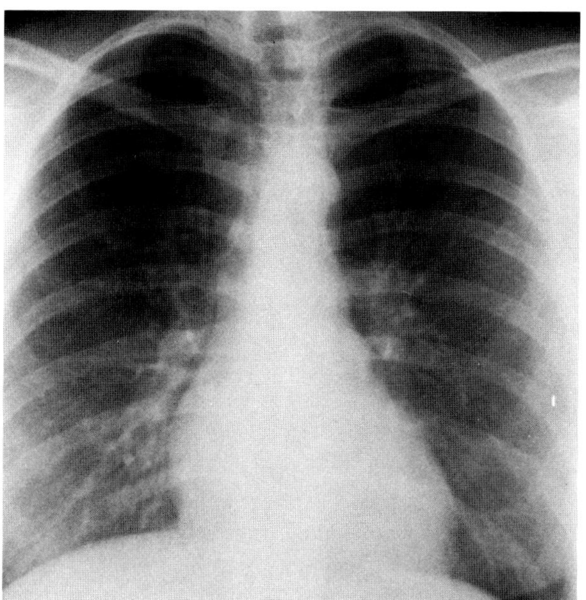

A

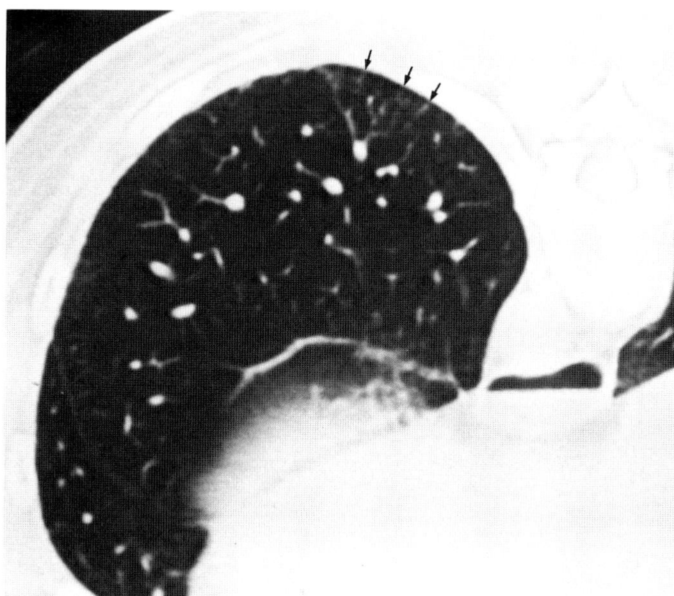

B

FIG. 2. PSS. **(A)** Chest radiograph is normal. **(B)** Prone HRCT scan shows mild thickening of interlobular septa consistent with early pulmonary fibrosis (*arrows*).

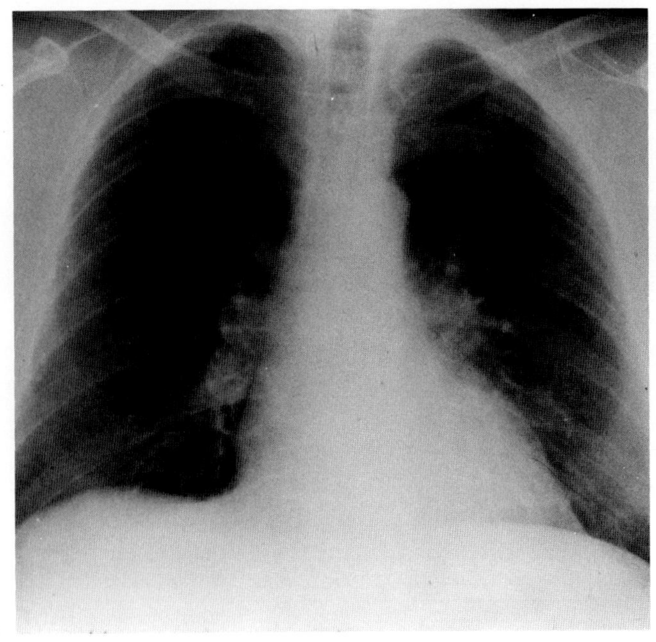
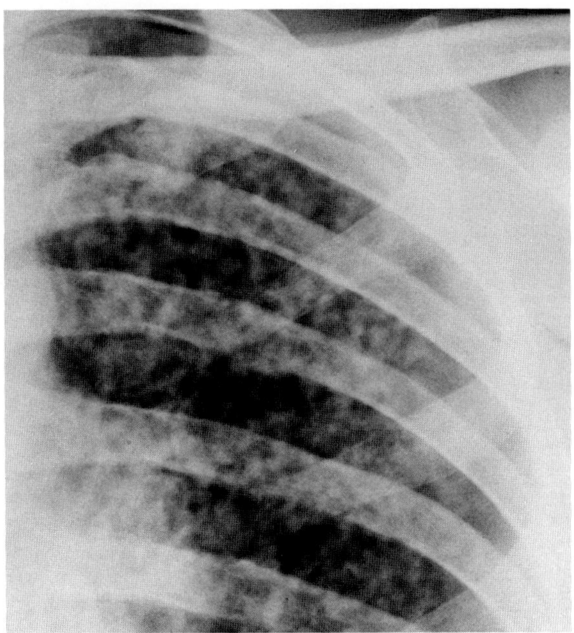

FIG. 3. Silicosis. **(A)** Chest radiograph shows scattered bilateral upper lobe nodules, associated with bilateral hilar lymphadenopathy. **(B)** Chest radiograph in another patient shows profuse 3–5 mm upper lobe nodules.

nodules of interstitial lung disease are usually smaller than those of airspace disease and are sharply defined (Fig. 3). The linear densities seen in interstitial lung disease are usually fine (less than 1 mm in thickness) and may form a reticular network (Fig. 4). They may represent thickened interlobular septa or linear areas of fibrosis. Thickened interlobular septa (Figs. 4 and 5) are char-

acteristically less than 2 cm long, straight, parallel, and are seen near the costophrenic angles (Kerley B lines). These lines are seen most commonly in pulmonary edema (cardiac or noncardiac) and lymphangitic spread of carcinoma.

Honeycomb cysts are identified as clusters of ring shadows 2 to 10 mm in diameter (Fig. 6). Recognition of

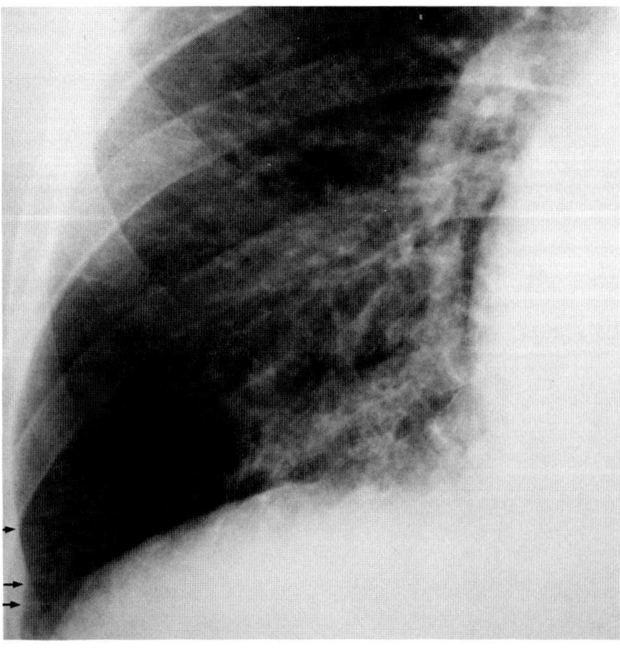
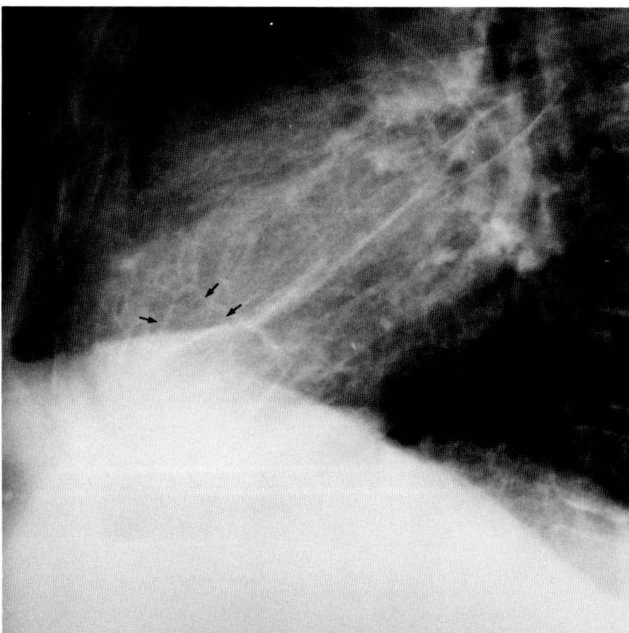

FIG. 4. Linear/reticular shadowing (interstitial pulmonary edema). **(A)** Chest radiograph (detail from right base) shows multiple septal lines (*arrows*, with reticular shadowing). **(B)** The network of lines seen on the lateral view corresponds to the septa between polygonal lobules (Kerley C lines) (*arrows*).

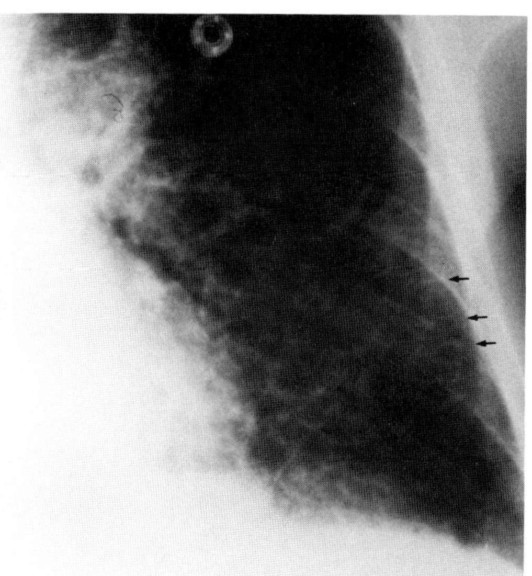
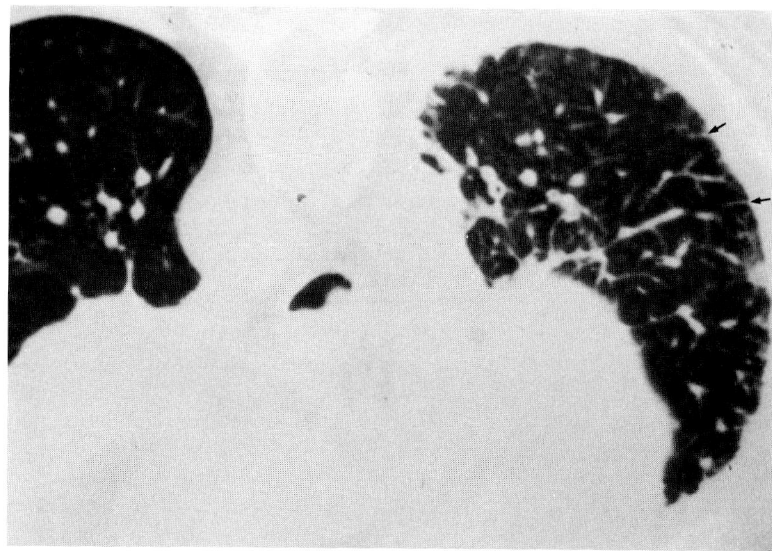

A

B

FIG. 5. Lymphangitic spread of carcinoma. (**A**) Chest radiograph shows multiple septal lines. (**B**) Prone HRCT scan in another patient demonstrates marked pleural thickening, with thickening of interlobular septa (*arrows*).

honeycombing is important because it is a sign of end-stage pulmonary fibrosis. Hazy (ground-glass) increase in lung density (Fig. 7) is most common in acute interstitial lung diseases, such as viral or opportunistic infections, desquamative interstitial pneumonitis, and hypersensitivity pneumonitis. It is well demonstrated on HRCT scanning, and may indicate active alveolitis.

Disease involving the pulmonary airspaces is characterized on the chest radiograph by homogeneous opacities with air bronchograms, or by ill-defined 5–10 mm nodular densities (acinar shadows) that tend to coalesce. Normal large airways are either not visible on the chest radiograph or are seen as thin-walled perihilar ring shadows. With disease of the airways the most common

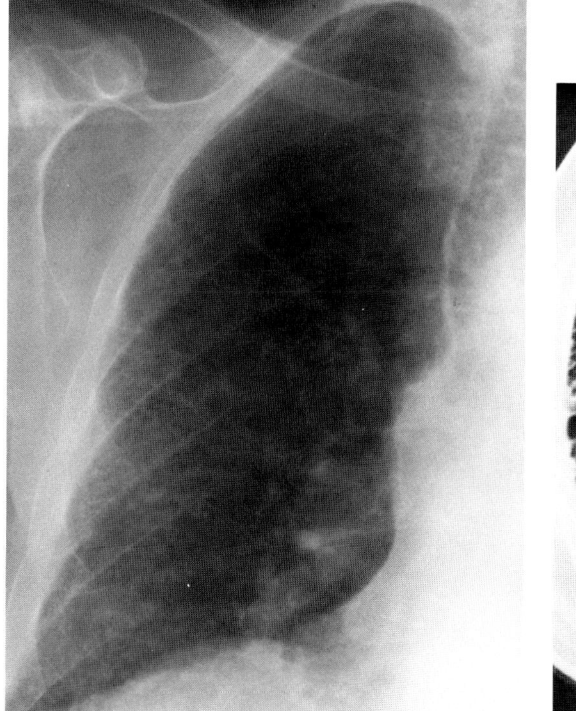
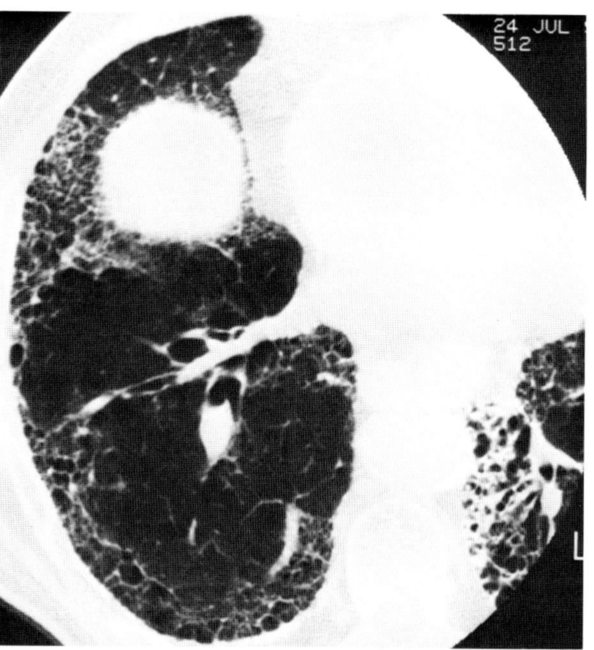

A

B

FIG. 6. IPF with honeycombing. (**A**) Chest radiograph shows honeycombing most evident at the left lung base. (**B**) HRCT scan shows a typical peripheral distribution of honeycombing and fibrosis in IPF.

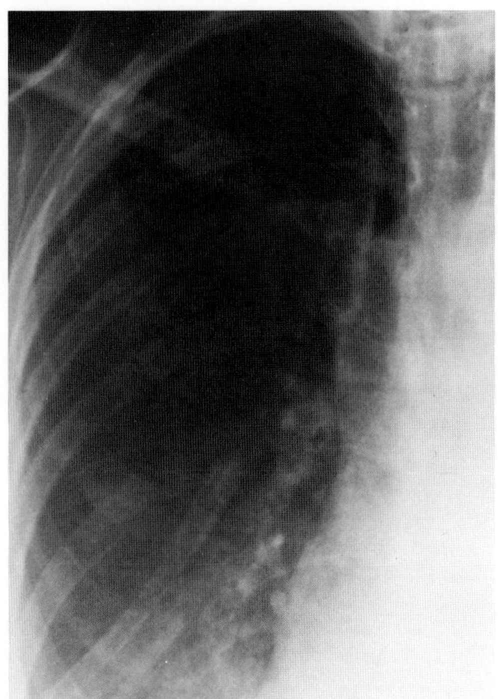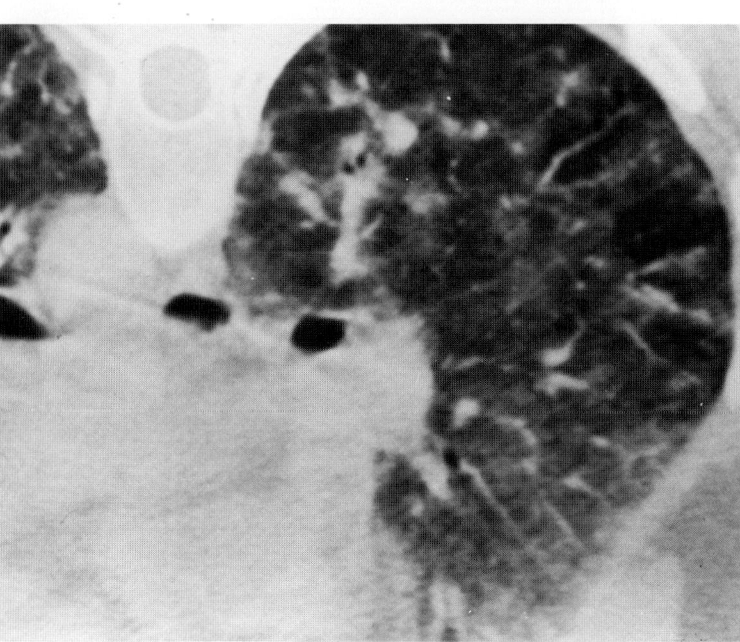

FIG. 7. Hypersensitivity pneumonitis. **(A)** Chest radiograph shows hazy (ground-glass) increased density over the lower half of the lung. **(B)** Prone HRCT scan makes it easier to appreciate the patchy, hazy increase in lung density, suggestive of active alveolitis.

finding is thickening of bronchial walls or the peribronchial interstitium, causing thick-walled ring shadows in airways that are running parallel to the x-ray beam or thin parallel lines (tramlines) in airways running perpendicular to the beam.

The pattern recognition approach previously outlined has significant and important limitations. Most interstitial diseases involve the airspaces to some extent, whereas many airspace diseases have an interstitial component. In these cases one should attempt to identify the dominant disease pattern. The pattern of hazy increase in lung density may be due to interstitial or early airspace disease. The distinction between airspace and interstitial nodules may be difficult and is sometimes unreliable. Sarcoidosis may have a pseudoalveolar appearance, with poorly defined nodules and air bronchograms. The chest radiograph represents a summation or superimposition of the radiographic opacities encountered by the x-ray beam as it traverses the lungs. In this way multiple linear densities may become superimposed to simulate an irregular nodule, and a group of nodules may coincide to simulate a line. This is why many interstitial diseases have a reticulonodular appearance on the chest radiograph. CT scanning demonstrates opacities in the axial plane and overcomes this summation effect. Proper use of the pattern recognition approach requires careful description of the radiographic abnormality and an awareness of the potential pitfalls (13).

RADIOLOGIC-PHYSIOLOGIC CORRELATIONS IN INTERSTITIAL LUNG DISEASE

The volume of the lungs on the chest radiograph correlates well with physiologic measurement of total lung capacity. Therefore, in following subjects with suspected or known interstitial lung disease, observation of changes in radiographic lung volumes is one of the most important indices of improvement or deterioration (Fig. 8). There have been many attempts to correlate the profusion of radiographic abnormalities with severity of symptoms and with pulmonary function abnormalities. The International Labor Organization has introduced a standardized grading scheme for profusion of chest radiographic abnormalities in pneumoconioses (14). Radiographic opacities are categorized as small round opacities, small irregular opacities, and large opacities. The scale is based on comparison with a set of standard radiographs and runs from 0/− to 3/+. The digit placed before the stroke represents the standard film that most closely corresponds to the profusion of the radiographic abnormality. The digit after the stroke corresponds to the next closest standard film. Therefore, a score of 2/1 means that the profusion of the radiographic abnormality is closest to the standard film, with a profusion of 2, and next closest to that with a profusion of 1. This scoring system has been modified by others to provide a system for scoring noninhalational interstitial lung diseases (15). Semi-

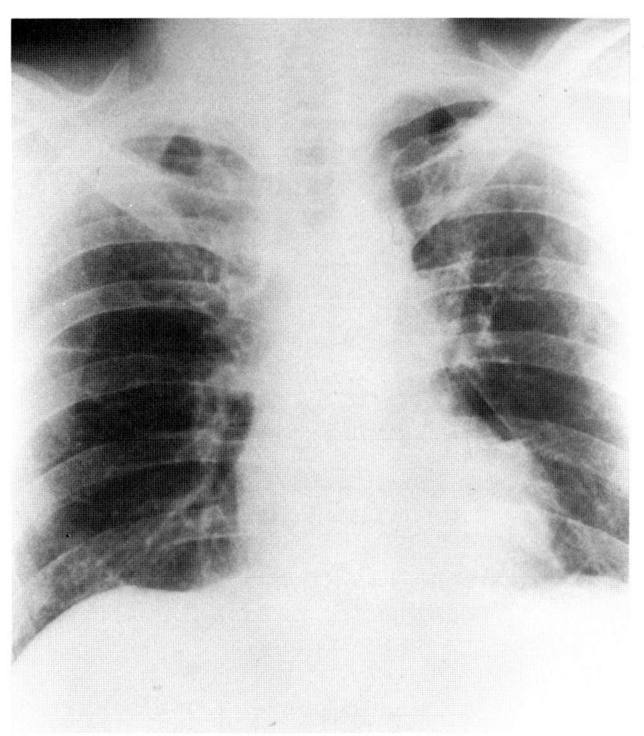
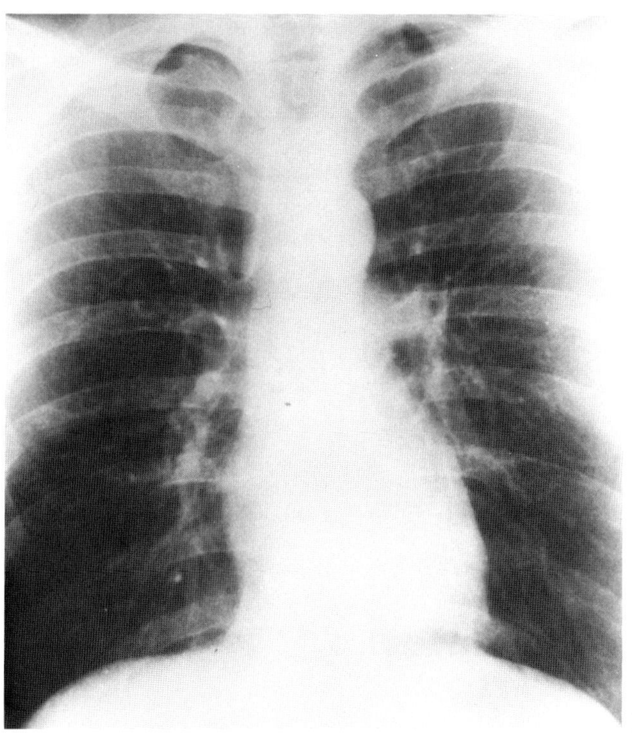

A

B

FIG. 8. Drug toxicity. **(A)** Chest radiograph shows no interstitial changes. However, comparison with the previous radiograph **(B)**, taken 5 years previously, demonstrates marked diminution in lung volumes, indicating severe restrictive lung disease. This is due to previous therapy with BCNU.

quantitative scores of profusion such as these achieve a modest correlation with measures of pulmonary function.

RADIOLOGIC-PATHOLOGIC CORRELATIONS IN INTERSTITIAL LUNG DISEASE

Correlation between chest radiographic appearance and pathologic appearance is limited by the summation effect. However, some useful general observations can be made. Round nodules, when seen on the chest radiograph, usually correlate with the presence of nodules (granulomatous, inhalational, or neoplastic) on pathology. Honeycombing seen on the chest radiograph correlates with honeycombing on pathology. Linear shadows correspond to thickened interlobular septa and linear bands of fibrosis.

HRCT scanning, by eliminating the summation effect, offers considerably better radiologic-pathologic correlation (16). Linear, nodular, or hazy opacities and honeycombing are readily recognized. The peripheral or central distribution of disease can be of considerable value in differential diagnosis. Diseases may also be categorized according to the distribution of abnormality within the secondary pulmonary lobule. Small airway diseases or granulomatous diseases often affect the center of the lobule and are termed centrilobular (17),

whereas lymphangitic spread of carcinoma, IPF, and asbestosis commonly affect the interlobular septa.

CATEGORIES OF INTERSTITIAL LUNG DISEASE

Idiopathic Pulmonary Fibrosis

IPF is the most common form of interstitial pulmonary fibrosis, but as the name implies it is a diagnosis of exclusion. This term is used to describe a clinical syndrome characterized by gradual onset of dyspnea, fine crackles on pulmonary auscultation, and digital clubbing. IPF is usually classified histologically into usual interstitial pneumonia (UIP) or desquamative interstitial pneumonia (DIP). UIP is characterized by fibrosis and thickening of the interstitium, and is often patchy in distribution. DIP is characterized by macrophage proliferation, especially in the alveolar airspaces associated with mild interstitial thickening. These pathologic appearances probably represent relatively acute (DIP) and chronic (UIP) patterns of lung injury.

The characteristic early radiographic pattern of IPF is of predominantly basal (often peripheral) reticular or reticulonodular shadowing. This may progress to diffuse honeycombing, again often most marked in the lower zones and sometimes associated with lower lobe volume

TABLE 3. Siltzbach staging system for sarcoidosis

Siltzbach stage 0	Normal chest radiograph
Siltzbach stage 1	Hilar and/or mediastinal lymphadenopathy, but normal lung parenchyma on chest radiograph
Siltzbach stage 2	Lymphadenopathy with abnormal lung parenchyma, but without evidence of fibrosis
Siltzbach stage 3	Abnormal lung parenchyma without fibrosis and without evidence of adenopathy
Siltzbach stage 4	Evidence of pulmonary fibrosis (upper lobe volume loss, decreased lung volumes, or honeycombing)

loss (Fig. 6). CT scanning demonstrates the peripheral distribution of the disease, shows the extent of honeycombing or associated emphysema, and may also show prominent ground-glass increase in lung density, perhaps indicating alveolitis (18). An acute or subacute variant of this clinical syndrome occurs in approximately 5 percent of subjects (the Hamman–Rich syndrome): this may be associated with either a normal chest radiograph or with ground-glass opacity; many of these subjects have pathologic changes of DIP.

Granulomatous Lung Diseases

The granulomatous lung diseases include infective and noninfective granulomata. Infective granulomatous diseases are discussed in Chapter 2. Noninfective granulomatous diseases include sarcoidosis, Wegener's granulomatosis, lymphomatoid granulomatosis, and pulmonary histiocytosis X. Pulmonary histiocytosis X (PHX) may cause nodules or cysts, and is discussed under cystic lung diseases.

Sarcoidosis is one of the most common interstitial diseases. Its pathologic hallmark is noncaseating granulomata usually occurring at more than one site in the body. The most common sites for sarcoidosis are the hilar and mediastinal lymph nodes and the lung parenchyma. Other possible sites for involvement include the eye, the brain, salivary glands, bones, muscles, skin, and gastrointestinal tract. Intrathoracic sarcoid may be staged by the Siltzbach radiographic staging system (Table 3). The importance of the Siltzbach staging system is that it is an important determinant of prognosis. Ninety-five percent of subjects with stage 0 or 1 sarcoidosis will have a normal chest x-ray at 5 years, whereas only 30 percent of stage III and 5 percent of stage IV will revert to a normal chest radiograph. In subjects with normal lung parenchyma on chest radiograph (stage 0 or I disease) granulomas will be found on transbronchial biopsy in about 80 percent.

The most common radiographic manifestation of sarcoidosis in the lungs is fine nodules (Fig. 9), but sarcoid may have multiple other appearances, including large nodules or masses, reticulonodular shadows, pseudoalveolar opacities, honeycombing, or thin-walled upper lobe cysts. Sarcoid may also present with endobronchial masses. Pleural disease is rare. When adenopathy is present it is usually symmetric and is usually most prominent in the pulmonary hila.

On HRCT scanning the nodules of sarcoidosis are characteristically distributed around the bronchovascular structures, in the subpleural region, and along interlobular septa (Fig. 10) (19). Hazy increase in lung density may be seen and may correlate with active alveolitis. CT is more sensitive than chest radiographs for detection of sarcoid lung disease, but occasional normal scans are encountered.

Inhalational Lung Disorders

Inhalation of organic or inorganic dusts may cause different patterns of parenchymal lung injury. Hypersensitivity pneumonitis is a pattern of lung injury that is usually related to inhalation of organic dusts (20). Pathologically this reaction is characterized by accumulation of lymphocytes and macrophages around bronchioles and small pulmonary vessels, and by granuloma formation. Pulmonary fibrosis may ensue. This disease is important because it is usually readily treatable by removing the offending antigen from the environment.

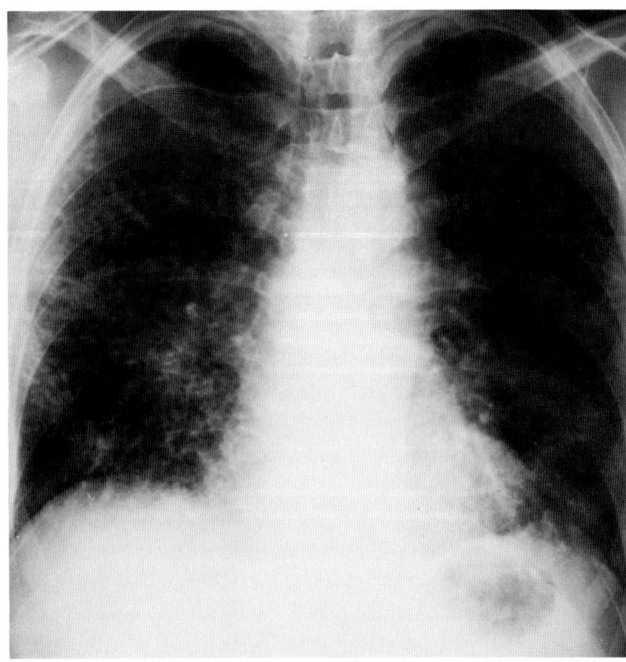

FIG. 9. Stage II sarcoidosis. Chest radiograph shows bilateral hilar and mediastinal lymphadenopathy, associated with profuse, predominantly nodular pulmonary densities.

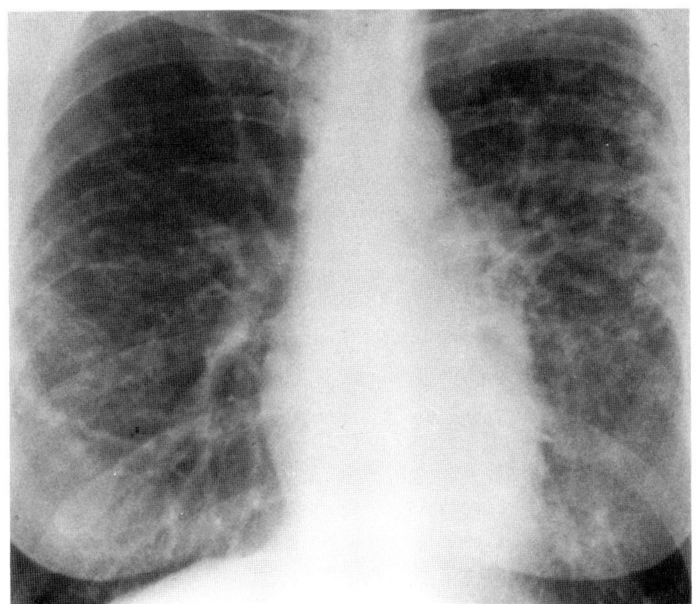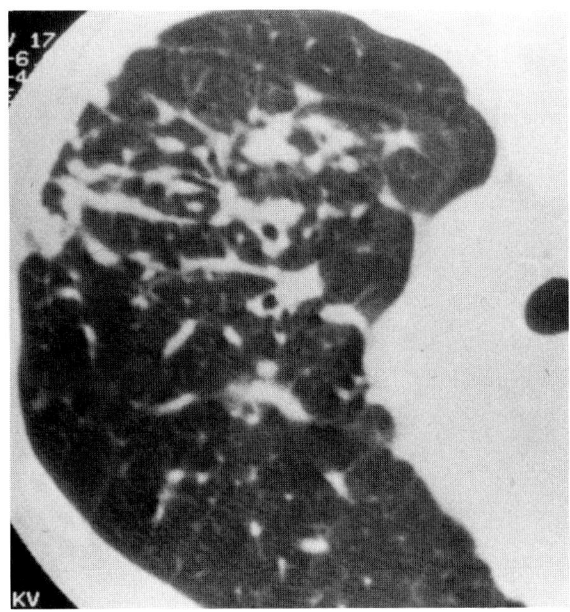

FIG. 10. Stage III sarcoidosis. **(A)** Chest radiograph shows bilateral lung nodules, left more than right. **(B)** Prone HRCT scan shows that the nodules are distributed along vessels and in the subpleural region, characteristic for sarcoidosis.

Hypersensitivity pneumonitis may present clinically in acute, subacute, or chronic phases. The acute phase is often manifested by diffuse hazy (ground-glass) increase in lung density obscuring the pulmonary vessels (Fig. 7) or by a diffuse nodular pattern. Alternatively, the chest radiograph may be normal. The acute phase usually occurs within 6–24 hours after exposure to the offending antigen. Radiographic manifestations of the chronic phase of hypersensitivity pneumonitis mimic those of many other fibrotic lung disorders. Common manifestations include reticulonodular shadowing, volume loss (especially in the upper lobes), and honeycombing. In these cases the clinical history of worsening in relationship to antigen exposure may not be clear. This diagnosis may require careful serologic and environmental assessments. The radiographs of subjects in the subacute phase of hypersensitivity pneumonitis tend to combine the features of acute and chronic disease.

Pneumoconiosis

The term pneumoconiosis is applied to the accumulation of abnormal amounts of inorganic dusts in the lungs and the pathologic response to this dust.

Silicosis

The characteristic pulmonary lesion of silicosis is the hyalinized nodule. Radiographically these nodules appear as 3–10 mm well-defined nodules, most profuse in the upper zones of the lungs (Fig. 3). In later stages, the nodules may coalesce to form larger masses, again characteristically in the upper lobes. This coalescence is called progressive massive fibrosis and radiographically is characterized by a sausage-shaped mass usually in the posterior segment of the upper lobe, often bilateral, and retracting toward the hila, leaving a zone of peripheral emphysema (Fig. 11). These masses may cavitate centrally due to ischemia. The masses are commonly associated with tuberculosis or atypical mycobacterial infection: this should be excluded by examination of the sputum in all cases. Another characteristic feature of silicosis is the presence of hilar lymphadenopathy, often with calcifications (Fig. 3). Eggshell calcification is characteristic but uncommon. Rarely, intense exposure to silica (especially in sandblasters) may cause an acute alveolar lipoproteinosis, similar to pulmonary alveolar proteinosis.

Coalworker's Pneumoconiosis

The characteristic pathologic lesion of coalworker's pneumoconiosis is the coal dust macule. Radiographically this appears as a regular nodule similar to but often slightly smaller than the silicotic nodule (Fig. 12A). Progressive massive fibrosis may also occur in coalworker's pneumoconiosis (Fig. 12B). Mixed dust exposures are common because many coal dusts contain silica. Other inhalational causes of nodular lung disease include talc inhalation.

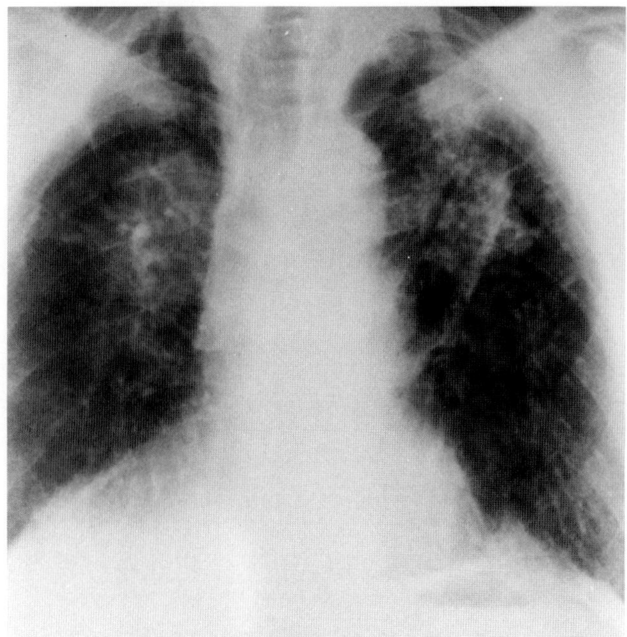

FIG. 11. Silicosis with progressive massive fibrosis. Chest radiograph shows large conglomerate masses in the posterior segment of each upper lobe. There is peripheral emphysema. These appearances are typical for progressive massive fibrosis, which in this case was complicated by infection with *Mycobacterium kansasii*. Mycobacterial infection should always be suspected in subjects with progressive massive fibrosis.

Asbestos-Related Diseases

Inhalation of asbestos mineral fibers causes a variety of pulmonary and pleural responses. The most common response is the development of calcified or noncalcified parietal pleural plaques (Fig. 13). Radiographically these are best seen when in profile as focal densities along the lateral chest walls, or as focal convexities along the smooth diaphragmatic surface. Pleural calcification is seen as a linear density following the chest wall. A plaque may be seen *en face* as a smoothly marginated area of increased density, sometimes with irregular calcifications. CT scanning is significantly more sensitive than chest radiographs for detection of asbestos-related pleural plaques (21).

Asbestos exposure may also cause a benign exudative pleural effusion, diffuse pleural thickening, malignant mesothelioma, or visceral pleural plaques.

Asbestos pleural disease is regarded as evidence of asbestos exposure, but does not usually cause significant disability. The term asbestosis is reserved for asbestos-related pulmonary fibrosis. The histologic appearance of asbestosis is similar to that of IPF or pulmonary fibrosis associated with collagen vascular disease. The radiographic features of these diseases are also similar. The characteristic features are small irregular or reticulonodular opacities, predominantly involving the lower lobes, leading to honeycombing and lower lobe volume loss.

HRCT scanning may show the features of asbestosis in subjects with normal chest radiographs. Early features include thickening of interlobular septa and prominence of the centrilobular core structures. These changes likely correspond to the early pathologic changes that characteristically first affect the distal bronchioles and subsequently affect the alveolar septa and interlobular septa. Subsequent changes are similar to those of IPF.

In addition to the fibrogenic affects of asbestos, asbestos may also cause a variety of intrapulmonary masses.

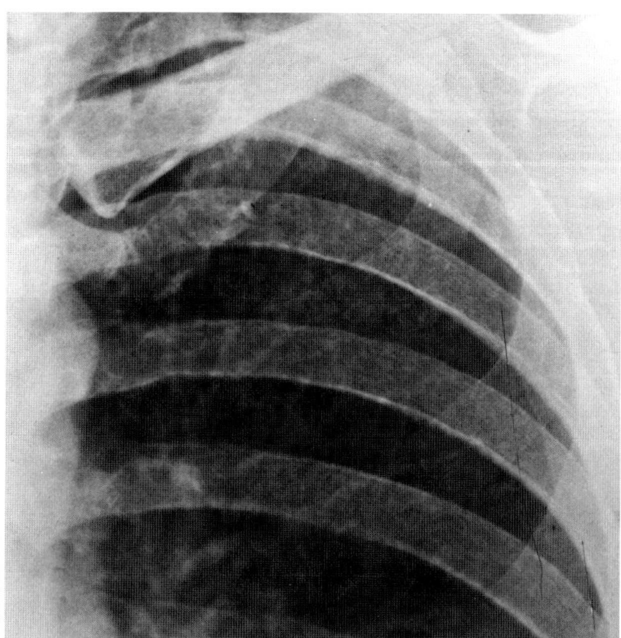

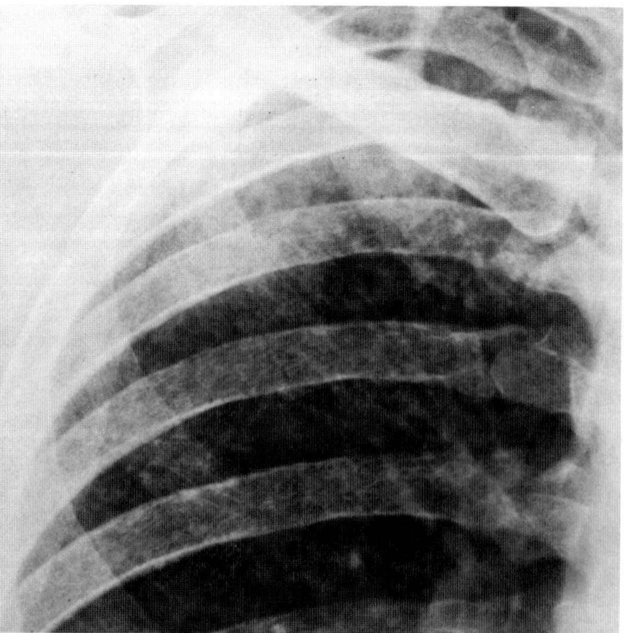

FIG. 12. Coalworker's pneumoconiosis. **(A)** Chest radiograph shows fine 2–4 mm nodules in the left upper lobe. **(B)** Chest radiograph in another patient shows an early conglomerate mass.

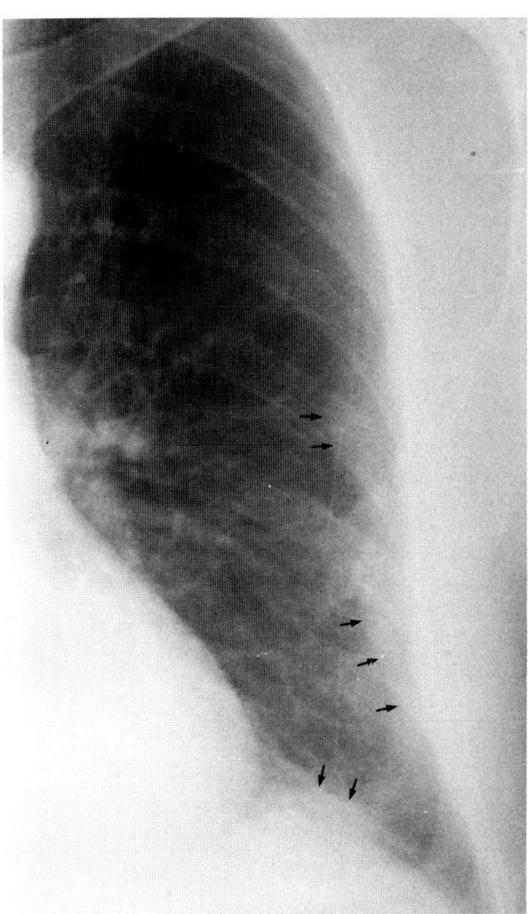

FIG. 13. Asbestos-related pleural disease. Chest radiograph shows multiple noncalcified pleural plaques along the lateral chest wall and diaphragm (*arrows*). The lung parenchyma is normal, so this patient does not have radiographic evidence of asbestosis.

The most important of these, of course, is bronchogenic carcinoma. Asbestos exposure appears to be synergistic with cigarette smoking for the development of lung cancer. Asbestos workers who are smokers have a 60-fold increase in lung cancer when compared with non-smoking nonexposed subjects. Carcinogenicity appears to vary with fiber type. Rounded atelectasis is a condition in which a cicatrizing pleural reaction causes the underlying lung to retract and form a mass. Typical cases are readily recognized radiographically by the "comet tail" of vessels and bronchi curving gently into the mass from the hilum. However, one must suspect broncho-genic carcinoma in any asbestos-exposed subject who has a pulmonary mass (22).

Collagen Vascular Disease

Most of the collagen vascular diseases can be associated with pulmonary fibrosis. The pulmonary fibrosis seen with these diseases is similar clinically, histologi-cally, and radiographically to that seen with IPF (7). Ninety percent of subjects with progressive systemic sclerosis (PSS) have pathologic evidence of pulmonary fibrosis at autopsy (Figs. 1, 2, and 4). However, only about 25 percent will have chest radiographic changes (Fig. 1), and symptoms of pulmonary disease will occur in only 16 percent. It must be remembered that because of esoph-ageal motility abnormalities (Fig. 1), these patients are also subject to recurrent or chronic aspiration pneumo-nia, which may also cause pulmonary fibrosis. Pulmo-nary arterial hypertension is a frequent feature of PSS. It has been suggested that PSS is associated with an in-creased risk of lung cancer but this association is proba-bly fortuitous.

Rheumatoid disease may be associated with pulmo-nary fibrosis. Other chest radiographic manifestations of rheumatoid disease include pleural effusions, pulmo-nary rheumatoid nodules, and bronchiolitis obliterans (sometimes related to penicillamine therapy). Patients who have pneumoconiosis and rheumatoid arthritis have a high frequency of pulmonary nodules. This rare association is called Caplan's syndrome.

The most common intrathoracic manifestation of sys-temic lupus erythematosus is pleural or pericardial effu-sion. Acute focal airspace infiltrates may occur, and diffuse pulmonary fibrosis is also seen. A rare manifesta-tion is progressive loss of lung volume (shrinking lungs) perhaps due to diaphragmatic dysfunction. Because many subjects with collagen vascular disease are on sys-temic immunosuppressive therapy, the possibilities of opportunistic infection and drug toxicity must always be considered in the differential diagnosis of lung disease occurring in this population.

Subjects with overlap syndromes such as CRST syn-drome and mixed connective tissue disease may also de-velop pulmonary fibrosis, as may patients with dermato-myositis (5–10 percent). In Sjögrens syndrome the most common abnormality is recurrent pulmonary infec-tions, likely related to drying of the airways, and im-paired mucociliary clearance. In addition, subjects with Sjögrens syndrome may develop lymphoproliferative disorders, including lymphoid interstitial pneumonitis (Fig. 14) and frank lymphoma.

Lymphoproliferative Disorders of the Lung

Lymphoid interstitial pneumonitis is characterized by a polyclonal proliferation of lymphocytes in the pulmo-nary interstitium. It may have a variety of radiographic appearances, including reticulonodular interstitial dis-ease, focal airspace opacities, and single or multiple lung masses. Although relatively uncommon, lymphoid in-terstitial pneumonitis is important because it may be a presenting feature of acquired immune deficiency syn-drome both in children and adults, and because it may progress to frank lymphoma.

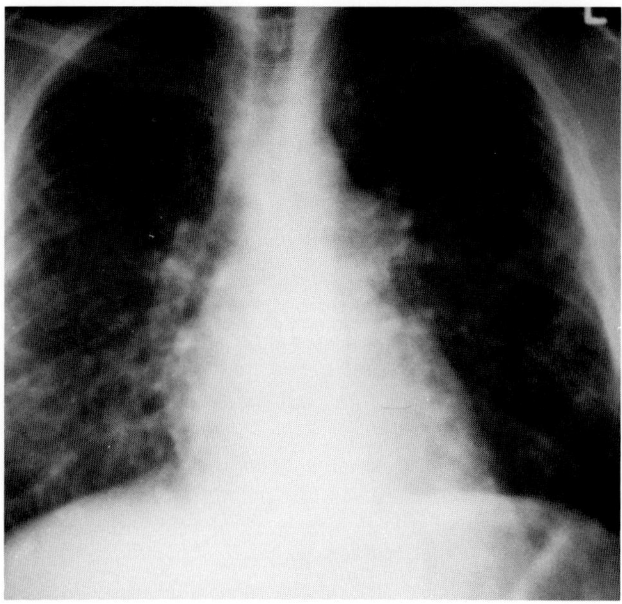

FIG. 14. Lymphoid interstitial pneumonitis. Forty-year-old male presents with Sjögren's syndrome. Chest radiograph shows a coarse nodular interstitial infiltrate.

Cystic Lung Diseases

Cystic diseases of the lung present radiographically with increased lung volumes and thin-walled cysts. The other common causes of interstitial disease with normal or increased lung volumes are bronchiolitis obliterans and the combination of IPF and emphysema. Neurofibromatosis is a rare cause of pulmonary cystic disease.

Lymphangiomyomatosis is a lung disease of young women characterized by abnormal proliferation of smooth muscle cells in lymph nodes and lymphatics, and by cyst formation. Chest manifestations include diffuse cystic lung disease, hyperinflation, pneumothorax, and chylous pleural effusions. A similar disorder occurs in male and female subjects with tuberous sclerosis. HRCT in these patients shows diffuse pulmonary cysts, usually less than 1 cm in diameter (Fig. 15) (23).

PHX is also called eosinophilic granuloma of the lung (Fig. 16). Although this lung disease is relatively uncommon, it is an important cause of interstitial lung disease with honeycombing in young people. It appears to be primarily related to cigarette smoking. Early PHX presents with poorly defined nodules that may remain stable, or may regress leaving a normal or near-normal radiographic appearance. The combination of nodules and cysts is virtually diagnostic of PHX.

Alternatively the nodules may progress, with formation of thin-walled cystic spaces and subsequent diffuse honeycombing. The nodules are most profuse in the mid and upper zones of the chest, with characteristic sparing of the costophrenic angles. About 15 percent of subjects present with pneumothorax. On HRCT there is often a characteristic combination of well-defined or poorly de-

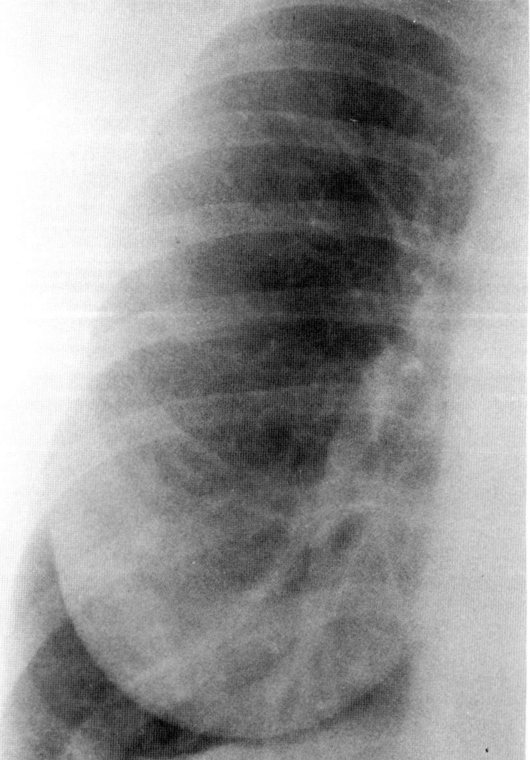

A

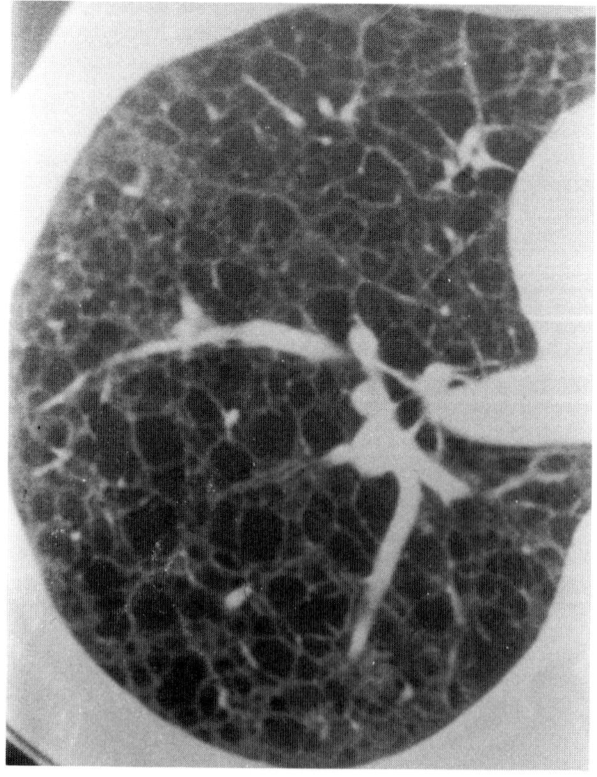

B

FIG. 15. Lymphangiomyomatosis. **(A)** Chest radiograph shows large lung volumes in a young female. Some scattered cysts are seen. **(B)** HRCT scan shows diffuse cystic lung disease with cysts of varying sizes.

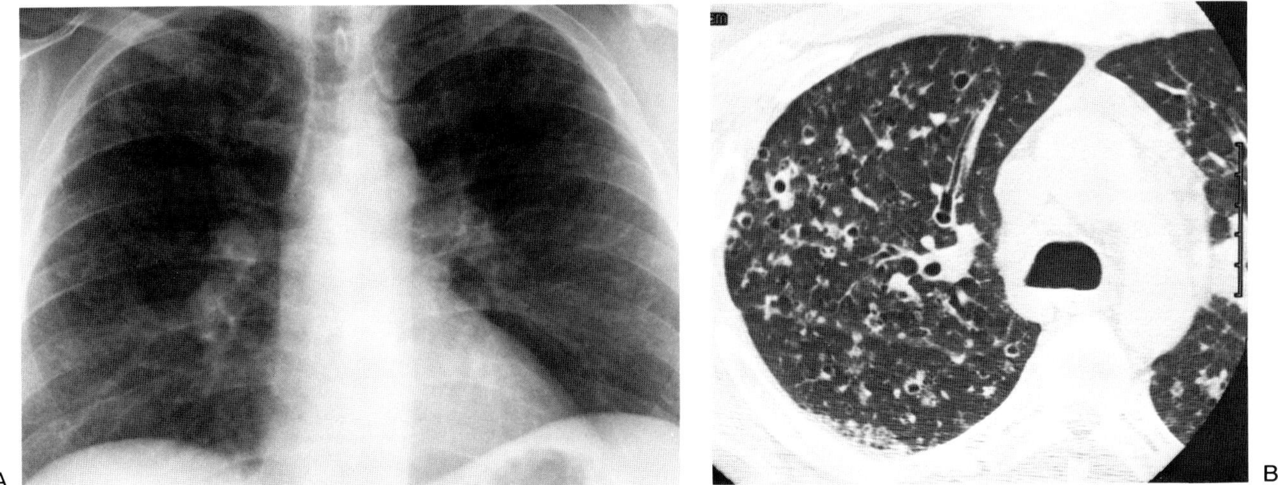

FIG. 16. PHX. (**A**) Chest radiograph shows nodules predominantly in the upper lobes. (**B**) HRCT scan shows multiple thick-walled cysts and scattered nodules.

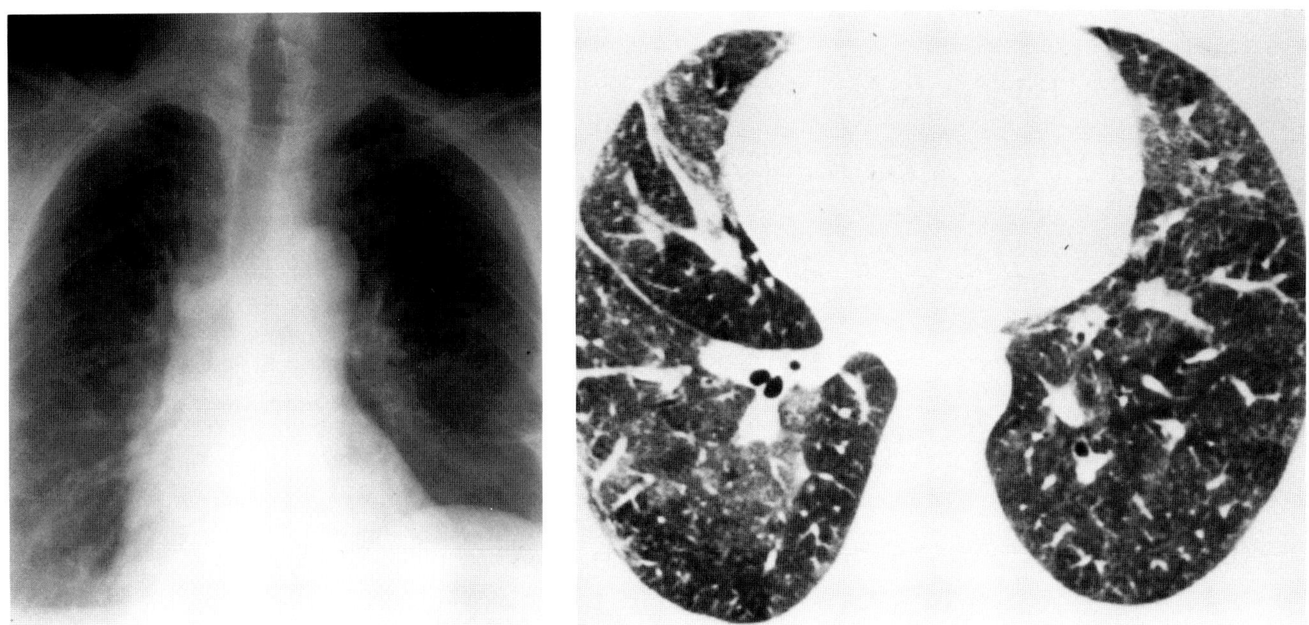

FIG. 17. Drug toxicity. (**A**) Chest radiograph in a subject with Wegener granulomatosis shows chronic bibasal scarring and elevation of left hemidiaphragm. (**B**) HRCT scan shows areas of hazy increase in density throughout both lungs, due to cyclophosphamide toxicity.

TABLE 4. *Common causes of drug-induced interstitial pneumonitis/fibrosis*

Noncytotoxic drugs	Cytotoxic drugs
Amiodarone	BCNU
Carbamazepine	Bleomycin
Gold	Busulfan
Nitrofurantoin	Chlorambucil
Sulfasalazine	Cyclophosphamide
	Methotrexate
	Procarbazine

fined nodules and cysts distributed throughout the lungs but most profuse in the upper zones (Fig. 16) (24).

Drug-Induced Lung Disease

Drugs are an important and increasingly common cause of interstitial pulmonary fibrosis (Fig. 17) (25). Table 4 lists some common cytotoxic and noncytotoxic drugs that are associated with pulmonary fibrosis. The syndrome of drug-induced pulmonary toxicity may be acute (diffuse alveolar damage or pulmonary edema) or chronic. Aspirin or narcotic overdose causes acute pulmonary edema, whereas antimetabolites such as bleomycin and carmustine (BCNU) tend to cause slowly progressive loss of lung volume and fibrosis (Fig. 8). The pulmonary toxic effect of bleomycin is facilitated by the administration of oxygen. Amiodarone may cause interstitial or airspace densities (often peripheral) or pleural effusions (Fig. 18).

Chronic Airspace-Filling Disorders

Clinical presentation of chronic airspace disorders often mimics that of chronic interstitial disease. The typical radiographic appearance of airspace disease, previously described, helps to identify this group. The appearance of airspace opacity is usually due to cellular or proteinaceous material occupying the air-containing spaces of the lung (Table 5). Pulmonary alveolar proteinosis is due to overproduction of surfactant-like material (Fig. 19). Perihilar airspace or granular pulmonary infiltrates that spare the diaphragms are characteristic. Pulmonary eosinophilia may be due to drugs, parasites, asthma, or allergic bronchopulmonary aspergillosis. Idiopathic pulmonary eosinophilia is categorized into acute or simple pulmonary eosinophilia (lasting less than 1 month), chronic pulmonary eosinophilia (more than 1 month) (Fig. 20), and hypereosinophilic syndrome (associated with cardiac and other manifestations). Pulmonary hemorrhage syndromes include idiopathic pulmonary hemosiderosis, collagen vascular diseases, and Goodpasture's syndrome, Wegener's granulomatosis, and other pulmonary-renal syndromes.

Bronchiolitis obliterans with organizing pneumonia is an idiopathic syndrome that is distinct radiographically, clinically, and pathologically from IPF. Clinically it is characterized by relatively acute onset of dyspnea, perhaps with flu-like symptoms. Radiographically one sees patchy unifocal or multifocal pulmonary opacities (Fig. 21) that correspond pathologically to areas of organizing pneumonia (26). The importance of recognizing bronchiolitis obliterans with organizing pneumonia is that it responds dramatically to steroids.

CONCLUSIONS

Recognition of the clinical syndromes associated with the various interstitial lung diseases should be of considerable value in their differential diagnosis. Identification

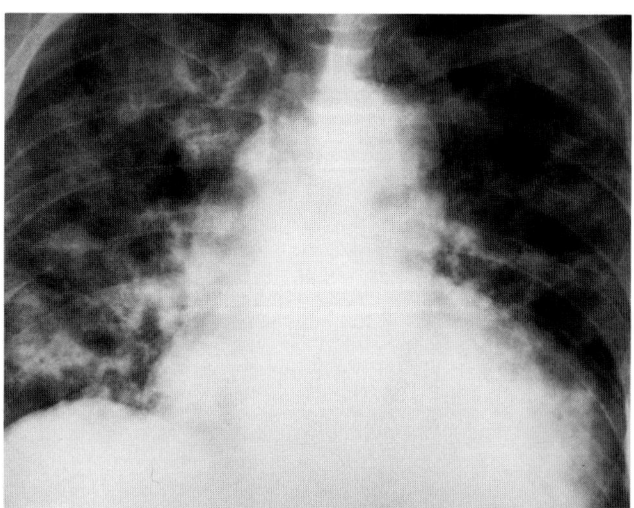
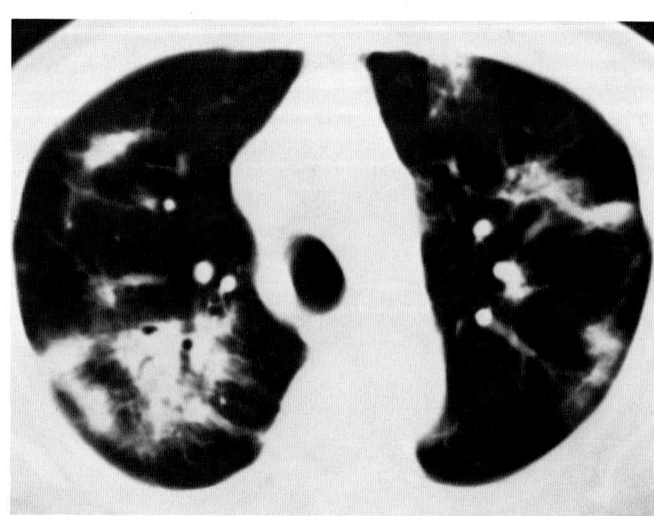

FIG. 18. Amiodarone toxicity. **(A)** Chest radiograph shows cardiomegaly and patchy, bilateral airspace opacities. **(B)** Ten millimeter CT scan shows patchy airspace opacities.

TABLE 5. *Chronic airspace–filling diseases*

Airspace disease[a]	Substance-occupying alveoli
Pulmonary alveolar proteinosis	Surfactant-like protein
Pulmonary eosinophilia	Eosinophils
Chronic infections (TB, fungus)	Inflammatory cells, microorganisms
BOOP	Inflammatory cells
Pulmonary vasculitis	Inflammatory cells, exudate, blood
Pulmonary renal syndromes	Blood (usually rapidly resorbed)
Sarcoidosis	Conglomerate granulomas
Lipid pneumonia, chronic aspiration pneumonia	Aspirated material
Bronchoalveolar carcinoma	Malignant cells, secretions
Lymphoma	Malignant cells

[a] TB, tuberculosis; BOOP, bronchiolitis obliterans with organizing pneumonia.

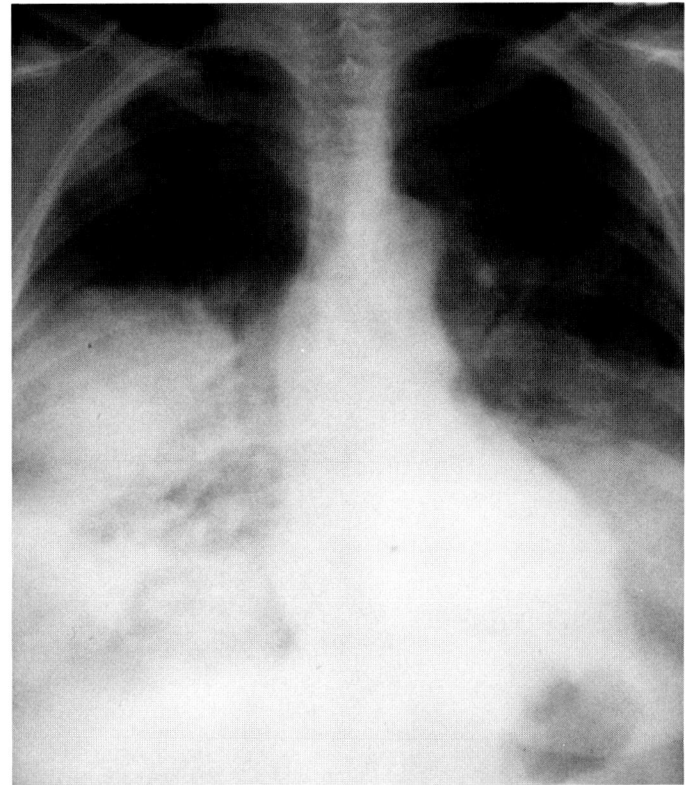

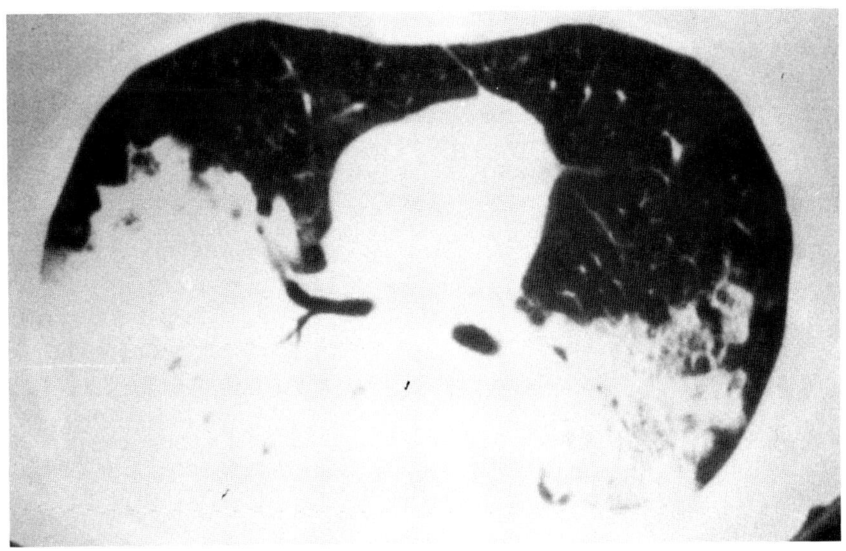

FIG. 19. Alveolar proteinosis. **(A)** Chest radiograph shows extensive airspace shadowing involving both mid and lower zones. **(B)** CT scan shows poorly defined opacities and air bronchograms, typical of airspace disease.

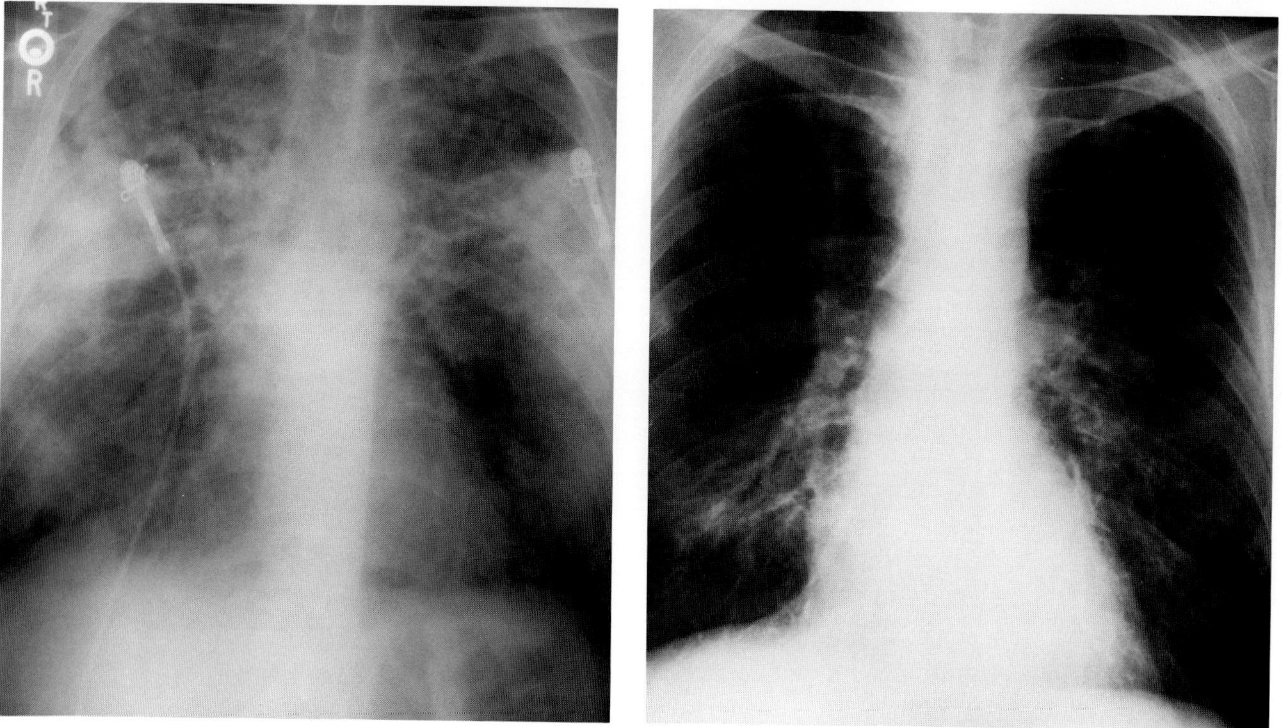

FIG. 20. Eosinophilic pneumonia. **(A)** A chest radiograph shows predominantly peripheral and upper lobe airspace pulmonary densities. **(B)** Chest radiograph 7 days later, following administration of steroids demonstrates near-complete resolution.

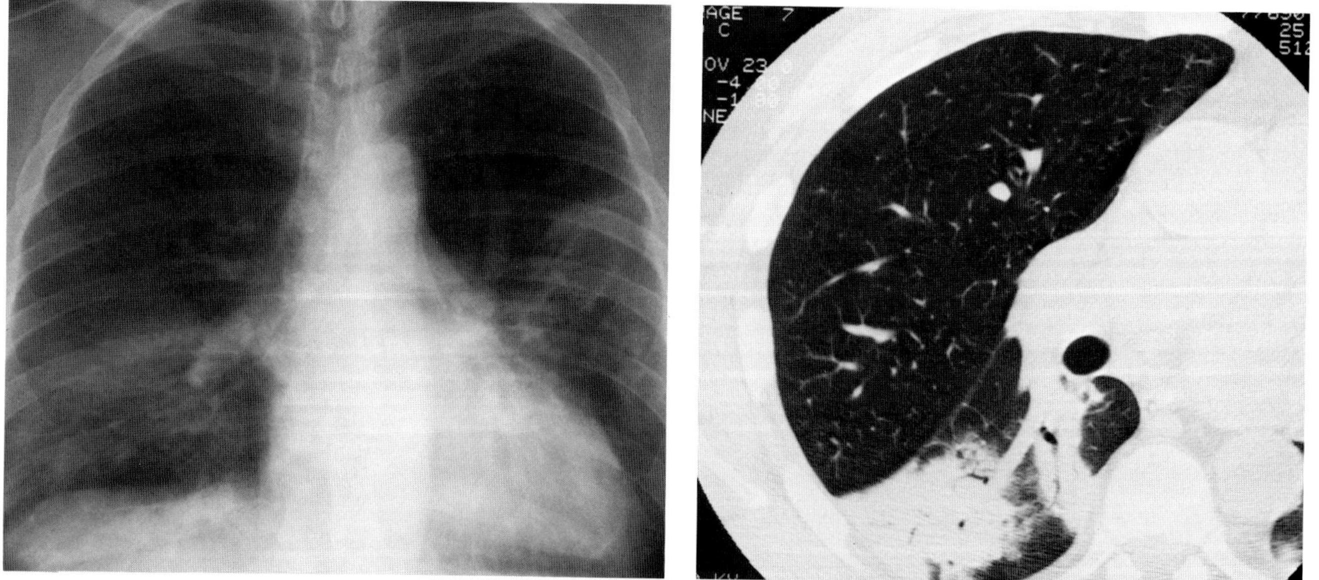

FIG. 21. Bronchiolitis obliterans organizing pneumonia. **(A)** A chest radiograph shows patchy airspace pulmonary densities. **(B)** HRCT shows focal airspace opacification, obscuring the pulmonary vessels. **(C)** Chest radiograph 2 months later, following treatment with steroids, demonstrates resolution of opacities. **(D)** Six months later, after stopping steroids, the patient's symptoms have recurred, and there is a new right midlung opacity of BOOP.

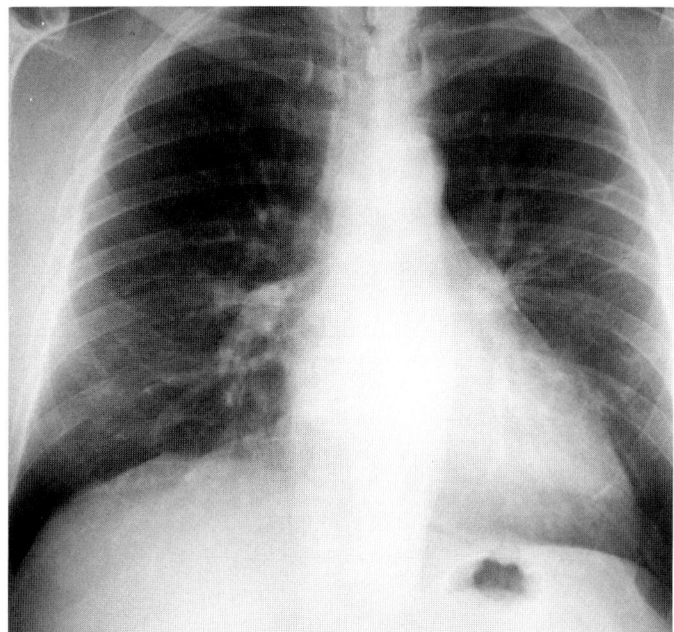

C

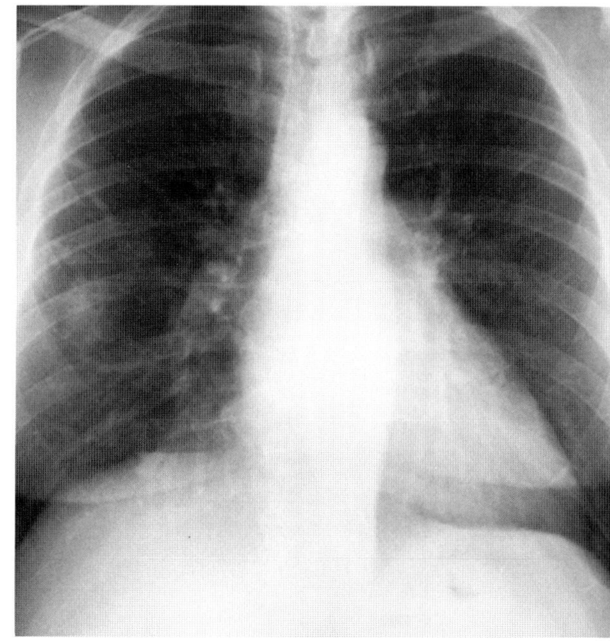

D

FIG. 21. *Continued.*

of a characteristic radiographic pattern is often helpful in narrowing the differential diagnosis. In particular HRCT scanning may be of value in confirming specific radiographic patterns. The radiologist has an important role in the detection, characterization, and follow-up of interstitial lung diseases.

REFERENCES

1. Crystal R, Bitterman P, Rennard S, Hance A, Keogh B. Interstitial lung diseases of unknown cause: disorders characterised by chronic inflammation of the lower respiratory tract. *N Engl J Med* 1984;310:154–166, 235–244.
2. Epler G, McLoud T, Gaensler E, et al. Normal chest roentgenograms in chronic diffuse infiltrative lung disease. *N Engl J Med* 1978;298:934–939.
3. Bekerman C, Hoffer PB, Bitran JD, Gupta RG. Gallium-67 citrate imaging studies of the lung. *Semin Nucl Med* 1980;10:286–301.
4. Line B, Fulmer J, Reynolds H, et al. Gallium-67 citrate scanning in the staging of idiopathic pulmonary fibrosis: correlation with physiologic and morphologic features and bronchoalveolar lavage. *Am Rev Respir Dis* 1978;118:355–365.
5. Line BR, Hunninghake GW, Keogh BA, Jones AE, Johnston GS, Crystal RG. Gallium-67 scanning to stage the alveolitis of sarcoidosis: correlation with clinical studies, pulmonary function studies, and bronchoalveolar lavage. *Am Rev Respir Dis* 1981;123.
6. Mayo J, Webb W, Gould R, et al. High-resolution CT of the lungs: an optimal approach. *Radiology* 1987;163:507–510.
7. Schurawitzki H, Stiglbauer R, Graninger W, et al. Interstitial lung disease in progressive systemic sclerosis: high-resolution CT versus radiography. *Radiology* 1990;176:755–759.
8. Mathieson J, Mayo J, Staples C, Muller N. Chronic diffuse infiltrative lung disease: comparison of diagnostic accuracy of CT and chest radiography. *Radiology* 1989;171:111–116.
9. Aberle DR, Gamsu G, Ray CS. High-resolution CT of benign asbestos-related diseases: clinical and radiographic correlation. *Am J Roentgenol* 1988;151:883–891.
10. Staples C, Muller N, Vedal S, Abboud R, Ostrow D, Miller R. Usual interstitial pneumonia: correlation of CT with clinical, functional, and radiographic findings. *Radiology* 1987;162:377–381.
11. Muller N, Mawson J, Mathieson J, Abboud R, Ostrow D, Champion P. Sarcoidosis: correlation of extent of disease at CT with clinical, functional, and radiographic findings. *Radiology* 1989;171:613–618.
12. McFadden RG, Carr TJ, Wood TE. Proton magnetic resonance imaging to stage activity of interstitial lung disease. *Chest* 1987;92:31–39.
13. Felson B. A new look at pattern recognition of diffuse pulmonary disease. *Am J Roentgenol* 1979;133:183–189.
14. International Labour Office. Guidelines for the use of ILO international classification of radiographs of pneumoconioses, rev. ed. Geneva: International Labour Office, 1980.
15. Epstein DM, Miller WT, Bresnitz EA, Levine MS, Gefter WB. Application of ILO classification to a population without industrial exposure: findings to be differentiated from pneumoconiosis. *Am J Roentgenol* 1984;142:53–58.
16. Meziane M, Hruban R, Zerhouni E, et al. High resolution CT of the lung parenchyma with pathologic correlation. *Radiographics* 1988;8:27–54.
17. Murata K, Itoh H, Todo G, et al. Centrilobular lesions of the lungs: demonstration by high-resolution CT and pathologic correlation. *Radiology* 1986;161:641–645.
18. Muller N, Staples C, Miller R, Vedal S, Thurlbeck W, Ostrow D. Disease activity in idiopathic pulmonary fibrosis: CT and pathologic correlation. *Radiology* 1987;165:731–734.
19. Lynch D, Webb W, Gamsu G, et al. Computed tomography in sarcoidosis. *J Comput Assist Tomogr* 1989;13:405–410.
20. Rose C, King TJ. Controversies in hypersensitivity pneumonitis. *Am Rev Respir Dis* 1992;145:1–2.
21. Lynch D, Gamsu G, Aberle D. Conventional and high resolution CT in the diagnosis of asbestos-related diseases. *Radiographics* 1989;9:523–551.
22. Lynch D, Gamsu G, Ray C, Aberle D. Asbestos-related focal lung masses: manifestations on conventional and high-resolution CT scans. *Radiology* 1988;169:603–607.

23. Aberle DR, Hansell DM, Brown K, Tashkin DP. Lymphangio-myomatosis: CT, chest radiographic, and functional correlations. *Radiology* 1990;176:381–387.

24. Moore A, Godwin J, Muller N, et al. Pulmonary histiocytosis X: comparison of radiographic and CT findings. *Radiology* 1989;172:249–254.

25. Gregory S, Grippi M. The clinical diagnosis of drug-induced pulmonary disorders. *J Thorac Imag* 1991;6:8–18.

26. Muller NL, Guerry FML, Staples CA, et al. Differential diagnosis of bronchiolitis obliterans with organizing pneumonia and usual interstitial pneumonia: clinical, functional, and radiologic findings. *Radiology* 1987;162.

Thoracic Radiology, edited by
J.D. Newell, Jr., and R.D. Tarver,
Raven Press, Ltd., New York © 1993.

CHAPTER 6

Pulmonary Angiography in Thromboembolism

Robert W. Holden and John T. Mail

The firm diagnosis of pulmonary embolism continues to be elusive in the absence of pulmonary angiography. The lack of specific clinical signs and symptoms combined with the insensitivity of chest radiography and the nonspecificity of abnormalities documented by both perfusion and ventilation lung scanning continue to promote the clinical utilization of pulmonary angiography in other than the most straightforward case.

PATHOPHYSIOLOGY

Whereas the vast majority of clinically significant pulmonary emboli originate from the deep veins of the lower extremity, other draining veins are cited as less common sites of origin for pulmonary emboli—upper extremity, pelvis, liver, and kidneys. The right heart may be the most frequent site of origin of nonlower extremity pulmonary emboli. In a recent autopsy series, Chakko and Richards (1) reported 80 percent of patients with right-sided cardiac thrombi (24 of 30 patients) demonstrated significant antemortem pulmonary emboli.

There is a long-standing argument about the propensity of calf vein thrombus to embolize. Although some authorities argue that calf deep vein thrombi seldom embolize, it seems more likely that approximately 15–20 percent of all thrombi embolize regardless of location in the upper or lower leg. However, the size of the vein of embolus origin is a determining factor in the caliber of the missile being embolized into the pulmonary circulation and subsequently its elicited symptoms. Clinicians frequently clear occluded indwelling venous lines by saline irrigation, producing small emboli that are well tolerated in almost every circumstance. Usually, the patient who becomes symptomatic from calf vein emboli has

multiple emboli. Thus, larger emboli or multiple small emboli are more likely to elicit symptoms. It has been estimated that 10–15 percent of the capillary bed must be obstructed to elevate pulmonary arterial pressures. A 40–50 percent obstruction of the pulmonary vasculature, usually called massive pulmonary embolism, produces acute right heart outflow obstruction with resultant systemic hypotension and death.

CLINICAL PRESENTATION

Pulmonary embolism presents with the same signs and symptoms as most other pulmonary or cardiac diseases. The acute onset of symptomatic pulmonary emboli is usually reported to have the following symptoms (incidence noted in parentheses): pleuritic chest pain (70 percent), dyspnea (85 percent), hemoptysis (30 percent), tachypnea (90 percent), tachycardia (40 percent), symptomatic deep venous thrombosis (DVT) (30 percent), and hypoxemia (90 percent). The classic triad of hemoptysis, dyspnea, and pleuritic chest pain occurs in less than 20 percent of patients with symptomatic pulmonary emboli.

This usual nonspecific presentation, even in life-threatening pulmonary emboli, accounts for their frequent autopsy demonstration in clinically unsuspected antemortem presentations. In 1858, Virchow (2) described the classic triad of endothelial injury, stasis, and hypercoagulable state. Subsequently, in 1865, Trousseau (3) noted an increase in DVT associated with malignant neoplasms. Currently, most believe that ovary, testicular, pancreatic, renal, and gastrointestinal malignancies have a definite predilection for DVT induction and, thus, an increased risk of pulmonary embolism. Interestingly, in our own experience, this relationship seldom presents in the occult malignancy, but the DVT at presentation is almost always accompanied by a clinically apparent malignancy. In our recent retrospective review

R. W. Holden: Department of Radiology, Indiana University Medical Center, Indianapolis, Indiana 46202.

J. T. Mail: Department of Radiology, Saint Francis Hospital Center, Indianapolis, Indiana 46107.

of 61 patients with iliofemoral DVT, 17 patients (27.9 percent) at the time of initial diagnosis were either known to have a malignancy or were found to have cancer during the hospitalization. Only one patient in the remaining cohort developed a malignancy in a mean follow-up of 38.7 months. Whereas this relationship is found in the adult patient, DVT and pulmonary embolism are extremely uncommon in the pediatric patient with or without neoplasm. Surgery, recent trauma, immobilization, advanced age, heart failure, previous venous thromboembolism, obesity, pregnancy, oral contraceptives, and selected clinical disorders are known to be risk factors for the development of venous thromboembolism (4).

PULMONARY ARTERIOGRAPHY

In 1923, Berberich and Hirsch (5) reported the visualization of the pulmonary arteries by using strontium bromide and a peripheral venous injection. Subsequently, in 1929, Werner Forssman (6) reported physiologic data from his own right heart and pulmonary arteries obtained by the intravenous passage of a ureteral catheter. In 1931, Moniz et al. (7) reported the first successful pulmonary arteriogram utilizing Forssman's catheter techniques. In the early 1960s, pulmonary angiography was shown to be accurate in the diagnosis of embolic disease (8).

In more recent years, the diagnostic accuracy and safety of pulmonary angiography has significantly improved. Advances in catheters, specifically utilization of the Grollman or pigtail catheter, has dramatically reduced cardiac perforations and enhanced selective pulmonary arterial catheterization (9). Diagnostic resolution has been improved by subselective angiography, adequate injections promoting the complete replacement of arterial blood by contrast, shorter exposure times made possible by better radiographic tubes and generators, increased acceptance of the diagnostic need to visualize intraluminal filling defects at right angles (Fig. 1), and magnification angiography. Pulmonary angiography is almost inevitably requested to establish a definitive diagnosis on which patient management decisions are based. Thus, pulmonary angiography must be performed with quality and precision to exclude or image emboli with a high degree of confidence. Such a

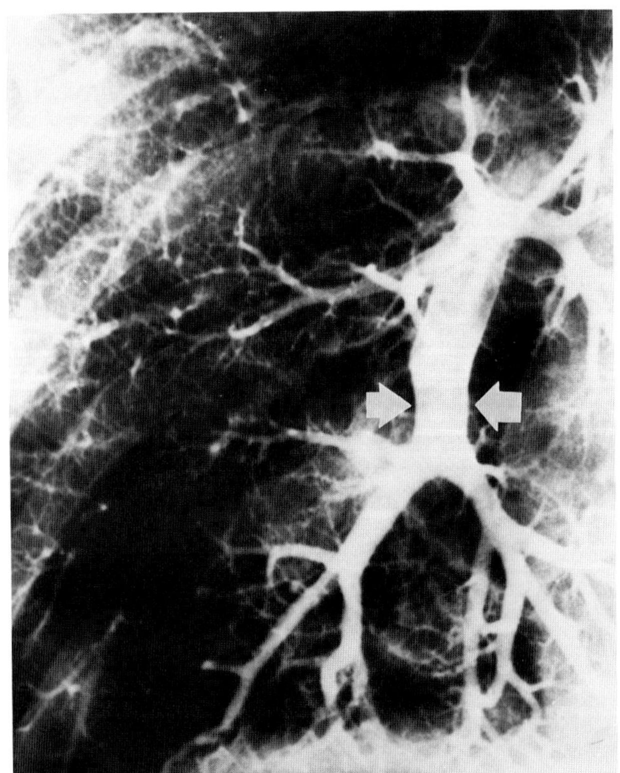
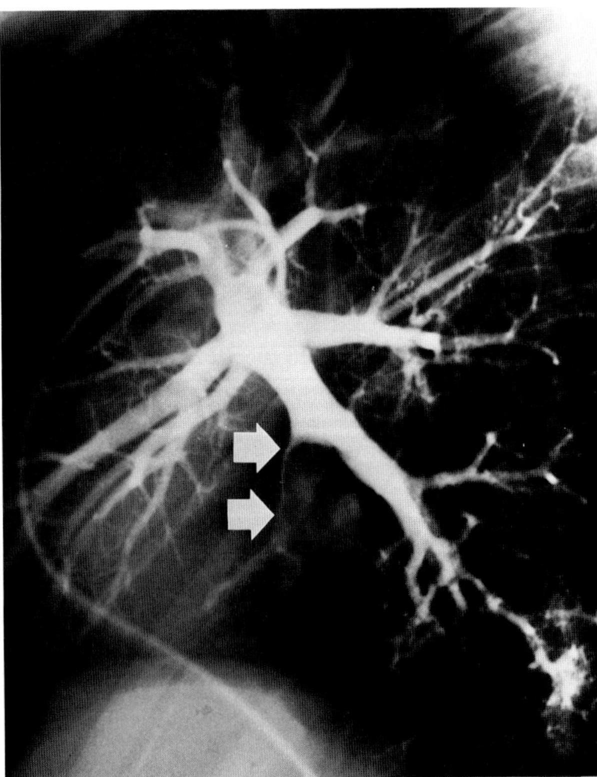

A   B

FIG. 1. A 32-year-old male with acquired immune deficiency syndrome complaining of acute onset of tachypnea, hypoxia, dyspnea, and right chest pain. Lung scan was indeterminate due to an infiltrate in the area of the perfusion defect. (**A**) Antero-posterior pulmonary angiogram with very subtle tapering of the interlobar pulmonary artery just prior to the bifurcation of the basilar segmental branches (*arrows*). (**B**) Lateral pulmonary angiogram provides a marked improvement in visualization of the almost completely occlusive embolus of the anterior basilar artery (*arrows*).

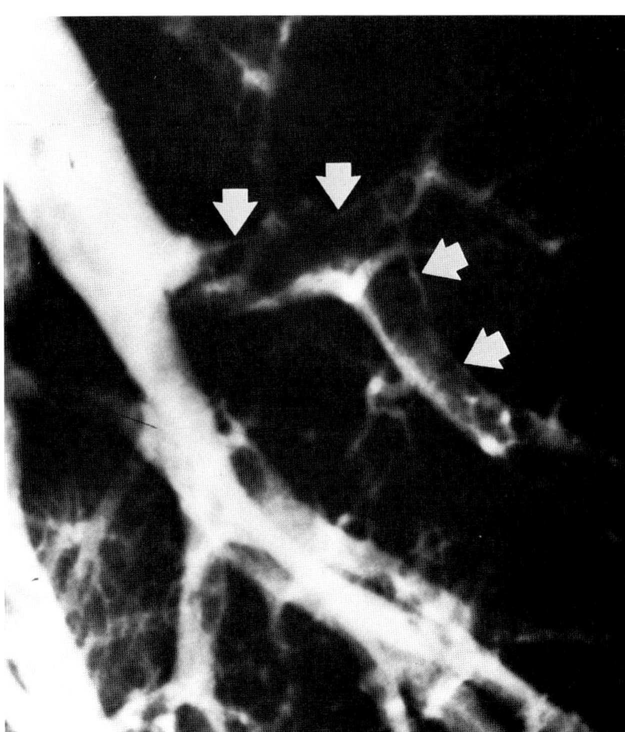

FIG. 2. A 44-year-old male reporting the acute onset of dyspnea who had hypoxia. Angiogram demonstrates delayed filling of the lingular artery and a large intraluminal filling defect caused by the embolus (*arrows*).

study requires intraluminal embolus visualization by angiographic evaluations with different obliques, selective and occasionally subselective injections, careful monitoring of injection rates, strict attention to technical detail to enable optimal film quality, and in some instances, magnification angiography.

Pulmonary arteriography directly visualizes the filling defect caused by thromboemboli. A diagnosis of pulmonary embolism is made by imaging a constant intraluminal defect with periembolus contrast flow or an intraluminal sharp cutoff with visualization of a trailing edge by the distal reconstitution of contrast material (Fig. 2). Other abnormalities, such as oligemia, vessel pruning, and loss of small vessel filling, are nonspecific and may occur in pneumonia, bronchiectasis, atelectasis, postinflammatory cicatrization (Fig. 3), emphysema, and pulmonary malignancies (Fig. 4). Known complications associated with pulmonary angiography include arrhythmias, endocardial or myocardial injury, cardiac perforation, cardiac arrest, and contrast reactions. A recent multicenter prospective evaluation of lung scanning and pulmonary angiography demonstrated a 0.3 percent death rate and a major complication rate of 1.6 percent (10). Thus, despite significant advances, pulmonary angiography remains an invasive procedure that should be properly utilized and when performed must achieve diagnostic accuracy.

PATIENT EVALUATION

Pulmonary angiography is not a painful procedure. Evaluation of the patient during the time required to obtain an informed consent allows the examiner to assess the patient's need for a sedative premedication (i.e., diazepam that can be given immediately prior to initiation of the procedure). Although the patient being evaluated is frequently anticoagulated, it is unnecessary to reverse the anticoagulation because venous compression of the femoral or antecubital veins provides easy and reliable hemostasis in all situations. Patients with bradycardia are unusual and merit careful consideration for pretreatment with 1 mg of intramuscular atropine prior to beginning the procedure. Prior to beginning the procedure, a recent electrocardiogram should be evaluated for a left bundle conduction abnormality, because passage of the catheter through the right heart can interrupt right bundle branch conduction and effect a complete heart block in the absence of left bundle branch conduction. A pacing catheter will be required to treat such an induced complete heart block.

All patients should have electrocardiographic, blood pressure, and pulse oximetry monitoring during the procedure. A defibrillator and emergency or crash cart should be immediately available to the laboratory. Right ventricular end-diastolic pressures and pulmonary artery pressures should be measured during the catheterization procedure, and any patient with elevated pressures should be examined with low osmolar contrast material. Low osmolar contrast agents produce less vasoconstrictive changes in the pulmonary vasculature and, thus, induce less of an increase in pulmonary arterial pressure (11). Mills et al. (12) demonstrated a significant increased mortality rate in patients with right ventricular end-diastolic pressures greater than 20 mm Hg using high osmolar contrast agents (12). They concluded that a 20 mm Hg or greater than right ventricular end-diastolic pressure contraindicated pulmonary angiography. With the more recent introduction of low osmolar contrast agents, the pressure changes induced by contrast administration may be less and allow a more liberal interpretation of this pressure contraindication; however, the grossly failing right ventricle will always be aggravated by an expansion of intravascular volume (13). In summary, all would agree that high osmolar agents should be avoided in all patients with pulmonary arterial hypertension and elevated right ventricular end-diastolic pressures.

PROCEDURAL METHODOLOGY

Percutaneous access into a peripheral vein of the antecubital fossa or inguinal area provides an adequate approach for pulmonary angiography, with the femoral

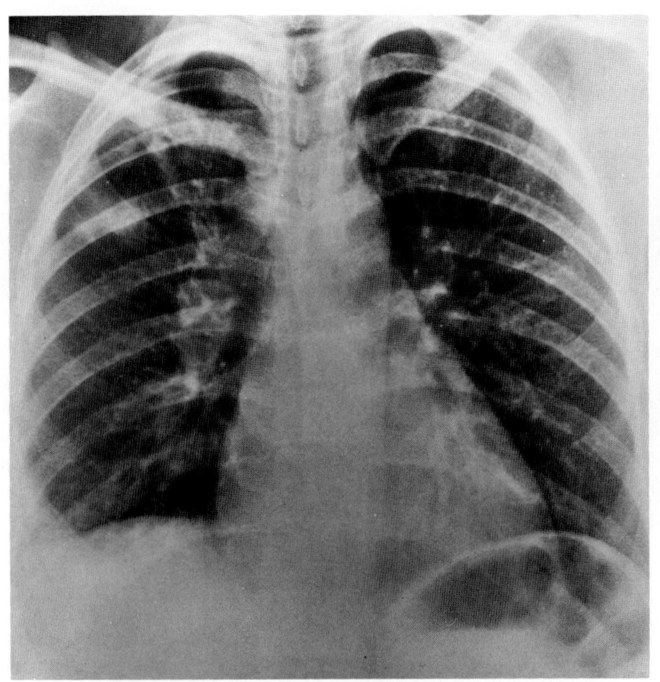
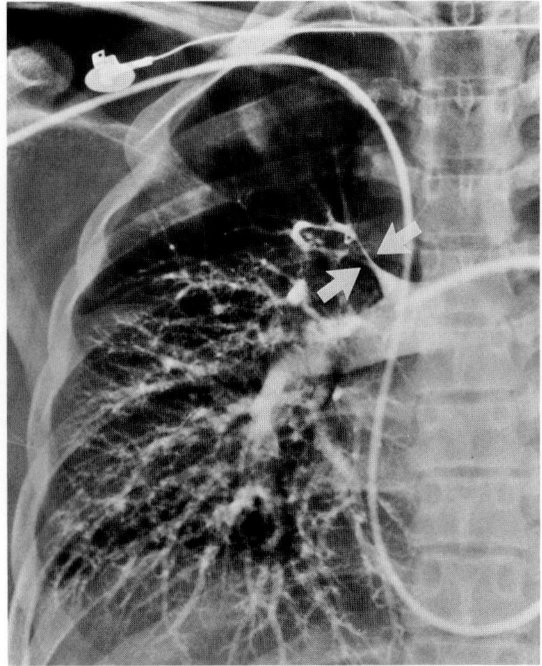

FIG. 3. A 28-year-old female with histoplasmosis. (**A**) Chest radiograph shows a right upper lobe alveolar infiltrate and right hilar enlargement. (**B**) Angiogram demonstrates no embolus, but does show severe stenosis of the proximal right upper lobe artery with severe pruning of the distal vessels (*arrows*). (**C**) Ventilation/perfusion scan demonstrates a large perfusion defect in the right upper lobe with late wash-in of xenon.

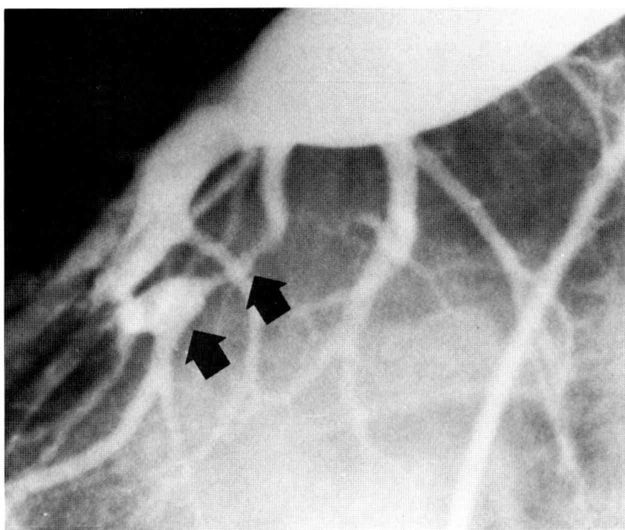

FIG. 4. A 62-year-old female with an indeterminate ventilation/perfusion scan. Note the constriction and distal dilation of a segmental artery caused by proven neoplastic encasement (*arrows*).

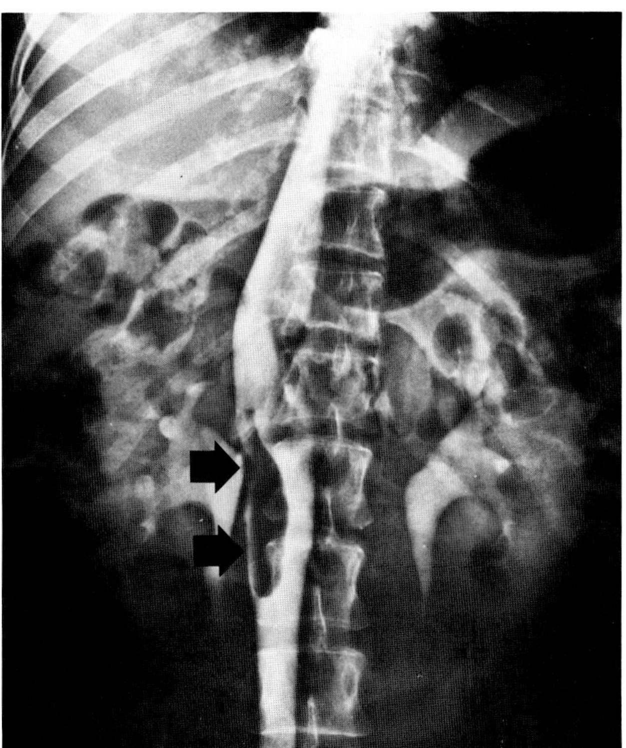

FIG. 5. Inferior vena cavagram demonstrating an ovarian vein thrombus extending into the abdominal cava (*arrows*).

vein being the larger vein and more popular approach for the procedure. The examiner should remember that venous canalization through either the upper or lower extremity offers the potential of dislodging and embolizing intraluminal thrombus (Fig. 5). To avoid this complication, the examiner should fluoroscopically monitor a contrast agent injection of the venous access site prior to catheter placement. We technically obtain this evaluation by advancing the needle over the guidewire following establishing a venous position with the wire. This establishes the needle in a stable intraluminal position and, with removal of the guidewire, contrast material may be injected through the needle and fluoroscopically monitored. Excellent opacification of iliofemoral veins and distal inferior vena cava is easily achieved with as little as 20 ml of contrast agent. The diagnostic catheter is then placed into the inferior cava, and a repeat injection of the catheter enables assessment of the more cephalad aspect of the inferior vena cava.

We most often use either a preformed Grollman or straight pigtail catheter in our laboratory. Despite the preformed character of the Grollman catheter (9), it requires deflection across the arteriovenous valve in approximately 50 percent of cases. This deflection is easily achieved with either the Grollman or straight pig by bending the distal 5–6 cm of the stiff end of a 0.038 fixed core guidewire into a very tight 360° curve. Placement of this guidewire curve into either catheter promotes deflection of the catheter across the tricuspid valve, allowing selection of the right ventricle. A right intraventricular position is recognized by the intrinsic ventricular motion producing a rhythmic deflection of the catheter.

Once this position is achieved, removal of the guidewire releases the enhanced catheter curvature and catheter advancement promotes selection of the pulmonary outflow tract. Engagement of the pulmonary outflow tract is recognized by the vertical course of the catheter as compared with the more oblique course of the coronary sinus. Because the catheter is passing through the tricuspid valve and the pulmonary outflow tract is anterior, the catheter should be rotated in a counterclockwise motion to facilitate pulmonary outflow tract selection. Once the searching tip of the catheter achieves a suprapulmonic valve position, the catheter should be advanced for subselection of either the right or left pulmonary artery. Occasionally, selection of the right pulmonary artery is difficult. When difficulty is encountered, the catheter should be advanced into a selective position in the descending ramus of the left pulmonary artery. The previously bent stiff end of the guidewire is then inserted into the distal catheter to approximate the distal catheter prior to the pigtail formation. (At no time should the stiff end of the bent wire be inserted out of any catheter.) With the guidewire in place, withdraw the catheter while clockwise rotating it to promote selection of the posteriorly and laterally directed right pulmonary artery. This maneuver has been much more successful for us than attempting the selection of the right pulmonary artery from the main pulmonary artery. It also has the advantage of avoiding the arrhythmias associated with the pigtail stimulating the pulmonary outflow tract and crossing the pulmonary valve. The sudden deflection of the catheter makes entry into the right pulmonary artery easily recognizable. Use of the pigtail catheter configuration is strongly recommended, because this configuration significantly reduces the incidence of myocardial injury, coronary sinus subselection, arrythmia induction, and cardiac perforation. When the catheter is properly positioned, the following injection volumes are recommended: 25 ml/second for a total volume of 40 ml into the right or left pulmonary artery; 12 ml/second for a total volume of 18 ml in the ascending ramus of either the right or left pulmonary artery; and 20 ml/second for a total volume of 30 ml in the descending ramus of either the right or left pulmonary artery.

Filming of the pulmonary circulation is performed at 4 frames/second for 3 seconds, and 1 frame/second for 5 seconds. Cut films are usually obtained in our laboratory despite state-of-the-art subtraction equipment. Digital subtraction angiograms can enhance acquired information even while using less contrast material than routine screen-film exams; however, even the slightest degree of patient motion generates a completely nondiagnostic study (Fig. 6). As previously described, all too frequently

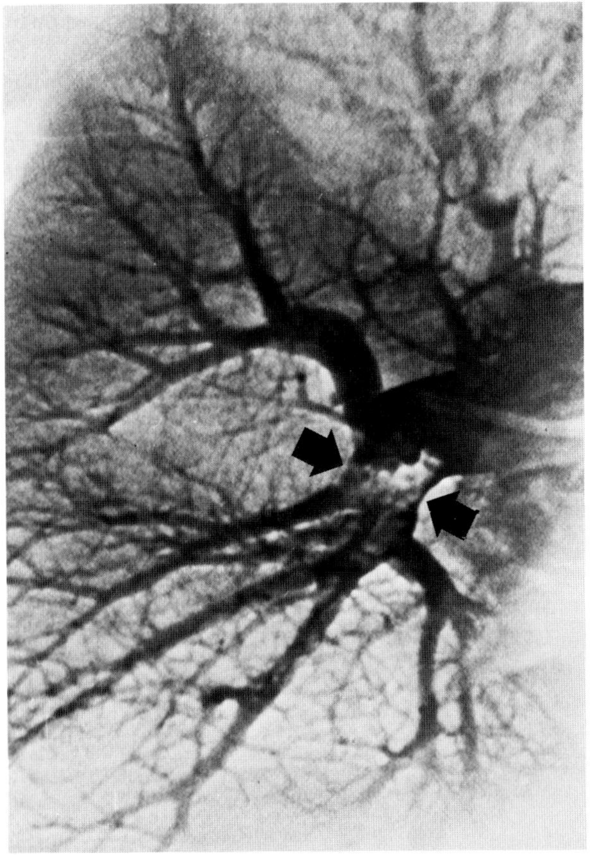

FIG. 6. A 65-year-old female with a high probability ventilation/perfusion scan with a relative contraindication to anticoagulation. Selective digital subtraction arteriography in this very cooperative patient demonstrates excellent visualization of a large embolus in the right interlobar artery (*arrows*).

the patient's symptoms preclude an extremely cooperative patient.

PULMONARY ANGIOGRAPHY'S ROLE IN PATIENT EVALUATION

Two recent large blinded prospective studies have significantly decreased the controversy about the correct approach for establishing the diagnosis of pulmonary embolism (10,14). Both studies reveal perfusion defects segmental or larger in size with normal ventilation have approximately a 90 percent probability of being caused by pulmonary embolism. However, only approximately 40 percent of pulmonary embolism demonstrates a high-probability scan. The high-probability scan found in a patient with asthma (Fig. 7) or previous pulmonary embolism has a markedly reduced accuracy as compared with that scan finding in other presentations. The symptomatic patient with an indeterminate scan has approximately a 33 percent chance of having a pulmonary embolism, and those patients with a low probability scan approximate a 12 percent chance. Near-normal/normal lung scans make the diagnosis of acute pulmonary embolism very unlikely. In the patient with a high clinical suspicion of pulmonary embolism and less than a high probability lung scan, one should consider venous duplex ultrasonography, impedance plethysmography, or venography. The demonstration of proximal thrombus in the thigh justifies the initiation of heparin therapy, in most instances, which prevents thrombus extension and the avoidance of additional embolization. Hull et al. (14) report a 30 percent incidence of normal venograms in their series of patients with angiographically proven pulmonary embolism. Thus, the positive venogram is very helpful, whereas the negative venous study will need to be followed by pulmonary angiography. The improving accuracy of duplex venous studies combined with Doppler examination avoids the complicating contrast volume required for bilateral lower extremity venography and allows one to move ahead to pulmonary angiography on the same day.

In the usual patient being studied to rule out pulmonary embolism, time is not a critical factor if heparin therapy has been initiated. The incidence of complications from heparin therapy is directly related to the number of days and the age of the patient. It is extremely uncommon to have a bleeding complication within the first 2 days of heparin therapy, and this time interval should allow the elective work-up of the patient. In the instance of questioned massive pulmonary embolism, the patient is inevitably felt to be too sick for angiography, and the primary care physician always wants to avoid the study; however, the patient is always put on a therapeutic path that is far more dangerous than the stress of angiography. The hypotensive patient should

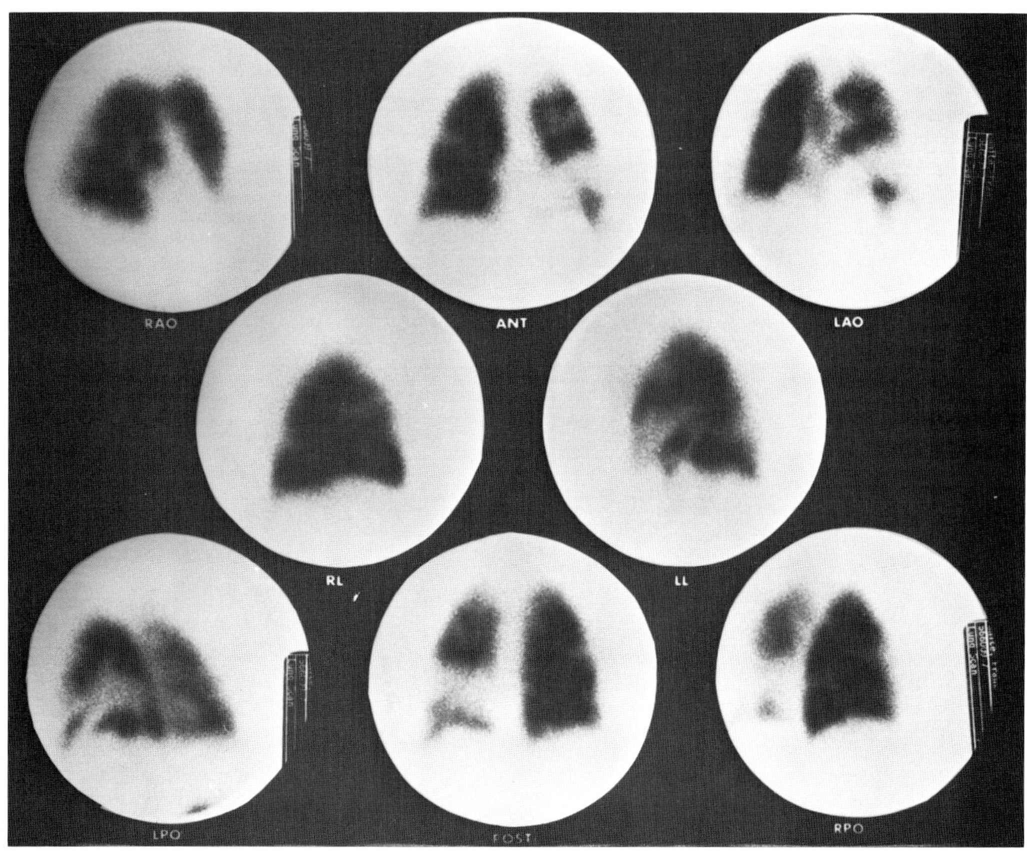

FIG. 7. Perfusion lung scan from a 39-year-old asthmatic smoker. Ventilation scan was normal. The perfusion defects, combined with a normal ventilation scan, define a high-probability scan. Bilateral pulmonary angiograms were normal.

have pressor therapy initiated and be transported to angiography. If the pressor therapy provides a hemodynamically stable patient, a portable perfusion lung scan can be done in the angiographic suite. Fibrinolytic therapy is recommended in patients with demonstrated emboli and the following: acute pulmonary arterial hypertension, controllable shock, and perfusion defects (single or multiple) equivalent to one or more lobes (15). It usually takes a minimum of 7 hours for intensive fibrinolytic therapy to promote sufficient embolic dissolution to improve the patient's right heart outflow obstruction (16,17). Patients with uncontrollable shock need documentation of emboli and emergency surgical embolectomy.

CONCLUSION

Although past controversy has focused on the over- and underdiagnosis of pulmonary embolism by nuclear lung scans, recent studies are increasingly revealing the proper use of lung scans, venous studies, and pulmonary angiograms. This more effective usage of pulmonary angiography is contributing to a definite improved accu-

racy of diagnosis that is accompanied by an appropriateness of therapy and, finally, both factors combined are effecting an enhanced quality of patient care.

REFERENCES

1. Chakko S, Richards F III. Right-sided cardiac thrombi and pulmonary embolism. *Am J Cardiol* 1987;59:195–196.
2. Virchow R. *Cellular pathology as based upon physiological and pathological histology.* London: Churchill, 1860;197–203.
3. Trousseau A. *Lectures on clinical medicine delivered at the Hotel-Dieu, Paris.* London: New Sydenham Society, 1865;282–332.
4. Hirsh J, Hull RD, Rsaskob GE. Epidemiology and pathogenesis of venous thrombosis. *J Am Coll Cardiol* 1986;8:104B–113B.
5. Berberich J, Hirsch S. Die roentgenographische darstellung der arterien und venen am lebenden menschen. *Klin Wochenschr* 1923;2:2226.
6. Forssman W. Die sondierung des rechten herzens. *Klin Wochenschr* 1929;8:2085.
7. Moniz E, deCarvalho L, Lima A. Angiopneumographie. *Presse Med* 1931;39:996.
8. Bjork L, Ansusinha T. Angiographic diagnosis of acute pulmonary embolism. *Acta Radiol Diag* 1965;3:129–137.
9. Grollman JH, Jr. Transfemoral selective bilateral pulmonary angiography with pulmonary-artery-seeking catheter. *Radiology* 1970;96:202–204.
10. The PIOPED Investigators. Value of the ventilation/perfusion scan in acute pulmonary embolism: results of the Prospective In-

vestigation of Pulmonary Embolism Diagnosis (PIOPED). *JAMA* 1990;263:2753–2759.

11. Tajima H, Kumazaki T, Tajima N, et al. Effect of iohexol and diatrizoate on pulmonary arterial pressure following pulmonary angiography; a clinical comparison in man. *Acta Radiol* 1988;29:487–490.

12. Mills SR, Jackson DC, Older RA, et al. The incidence, etiologies and avoidance of complications of pulmonary angiography in a large series. *Radiology* 1980;136:295–299.

13. Belenkie I, Dani R, Smith ER, et al. Effects of volume loading during experimental acute pulmonary embolism. *Circulation* 1989;80:178–188.

14. Hull RD, Hirsh J, Carter CJ, et al. Pulmonary angiography, ventilation lung scanning, and venography for clinically suspected pulmonary embolism with abnormal perfusion lung scan. *Ann Intern Med* 1983;98:891–899.

15. Sherry S, Gustafson E. The current and future use of thrombolytic therapy. *Ann Rev Pharmacol Toxicol* 1985;25:413–431.

16. Holden RW. Plasminogen activators: pharmacology and therapy. *Radiology* 1990;174:993–1001.

17. Verstraete M, Miller GAH, Bounameaux H, et al. Intravenous and intrapulmonary recombinant tissue-type plasminogen activator in the treatment of acute massive pulmonary embolism. *Circulation* 1988;77:353–360.

Thoracic Radiology, edited by
J.D. Newell, Jr., and R.D. Tarver,
Raven Press, Ltd., New York © 1993.

CHAPTER **7**

The Chest Wall and Pleura

Normal and Abnormal

Caroline Chiles

THE CHEST WALL

The Normal Chest Wall

The chest wall serves a variety of purposes, ranging from respiration to protection of the intrathoracic contents. The chest wall is very difficult to evaluate on conventional chest radiographs, and it is only with the advent of computed tomography (CT) and magnetic resonance (MR) that radiologists have been able to contribute significantly to the work-up of a patient with a chest wall lesion. As with any part of the body, a thorough knowledge of normal anatomy facilitates recognition and diagnosis of pathologic conditions (1–3).

The first layer of the chest wall, beginning within the chest, and working one's way out, consists of the ribs and intercostal muscles. The deepest layer of muscle is the transverse thoracis muscle, which is the thoracic equivalent of the transversus abdominis muscle in the anterior abdominal wall. The next layer is the internal intercostal muscle, which is in turn covered by the external intercostal muscle. These three muscles extend from the inferior border of the rib above to the superior border of the rib below. The intercostal vessels and intercostal nerves run along the undersurface of the rib, between the internal and external intercostal muscles.

The serratus anterior muscle is a broad sheet that originates from the outer surfaces of the first through eighth ribs and extends posteriorly to insert into the medial border of the scapula (Fig. 1). On chest radiographs, the serratus anterior muscle may be seen as a bowling-pin-shaped opacity overlying the lateral ribs (4). This may cause confusion with pleural plaques or pleural thickening.

Over the anterior chest wall lie the pectoralis major and pectoralis minor. Lymph nodes may lie between the pectoralis major and pectoralis minor muscles (5). At the level of the scapula are seen the subscapularis muscle, lying between the serratus anterior muscle and the scapula. External to the scapula are the teres minor muscle laterally and the infraspinatus muscle medially. The larger teres major lies laterally, originating from the lateral border of the scapula on its way to inserting into the bicipital groove of the humerus. Superficial to the teres major lies the latissimus dorsi muscle. It originates from the iliac crest and spinous processes of the seventh through twelfth thoracic vertebrae. The tendon of the latissimus dorsi wraps around the lower border of the teres major muscle to insert on the bicipital groove of the humerus.

Medial to the scapula lies the rhomboid major, which originates from the spinous processes of the second through fifth thoracic vertebrae, and extends to insert on the medial border of the scapula. On either side of the spinous processes of the thoracic spine lie the deep muscles of the back, the erector spinae, which include the sacrospinalis and transversospinalis muscles. The trapezius muscle lies superficial to the spinal muscles, and extends to insert on the upper and medial borders of the scapula.

The muscles of the chest wall are covered by a layer of subcutaneous fat. Both CT and MR provide sufficient contrast resolution to allow recognition of the normal structures of the chest wall, as well as a number of pathologic processes (Fig. 2).

C. Chiles: Department of Radiology, Medical College of Virginia, Richmond, Virginia 23298.

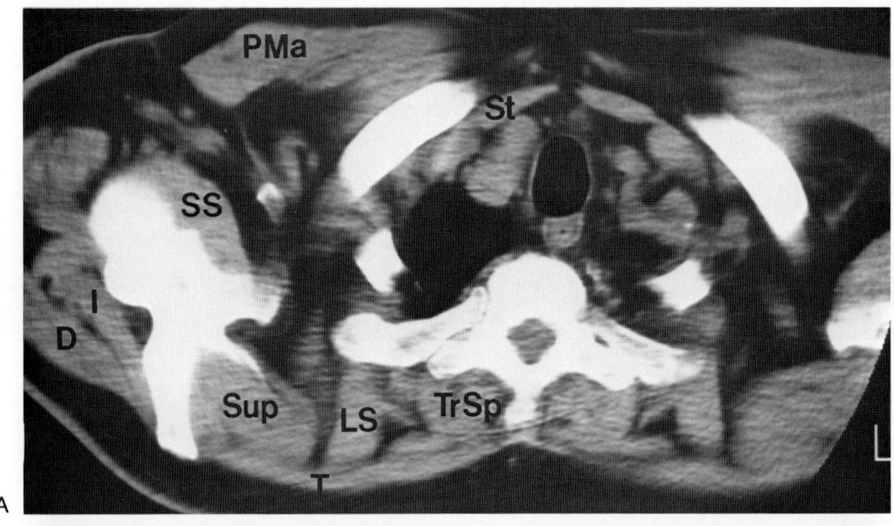

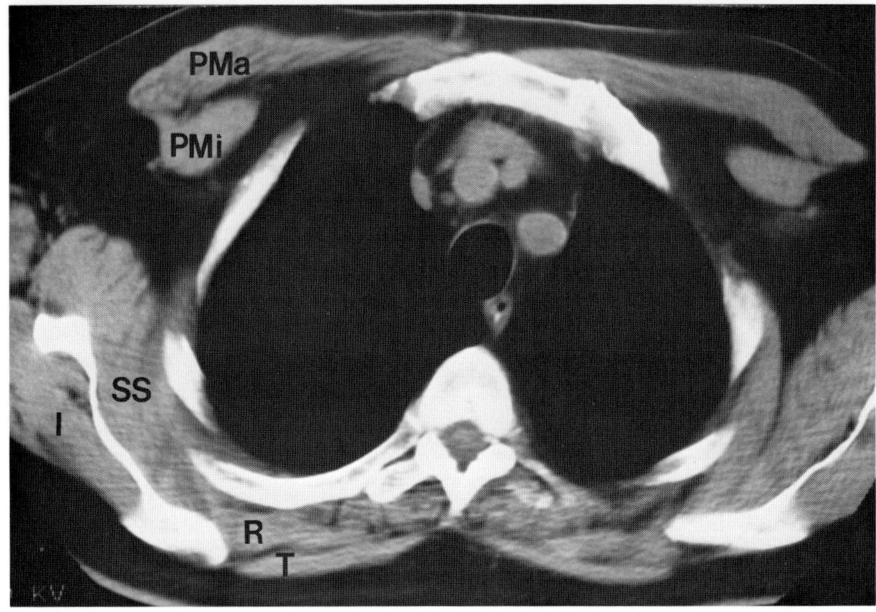

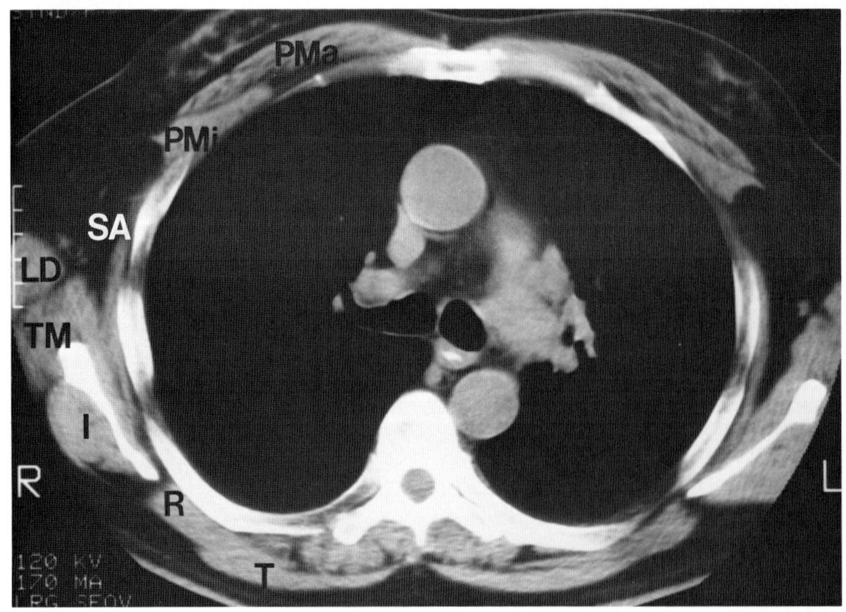

FIG. 1. (A–E) The muscles of the chest wall. D, deltoid; I, infraspinatus; LD, latissimus dorsi; LS, levator scapuli; PMa, pectoralis major; PMi, pectoralis minor; R, rhomboid major; SA, serratus anterior; Sc, sacrospinalis; SS, subscapularis; St, sternohyoid and sternothyroid; Sup, supraspinatus; T, trapezius; TM, teres major; TrSp, transversospinalis.

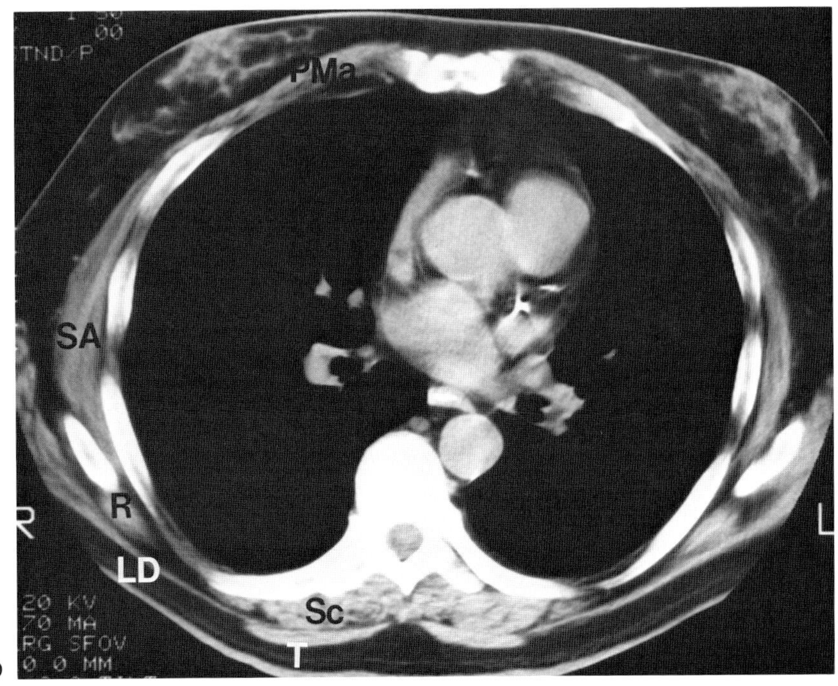

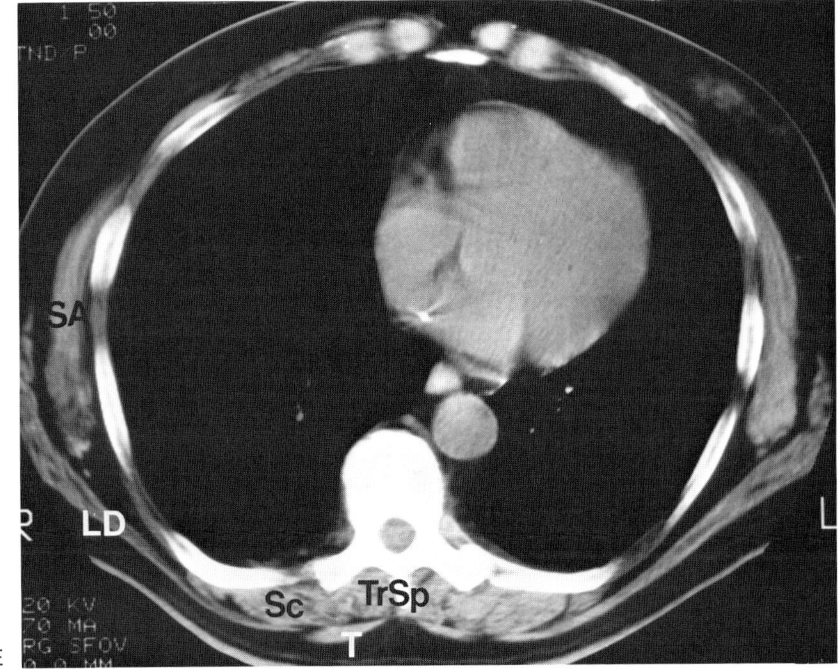

FIG. 1. *Continued.*

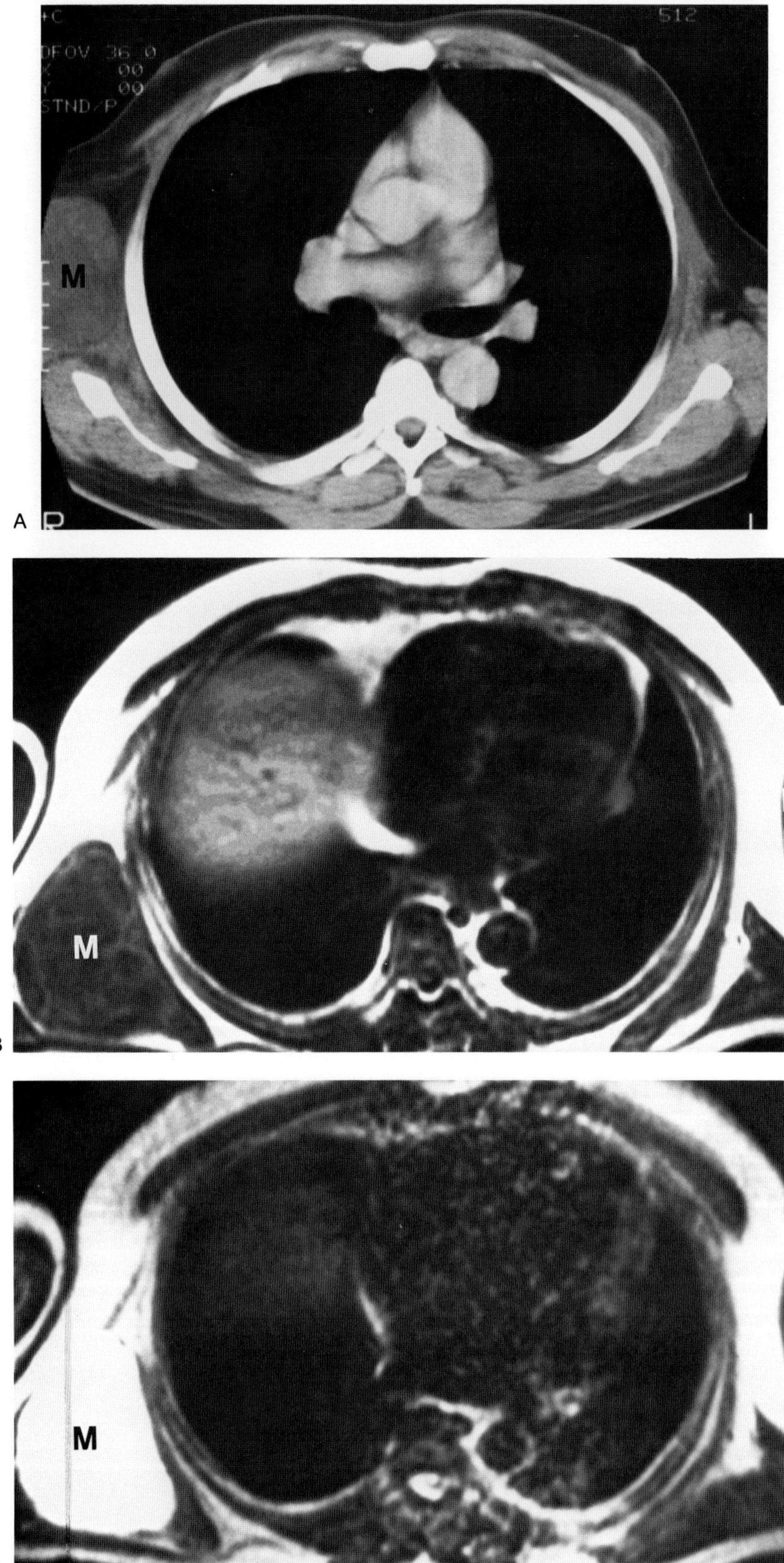

FIG. 2. **(A)** A mass (*M*) in the right lateral chest wall can be distinguished from lower attenuation subcutaneous fat on axial CT. **(B)** Contrast resolution of MR is superior to that of CT. On a T1-weighted axial MR image, the mass (*M*) is visible as an inhomogeneous low-signal mass separated by high-signal subcutaneous fat from the serratus anterior and latissimus dorsi muscles. **(C)** A T2-weighted axial MR image shows high-signal intensity within the mass (*M*), which was diagnosed as a myolipoma after surgical resection. The difference in the position of the mass on the axial CT and MR images is due to the change in position of the patient's arms on the two studies.

The Abnormal Chest Wall

Primary Tumors

Benign

An enchondroma is a benign cartilaginous tumor that can occur in any bone preformed in cartilage. An enchondroma appears as a round or oval radiolucency, which may cause expansion of the bone as the lesion grows, thinning the cortex of the bone. An enchondroma may arise within a rib. If large enough, it may be noted by the patient as a focal mass in the chest wall. Otherwise, an enchondroma may be discovered on a routine chest radiograph. If an enchondroma exceeds 4 cm in diameter, or if the lesion is painful, the possibility of malignant degeneration into chondrosarcoma should be considered (6).

Osteochondromas also occur in any bone that develops by enchondromal ossification and can be found in the ribs or clavicles. The osteochondroma protrudes from the rib or clavicle, growing at right angles to the bone. The cortex of the normal bone is continuous with the cortex of the osteochondroma. Enlargement of the tumor or pain within the lesion again suggests malignant degeneration into chondrosarcoma, or less commonly, osteosarcoma.

In fibrous dysplasia, the medullary cavities of the bones are replaced by fibrous tissue. In the ribs, fibrous dysplasia may produce increased density or sclerosis within the rib, obscuring the normal definition of the bony cortex. Fibrous dysplasia can also produce lytic lesions, with thinning of the cortex and expansion of the rib.

Malignant

Many malignant tumors of the chest wall present as painful, enlarging masses and are often initially misdiagnosed as benign (7). Malignant fibrous histiocytoma is the most common malignant soft tissue tumor of the chest wall; chondrosarcoma is the most common malignant bone tumor of the chest wall (7). Although malignant fibrous histiocytoma most commonly arises in a lower extremity, 10 percent of cases involve the chest wall. Because of the variable morphologic pattern of this tumor, it may be confused with other sarcomas, including fibrosarcoma, liposarcoma, and rhabdomyosarcoma (8).

Chondrosarcomas of the chest wall most commonly arise from the anterior costochondral or sternochondral junction of the upper four ribs. The tumor may also arise from the posterior head of the ribs, as well as from the body of the sternum or manubrium (9). Secondary chondrosarcomas arise in preexisting lesions, including enchondromas and osteochondromas. Chondrosarcoma is a tumor of adulthood, with the peak incidence in the sixth decade of life. Patients typically notice a palpable mass, which may or may not be painful. The tumor generally exceeds 4 cm in size at the time of its discovery (10).

Radiographic features that suggest a malignant chondrosarcoma over a benign chondroma are ill-defined margins, cortical thickening, and breakthrough of the cortex (11). On chest radiographs, as well as on CT, the amorphous, speckled calcification characteristic of chondroid matrix may help in the recognition of this tumor (Fig. 3) (12,13).

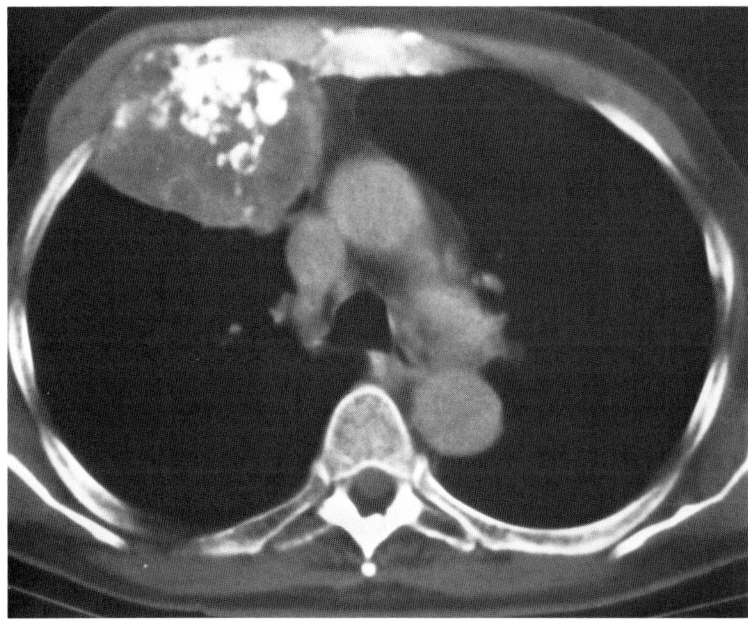

FIG. 3. Amorphous calcification is present within a chondrosarcoma. Chondrosarcoma arose from the anterior aspect of the right second rib and extended inferiorly to invade the right upper lobe. From Chiles (6), with permission.

The surgeon may elect to perform a local excision, a wide resection, or in the case of very large tumors, a palliative excision. The likelihood of recurrent chondrosarcoma at 10 years after palliative excision is 94 percent, but decreases to 50 percent after local excision, and 17 percent after wide resection. Pulmonary metastases are almost invariably associated with local recurrence.

Ewing sarcoma is primarily confined to the pediatric population, rarely affecting patients over 30 years old. Ewing sarcoma may occur in the scapula, clavicle, or ribs. The lesions are usually lytic and may produce lamellar periosteal reaction. The lesions of the thorax often have a permeative appearance similar to metastatic disease seen in adults (Fig. 4).

Multiple myeloma is the most common primary malignant neoplasm of bone and often involves the ribs and thoracic vertebrae (Fig. 5). Multiple lytic lesions are seen scattered throughout the skeletal system. In the ribs, the lesions of multiple myeloma expand the rib, with complete erosion of the cortex. Pathologic fractures of the ribs and vertebrae are common.

Metastatic Disease

Metastatic carcinoma may involve the thoracic skeleton hematogenously, via the lymphatic system, or by di-

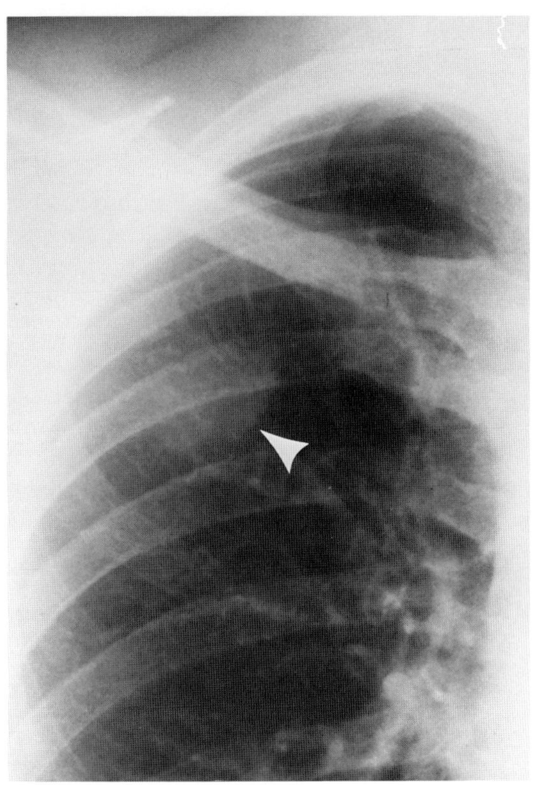

FIG. 5. Multiple myeloma in the anterior aspect of the right second rib (*arrowhead*) causes destruction of the rib cortex. Indistinct margins of this lesion help to distinguish this as a pleural or chest wall lesion, instead of a pulmonary nodule.

rect extension. The most common primary tumors with skeletal metastases are breast, lung, prostate, thyroid, and kidney. The thoracic vertebrae and ribs contain red marrow and are frequent sites of involvement. Both osteolytic and osteoblastic metastases may be seen in the bony thorax. Radionuclide bone scanning, however, remains the most sensitive imaging modality for evaluation of skeletal metastases.

Direct extension into the chest wall may occur in bronchogenic carcinoma, as well as in breast cancer and lymphoma (14,15). Chest wall invasion occurs in 8 percent of patients with a contiguous bronchogenic carcinoma and categorizes the patient as having stage IV disease, which is usually considered unresectable (Fig. 6). CT is inaccurate in the diagnosis of chest wall invasion, unless there is frank rib destruction (16,17). The CT signs of pleural thickening, the angle the tumor forms with the chest wall, the amount of contact between the tumor and the adjacent pleural surface, and the appearance of the extra pleural fat are nonspecific, and can be seen in patients with or without histologic evidence of chest wall invasion (16,18). Although pleural thickening occurs in all patients with chest wall invasion, it is also present in 44 percent of those in whom there is no evidence of chest wall invasion at surgery. The clinical symptom of chest wall pain is a more accurate indicator

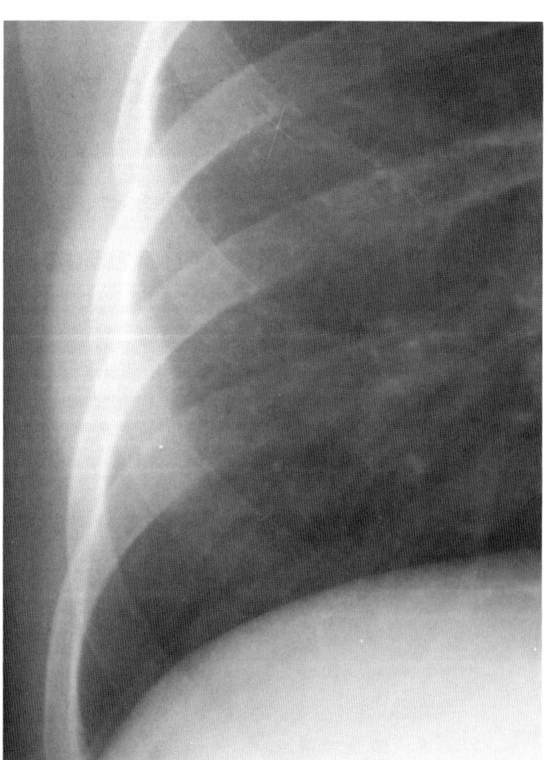

FIG. 4. Ewing sarcoma in the lateral right eighth rib is visible as an expansile, permeative lesion, with an associated soft tissue mass.

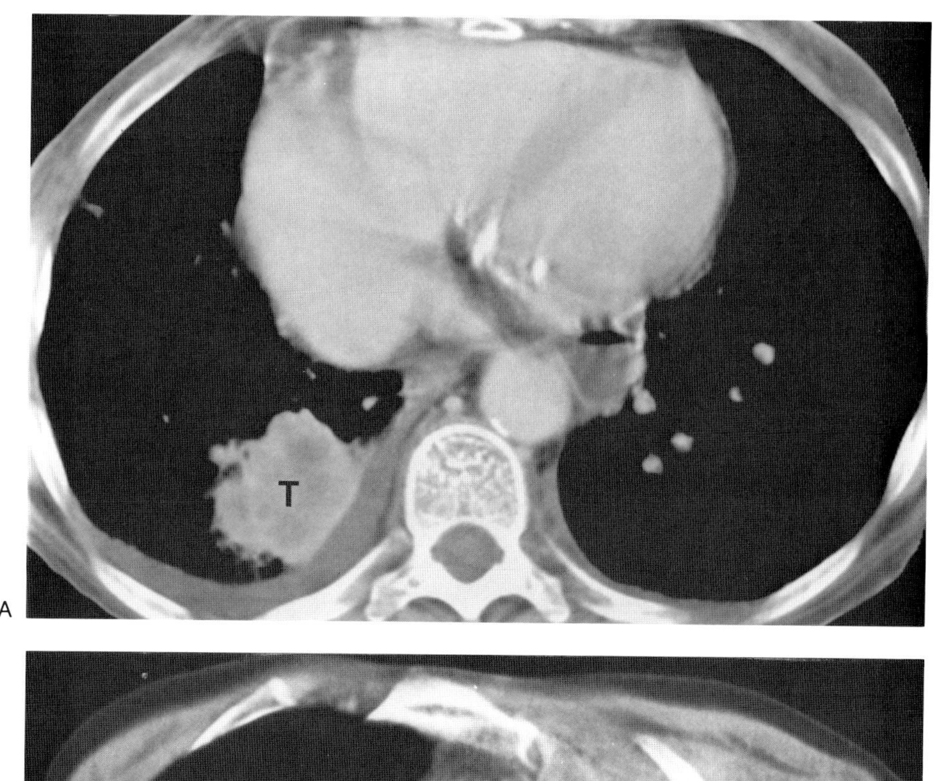

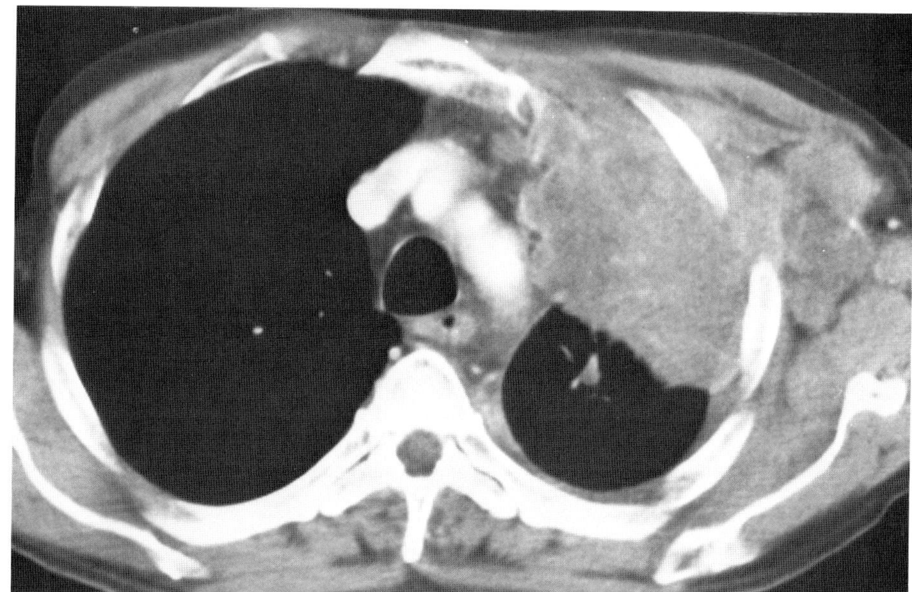

FIG. 6. (**A**) Pleural thickening and the length of contact between the tumor (*T*) and the pleura are not reliable indicators of pleural or chest wall invasion by bronchogenic carcinoma. (**B**) Small cell bronchogenic carcinoma has involved the chest wall by direct extension from a left upper lobe mass. Bulky adenopathy is present in the left axilla.

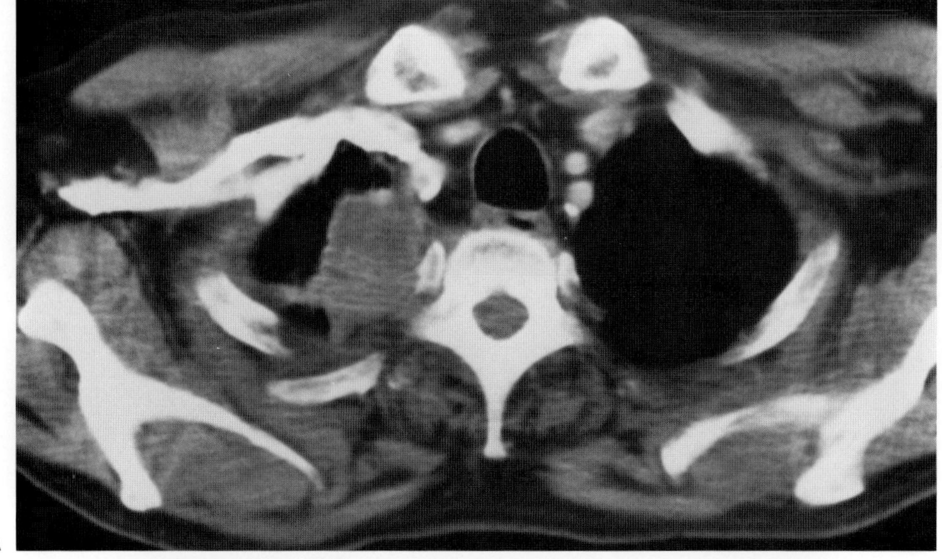

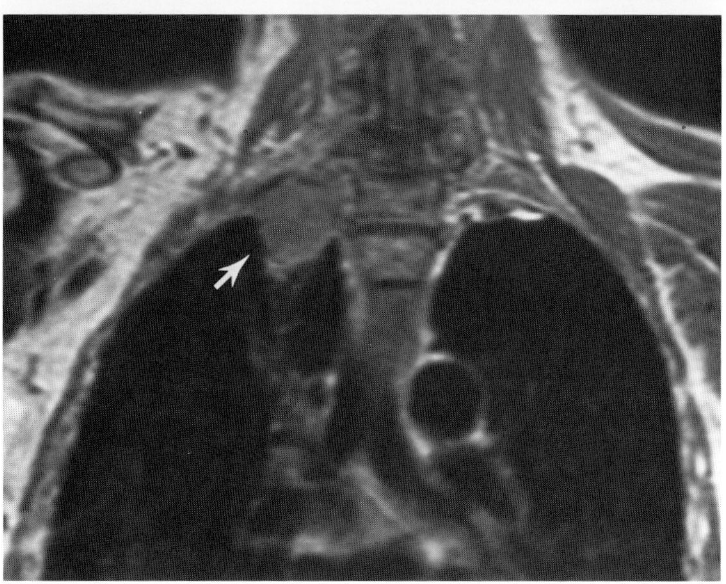

FIG. 7. (**A**) Axial CT in a patient with numbness in the medial aspect of the right arm shows a soft tissue mass at the right lung apex. (**B**) Coronal MR (TR = 2000 msec, TE = 20 msec) demonstrates the relationship of this Pancoast tumor (*arrow*) to the chest wall. At surgery, there was invasion of the first rib and thoracic vertebra.

than CT in the diagnosis of chest wall extension of tumor.

MR may prove to be more accurate than CT in this diagnosis. Chest wall abnormalities are best seen on T2-weighted images (long TR/TE pulse sequences). Coronal or sagittal imaging planes are useful for apical lesions; axial imaging planes are better for lesions in the remainder of the chest (Fig. 7). MR criteria for chest wall invasion include focal areas of increased signal intensity extending into the chest wall from the adjacent lung tumor and diffuse chest wall thickening with diffuse increased signal (19).

Chest wall involvement has been seen in 10 to 14 percent of patients with Hodgkin disease and non-Hodgkin lymphoma undergoing chest CT as part of initial staging procedures or because of suspected recurrence. Chest wall involvement may occur due to direct extension from contiguous mediastinal or pulmonary disease. A more common manifestation of chest wall disease is a mass arising within the thoracic wall tissues, independent of any contiguous mediastinal or parenchymal involvement (Fig. 8) (20). The masses are typically in the anterior chest wall and may lie beneath or within the pectoralis muscles (21). The lesions may also be centered in the ribs and sternum, where they produce lytic destruction. Chest wall involvement may not be recognized on physical examination, and, when present, often causes a modification of radiation treatment ports.

Subcutaneous metastases may be palpated initially by the patient or clinician. CT is useful in demonstrating occult subcutaneous metastases, due to the contrast between the soft tissue nodule and the lower attenuation subcutaneous fat (22) (Fig. 9). Mimics of subcutaneous metastases include sebaceous cysts, injection granulomata, subcutaneous blood vessels, and the residua of

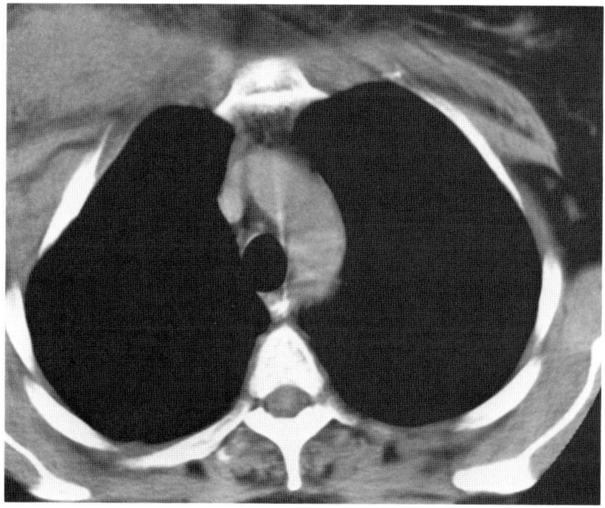

FIG. 8. Axial CT reveals enlargement of the right pectoral muscles and axillary adenopathy. Biopsy showed recurrent Hodgkin disease involving muscle and connective tissue.

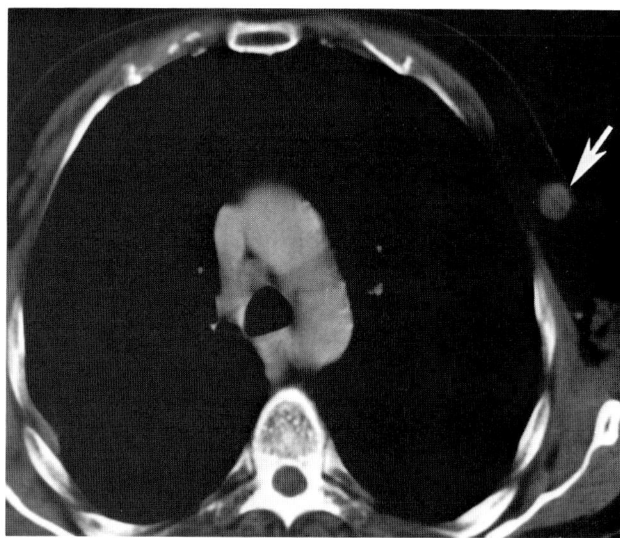

FIG. 9. A soft tissue nodule (*arrow*) within the subcutaneous fat of the left lateral chest wall represents metastatic melanoma.

prior intravenous catheter insertion. Subcutaneous vessels may be especially prominent when recruited as the collateral pathway in obstruction of the superior or inferior vena cava (Fig. 10) (23). Removal of a Hickman catheter, which is tunneled subcutaneously before insertion into the subclavian vein, usually leaves a Dacron felt cuff in the subcutaneous tissue of the anterior chest wall (24). This cuff produces a soft tissue nodule on CT that mimics a subcutaneous metastasis.

Trauma to the Chest Wall

Sternal fracture after blunt trauma to the chest may occur as an isolated phenomenon, with a benign outcome. The heart's anatomic position immediately beneath the sternum makes it vulnerable to injury, however, and a sternal fracture should increase the awareness of possible cardiac injury as well (25).

Rib fractures also occur after blunt trauma to the chest, but are frequently not seen on initial chest radiographs. Therapy is aimed at relief of pain and is not significantly altered by the ability to document rib fractures radiographically (26). The goal of the chest film, instead, is to assess pulmonary or pleural complications of rib fracture, such as pneumothorax.

There has been an attempt to use the specific rib fractured to guide further work-up. In 1971, Richardson et al. (27) reported 55 patients with fractures of the first rib. Thirty-five of those patients had a major chest injury, including pneumothorax, hemothorax, pulmonary contusion, and flail chest. Three patients had an associated injury of the subclavian artery, and they concluded that a first rib fracture is a hallmark of severe trauma. The

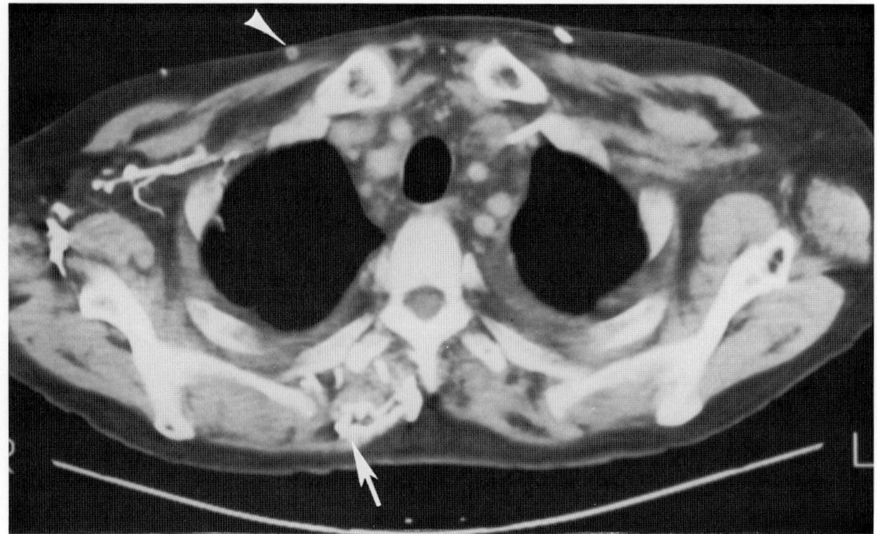

FIG. 10. Mimics of subcutaneous metastases. Collateral vessels in the chest wall (*arrow*) were recruited because of brachiocephalic vein thrombosis around an indwelling venous catheter. The Hickman catheter, which is now visible in the left anterior chest wall, had previously been placed into the right subclavian vein. The Dacron felt cuff (*arrowhead*), which remains in the subcutaneous tissues of the right anterior chest wall after catheter removal, mimics a soft tissue nodule.

presence of fractures of the first and second ribs became an indication for emergency thoracic aortography. Subsequent studies have shown that the sole presence of a rib fracture, in the absence of other signs of arterial injury, such as widening of the superior mediastinum, indistinctness of the aorta, or displacement of the trachea or nasogastric tube, is not by itself an indication for aortography (28,29). Additionally, the type of rib fracture (posterior, lateral, or anterior) has not been found to be a useful predictor of arterial injury (30).

Appearance of the Chest Wall After Surgery

The Chest Wall After Mastectomy

The appearance of the chest wall is distorted after mastectomy for breast cancer (31). The surgeon may opt to perform a radical mastectomy, with resection of the breast tissue, both pectoralis major and minor, and an *en bloc* resection of the axillary contents. The most common surgical procedure for breast cancer is currently the modified radical mastectomy, which resects the breast tissue, but leaves the pectoralis muscles intact. The axilla is dissected, with less deformity than the *en bloc* resection. A simple mastectomy removes the breast tissue only; dissection of the axilla may or may not be performed as part of this procedure. A subcutaneous mastectomy is performed for *in situ* carcinoma, or as a prophylactic procedure in patients at high risk for developing breast cancer. In a subcutaneous mastectomy, the breast tissue is removed, leaving sufficient subareolar tissue for blood supply to the nipple.

The type of breast reconstruction performed after mastectomy depends to some extent on the type of mastectomy performed. In the case of subcutaneous mastectomy, a saline prosthesis can be inserted behind the subareolar breast tissue, similar to a breast augmentation. After simple or modified radical mastectomy, the saline prostheses are placed superficial to the pectoralis muscles. After radical mastectomy, breast reconstruction is more difficult. One surgical approach is the latissimus dorsi flap, which rotates the latissimus dorsi muscle through a subcutaneous tunnel anteriorly to cover the saline prosthesis in the mastectomy site (Fig. 11a). On CT, this surgical procedure can be recognized by the absence of the latissimus dorsi from its normal position, and by the thin strip of muscle that wraps laterally around the chest wall and over the prosthesis (Fig. 11b). An alternative surgical repair is the transverse abdominis flap, which swings subcutaneous fat on a vascular pedicle, from the anterior abdominal wall through a subcutaneous tunnel into the mastectomy site (Fig. 12a). The fat is used to simulate the breast tissue. On CT, this can be recognized by the absence of breast tissue within the fatty area (Fig. 12b). The fat can undergo necrosis if the vascular supply is not well maintained, producing calcifications within the tissue (Fig. 12c).

The Chest Wall After Thoracotomy

Lateral thoracotomy is a common surgical approach to lesions of the lungs or esophagus. The surgeon may spread the ribs to obtain access, and ribs may be inadvertently fractured. Ribs may be resected for better access

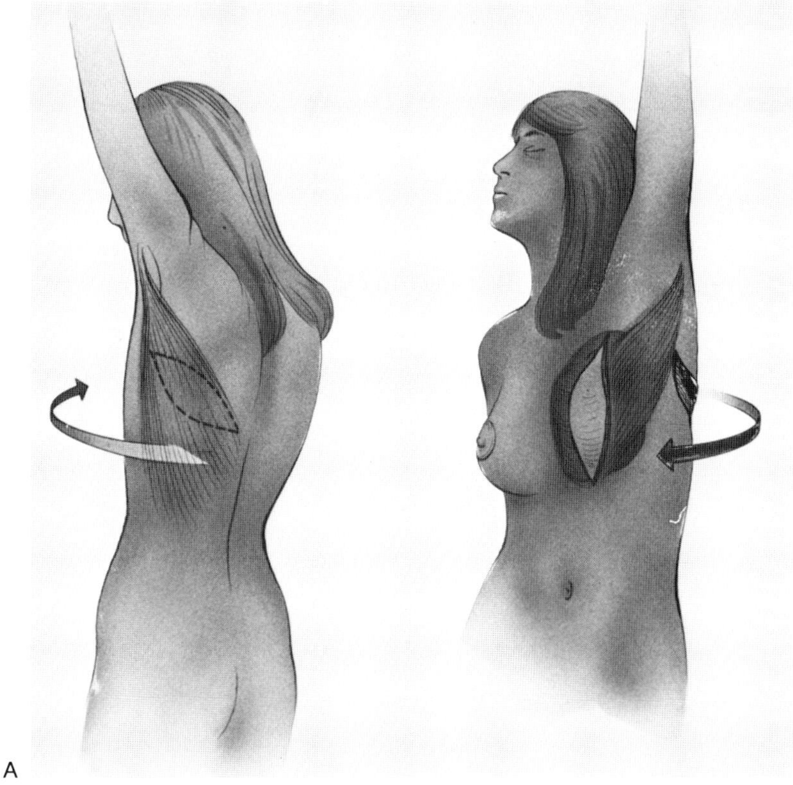

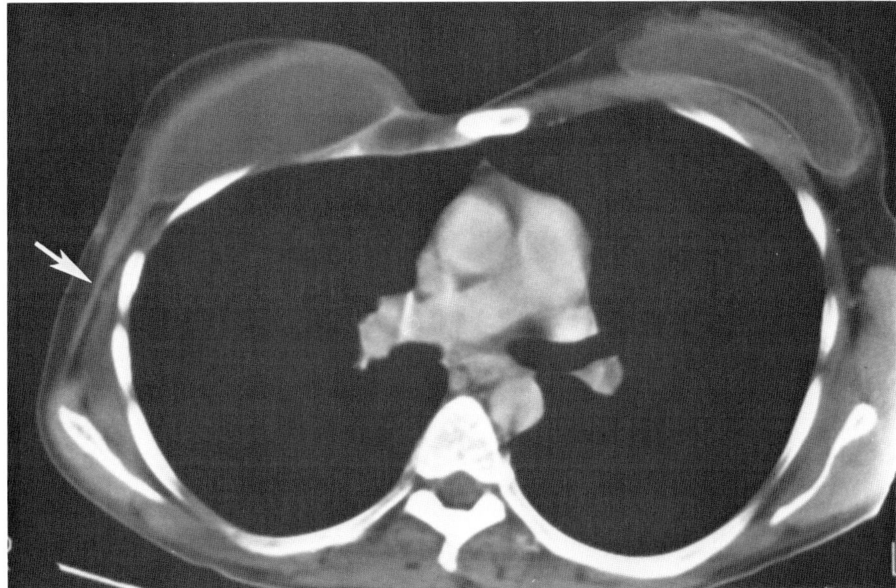

FIG. 11. (A) A latissimus dorsi flap may be used for breast reconstruction after radical mastectomy. The muscle is rotated anteriorly to cover a saline prosthesis. (B) On CT, the latissimus dorsi flap is seen as a thin strip of muscle (*arrow*) wrapping laterally around the right chest wall. A saline prosthesis has been placed behind the left breast tissue for augmentation. From Chiles (6), with permission.

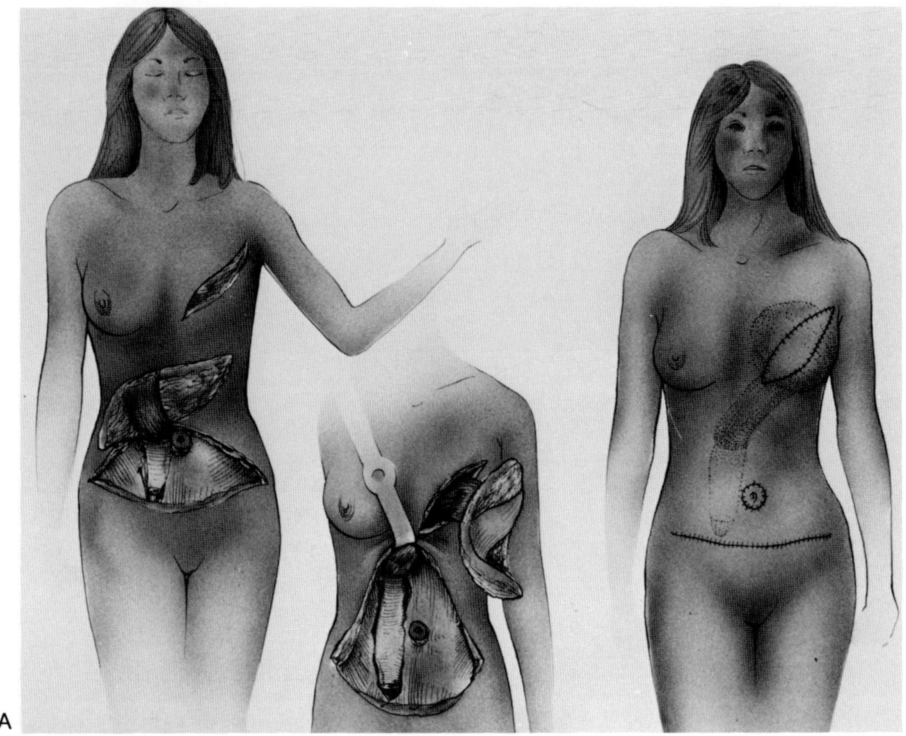

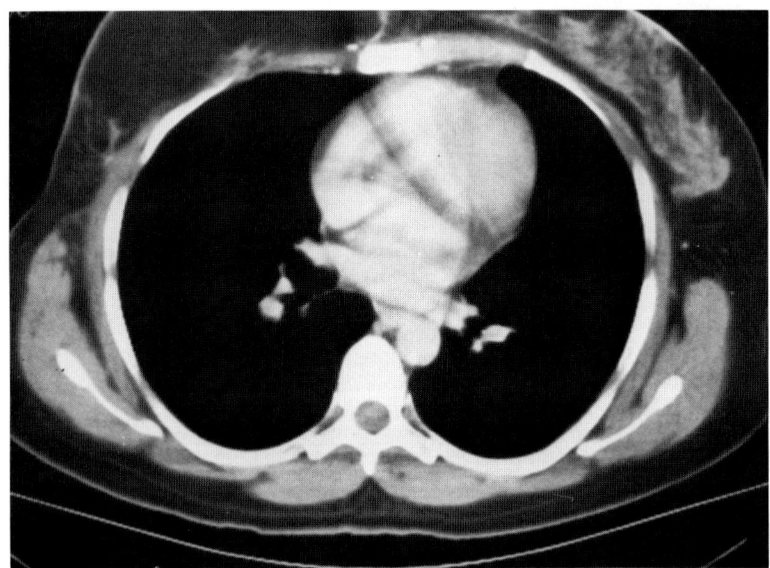

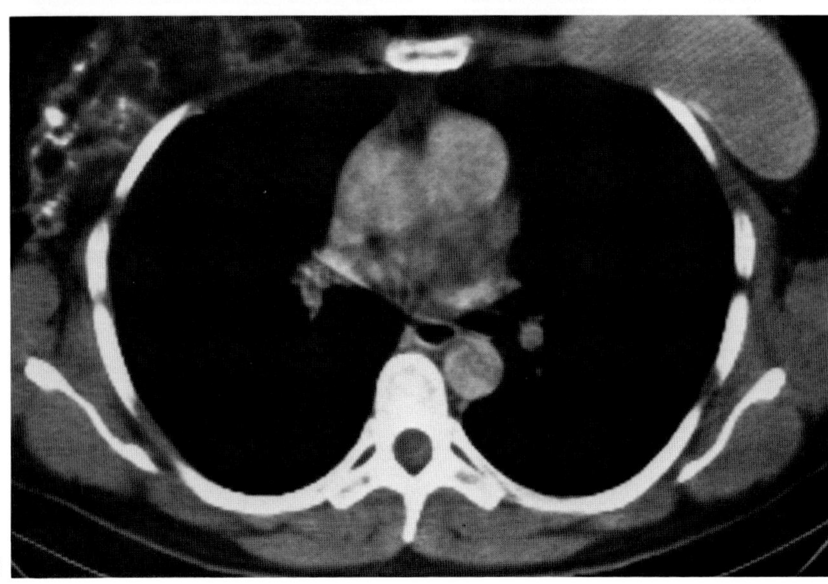

FIG. 12. (A) A transverse abdominis flap uses subcutaneous fat to replace the resected breast tissue after radical mastectomy. The fat and muscle are rotated through a subcutaneous tunnel to the mastectomy site. From Chiles (6), with permission. **(B)** On CT, fat is seen within the reconstructed right breast. **(C)** Fat necrosis has occurred within a right transverse abdominis flap breast reconstruction as a result of ischemia, producing calcification. A saline prosthesis has been placed in the left breast. From Chiles (6), with permission.

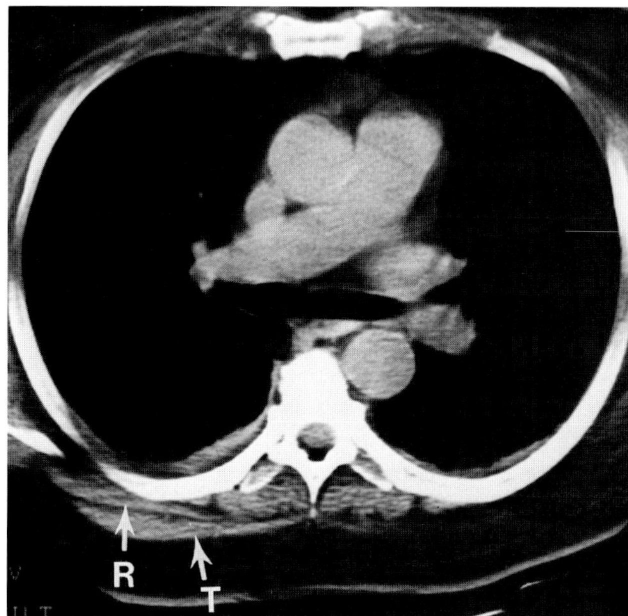

FIG. 13. After surgical intervention for thoracic outlet syndrome, there is atrophy of the trapezius (*T*) and rhomboid (*R*) muscles of the left chest wall. The normal muscles of the right chest wall are labeled for comparison.

during surgery. If there is damage to thoracic nerves at the time of surgery, postoperative studies may show atrophy of the muscles of the chest wall (Fig. 13).

Herniation of the lung through the chest wall is an uncommon condition that can occur congenitally, or after thoracotomy or trauma. The patient typically notices a spongy, crepitant mass that changes in size with inspiration or coughing. The congenital herniations are more often in the cervical area; posttraumatic herniations are usually along the lateral chest wall.

Diagnosis of lung herniation is usually made clinically. Confirmation of the diagnosis may be difficult on routine chest radiographs, unless the x-ray beam is tangential to the lesion. CT is helpful not only in confirming the diagnosis, but also in evaluating the size and extent of the herniation (Fig. 14). Strangulation and incarceration of the herniated lung are uncommon events.

The Chest Wall After Median Sternotomy

The median sternotomy has become the principal surgical approach to the heart and great vessels. On the normal postoperative chest, a lucent stripe may be seen in the midsternum. This was initially felt to be indicative of sternal dehiscence, but is now recognized as a normal finding. Periosteal elevation may be present in the normal postoperative patient as well. Sternal wound infections occur in 3 percent or less of all patients following median sternotomy, but the mortality of sternal dehiscence, mediastinitis, and osteomyelitis exceeds 50 percent. The clinical signs of sternal infection (including pain, erythema, sternal discharge, fever, elevated white blood cell count, and sternal separation) are usually apparent before the radiographic signs. Sternal dehiscence is indicated by a progressive increase in the width of the midsternal stripe, which breaks or changes the position of the sternal suture wires (32). Air may be seen in the subcutaneous tissue of the chest wall, or in the anterior mediastinum, but an increase in the amount of air suggests sternal wound infection (33,34). CT helps to identify drainable fluid collections in the anterior mediasti-

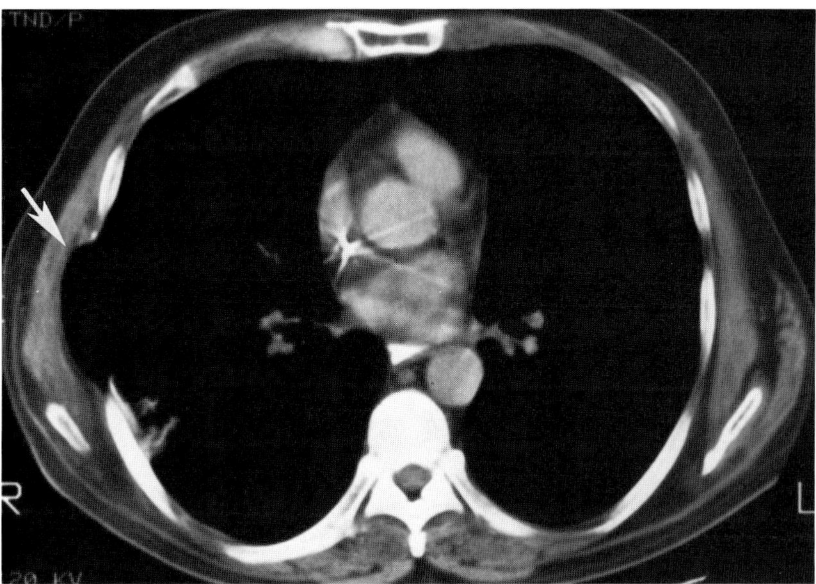

FIG. 14. Herniation of the lung (*arrow*) can occur after thoracotomy. The patient typically notices a crepitant mass that changes in size with respiration.

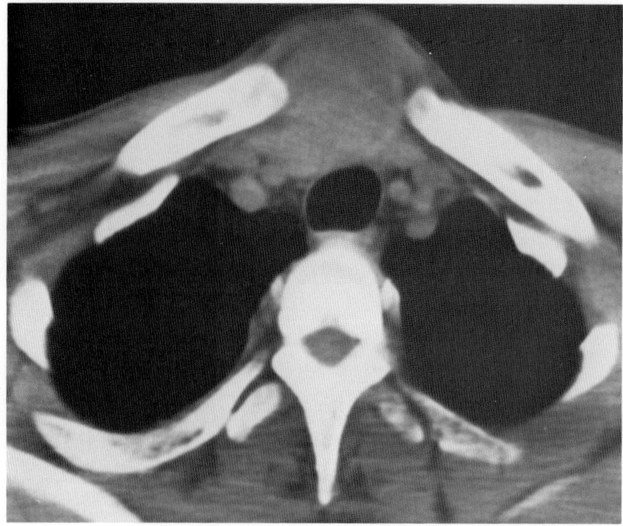

FIG. 15. After median sternotomy for aortic valve replacement, a soft tissue mass in the jugular notch represented hematoma.

num (35). Fluid collections with CT attenuation values higher than water are likely to represent hematomas, which may occur in the anticoagulated patient (Fig. 15).

Infections of the Chest Wall

Actinomycosis may involve the chest wall as extension from the neck or abdomen, or, more commonly, direct extension from pulmonary involvement. *Actinomyces israelii* is commonly found in the normal oral flora, particularly in patients with poor dental hygiene. Aspiration of the organisms from the mouth can pro-

duce pulmonary infection. Mediastinal involvement is felt to be the result of contiguous spread or lymphatic drainage from the oral cavity.

The typical radiographic pattern of acute pulmonary actinomycosis is a mass or alveolar opacity that may extend across interlobar fissures (36). Pleural involvement occurs in most patients as either pleural effusion, empyema, or pleural thickening. Chest wall involvement can be recognized as soft tissue swelling, sinus tracts, wavy periostitis of ribs, or frank destruction of ribs or vertebral bodies (36). On CT, thickened soft tissues of the chest wall and periosteal new bone formation may be seen in the ribs adjacent to pulmonary consolidation (37) (Fig. 16). The differential diagnosis includes other infections, such as tuberculosis, blastomycosis, cryptococcocis, and nocardiosis, as well as lymphoma, bronchogenic carcinoma, and mesothelioma.

Thoracic Outlet Syndrome

The majority of patients with thoracic outlet syndrome present with neurologic symptoms due to brachial plexus impingement. Compression of the subclavian artery or vein occurs much less frequently. Skeletal radiographs that demonstrate cervical ribs or abnormally long C7 transverse processes, or previous fractures of the first rib or clavicle, confirm the etiology of the thoracic outlet syndrome. No osseous abnormalities are apparent, however, in as many as 45 to 70 percent of patients with thoracic outlet syndrome. CT has been shown to be useful in patients with normal radiographs and thoracic outlet syndrome. In 8 of 12 patients (67 percent), CT showed impingement of the C7 transverse

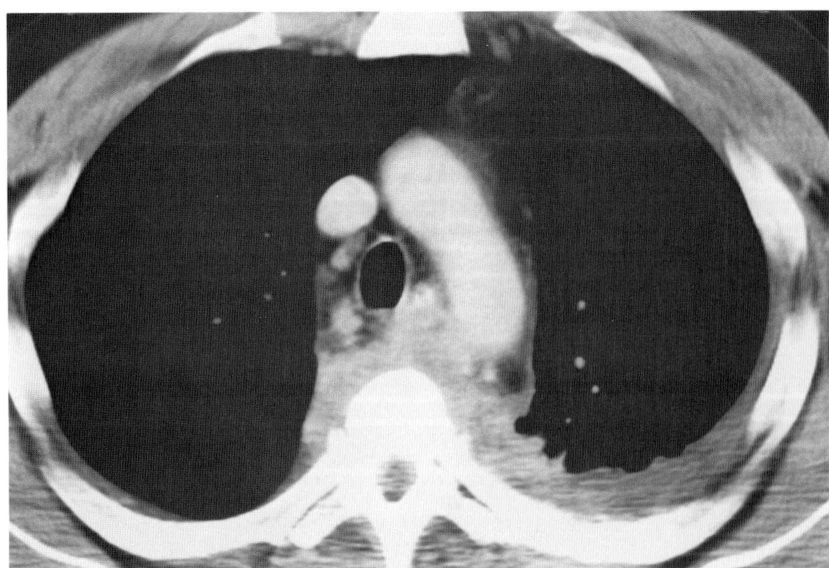

FIG. 16. Actinomycosis involves the pleura, mediastinum, and chest wall. Note the pleural thickening in the left hemithorax, the thickened adjacent rib, the obliteration of the fat planes between the rhomboid and trapezius muscles, and the retrotracheal extension across the mediastinum.

process on the scalene triangle or anteromedial aspect of the middle scalene muscle (38). This was seen in only 2 of 21 (9.5 percent) of the control population.

Congenital fibromuscular bands that compress the brachial plexus or the subclavian vessels have been identified at surgery in 98 percent of patients with thoracic outlet syndrome (39). This suggests that MR may be of greater value than CT in thoracic outlet syndrome, due to the superior soft tissue contrast of MR relative to CT (40).

Congenital Anomalies of the Chest Wall

An intrathoracic rib is an extremely rare congenital anomaly of the thoracic cage, which is significant only because of its potential to mimic pathology (Fig. 17). The intrathoracic rib is usually single, and can arise from either a vertebral body, or from the posteroinferior margin of an otherwise normal rib. The rib extends into the substance of the lung, but remains covered by both visceral and parietal pleura. This pleural covering may render it more opaque and less well-defined than other ribs, which may complicate its recognition.

Another chest wall anomaly is the midline sternal foramen, which is most easily recognized on CT. The foramen represents incomplete fusion of one pair of sternal primordia, resulting in a circular defect in the middle of the lower part of the sternal foramen (41,42). Familiarity

with the normal CT anatomy of the sternum helps to prevent misdiagnosis as a destructive lesion (43).

Episternal ossicles lie medial to the proximal end of the clavicles and can mimic pulmonary nodules on chest radiographs. On CT, they are clearly calcified, but can mimic vascular calcifications or calcified lymph nodes (44).

THE PLEURA

The Normal Pleura

The pleural space is a potential space that exists between the visceral and parietal pleura. The visceral pleura is a serous membrane covering the lung and extending between the lobes into the interlobar fissures. The parietal pleura lines the internal thoracic cavity, covering the surface of the ribs and intercostal muscles, and extending inferiorly over the diaphragm and medially along the mediastinum. The visceral and parietal pleura reflect over the pulmonary hilum, representing a continuous membrane. Inferior to the hilum, a double fold of pleura forms the inferior pulmonary ligament, tethering the medial aspect of the lower lobe to the mediastinum (45).

In a normal subject, 1–5 ml of fluid are present within the pleural space (46). The amount of fluid increases after exercise and as much as 15 ml of fluid may be pres-

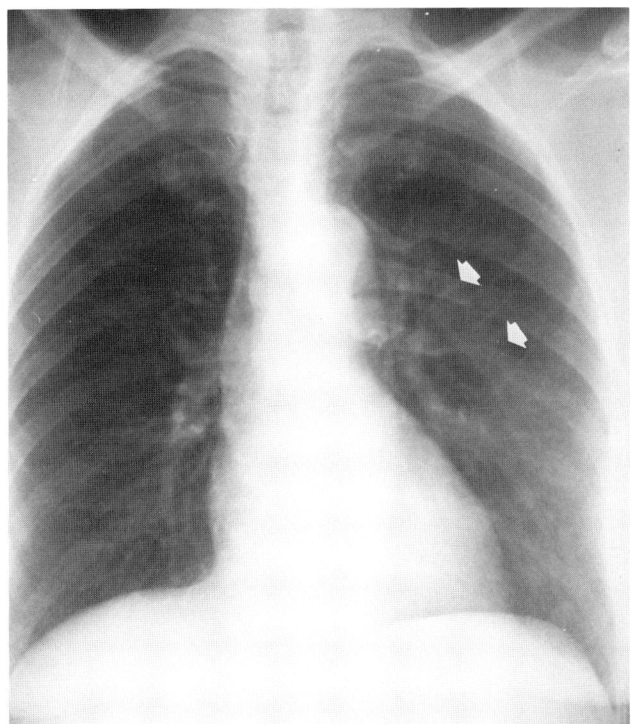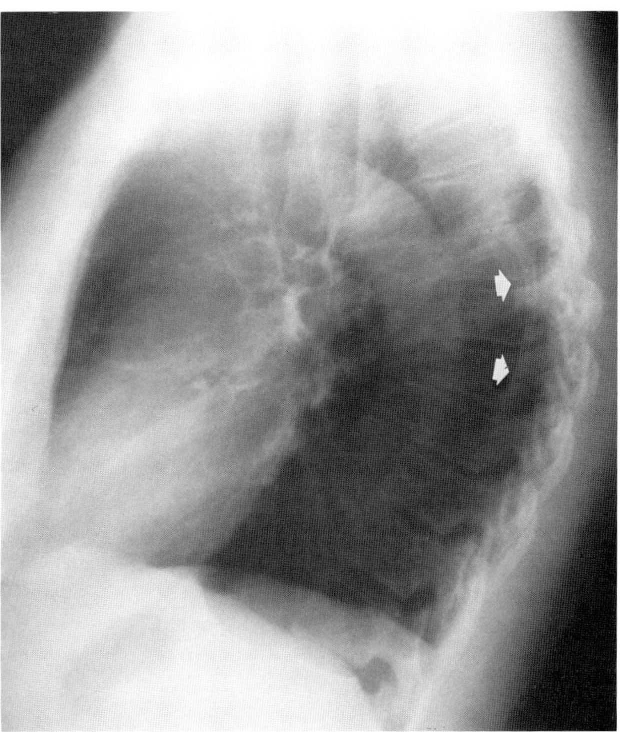

A

B

FIG. 17. On the frontal (**A**) and lateral (**B**) radiographs, an intrathoracic rib (*arrowheads*) arises from an anomalous vertebral body and extends into the lung.

ent in a normal individual. The combined thickness of the layers of visceral and parietal pleura and the fluid-containing pleural space is 0.2 to 0.4 mm. On high-resolution computed tomographic images, the visceral and parietal pleura, fluid-containing pleural space, endothoracic fascia, and innermost intercostal muscles are visible as a 1- to 2-mm–thick line of soft tissue attenuation in the anterolateral and posterolateral intercostal spaces (47).

The Abnormal Pleural Space

The pleural space may be filled by large amounts of fluid in a variety of diseases. Pleural effusion creates a characteristic appearance on chest radiographs, as well as on CT, MR, and ultrasound images. Pleural fluid is heavier than the air-filled lung, and therefore collects in dependent areas of the thorax. In the upright patient, pleural fluid initially collects between the base of the lung and the hemidiaphragm. The lung recoils from the chest wall, but tends to preserve its shape as the pleural fluid displaces it from the chest wall and diaphragm.

On chest radiographs, pleural fluid in this subpulmonic, or infrapulmonary, location mimics an elevated hemidiaphragm. On the left side, subpulmonic fluid can be recognized as an increase in the distance from the lung base to the gastric air bubble. This distance is usually a few millimeters to as much as 1 cm in the normal individual.

In the right hemithorax, subpulmonic fluid lifts the lung base away from the hemidiaphragm. Because the medial aspect of the right lower lobe is tethered to the mediastinum, only the lateral aspect of the right lower lobe is free to float on top of the pleural fluid. This creates a lateral peak in what initially appears to be the right hemidiaphragm, but is actually subpulmonic pleural fluid.

As much as 1 liter of pleural fluid can collect in a subpulmonic location. Typically, the lateral costophrenic angles appear blunted when the volume of pleural fluid reaches 175 ml, which aids in the radiographic recognition of pleural fluid.

To confirm the free-flowing nature of a pleural effusion, lateral decubitus radiographs can be obtained. Lateral decubitus radiographs can also be used to allow detection of small amounts of pleural fluid, because as little as 5 ml of fluid can be seen on these views (48).

In the supine patient, pleural fluid is apparent on axial CT images as crescentic areas of water attenuation in the posterior aspects of the thorax. The pleural effusions compress the lower lobes, and atelectatic basilar segments are typically present anterior to the fluid collections. The atelectatic bands of lung can create confusion. An atelectatic band of lung can simulate the diaphragm on axial CT images, and pleural effusion lying anterior to the atelectatic lung can be mistaken for ascites lying beneath the diaphragm (Fig. 18).

Differentiation of pleural fluid from intraperitoneal fluid is possible in most cases, however (49,50). A basic principle is that pleural fluid lies peripheral to the convexity of the diaphragm, whereas ascites lies centrally. Pleural effusion displaces the crus of the diaphragm laterally, away from the vertebral column (51). The dia-

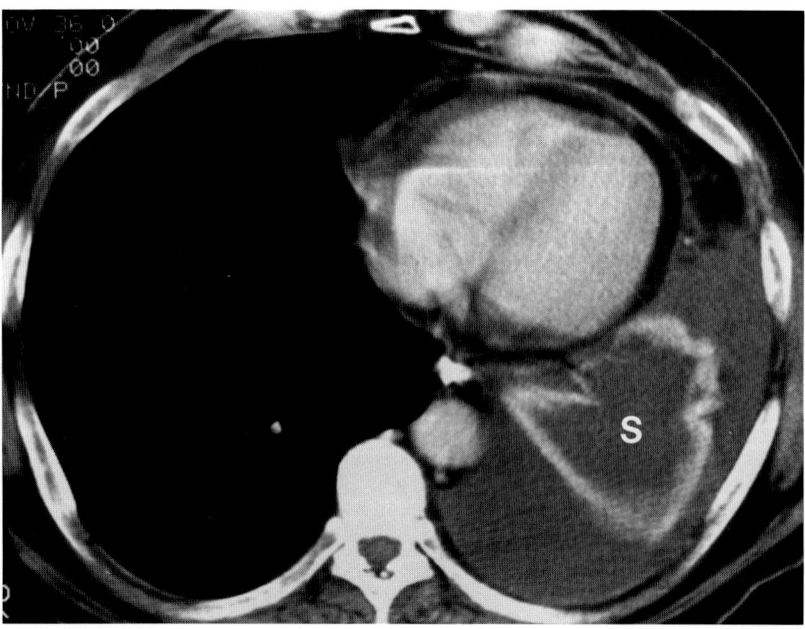

FIG. 18. Subpulmonic pleural fluid (S) beneath the atelectatic left lower lobe may be mistaken for ascites beneath the diaphragm.

phragm is usually a continuous band of uniform thickness. Atelectatic lung is usually thicker than the diaphragm and is interrupted. Following the band of atelectatic lung on more cephalad scans may demonstrate contiguity with air-containing structures that are easily recognized as lung (52).

The interface the fluid creates with the margin of the liver also provides a clue to the distinction of ascites from pleural fluid (53). Pleural fluid produces an indistinct interface with the liver. In the patient with ascites, the margin of the liver is distinct.

A portion of the right lobe of the liver is directly attached to the posterior hemidiaphragm. Ascites is restricted from this bare area of the liver due to coronary ligaments. Fluid that is in direct contact with the bare area of the liver must, therefore, lie within the pleural space (54).

Ultrasonography is frequently used to localize pleural fluid collections for thoracentesis. Pleural effusion appears as a hypoechoic or anechoic area above the diaphragm. Septations may be seen within the fluid collections and are more commonly seen with exudative effusions than with transudative effusions (55).

Ultrasonography can also be use to differentiate pulmonary parenchymal consolidation from pleural fluid (56). Fluid bronchograms or echoes from air bronchograms may be identified in consolidated lung on ultrasound.

There have been efforts to categorize pleural effusions based on their appearances on MR images. On T1-weighted images, pleural effusions show low signal intensities; on T2-weighted images, pleural effusions show medium to high signal intensity (higher than muscle) (57) (Fig. 19). The images are improved by electrocardiogram-gating, but cardiac and respiratory motions nevertheless create artifactual changes in the signal intensities in the effusions, precluding categorization as transudates or exudates. Hemothorax, however, does produce higher signal intensity on T1-weighted images.

Pleural Tumors

Primary Tumors

Benign

A localized pleural fibroma is typically a solitary, poorly vascular, nodular mass that arises from the visceral pleura. Less commonly, a localized pleural fibroma is larger and arises from the parietal pleura on a highly vascular pedicle. The localized pleural fibroma has also been called solitary or localized pleural mesothelioma, but this term is apt to cause confusion with the malignant form of mesothelioma. A solitary pleural fibroma has no known association with asbestos exposure, and there is a good prognosis after local excision (58,59).

The majority of pleural fibromas are discovered incidentally on routine chest radiographs in asymptomatic individuals (Fig. 20a). A change in the position of the mass is an indirect sign of pedunculation of the tumor (60). On CT, the mass is a soft tissue attenuation mass, which, because of its nodular configuration, does not create an obtuse angle with the chest wall (61) (Fig. 20b).

A localized pleural fibroma may occur in a patient of

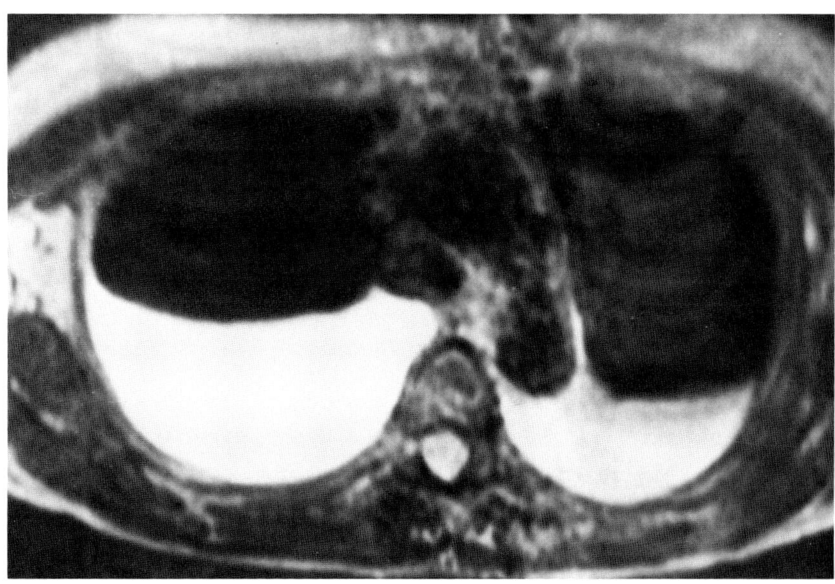

FIG. 19. Pleural effusion on T2-weighted (TR = 2500 msec, TE = 70 msec) MR images are visible as crescentic areas of high-signal intensity in the dependent regions of the thorax.

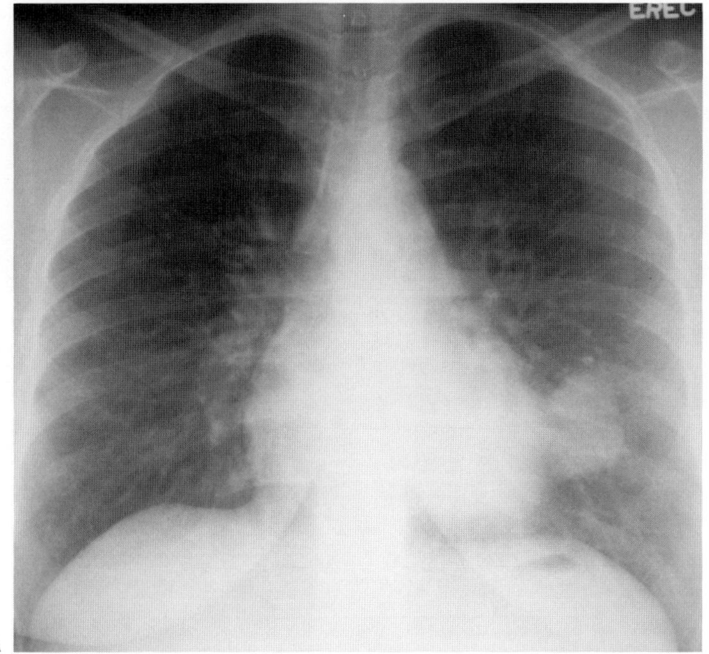

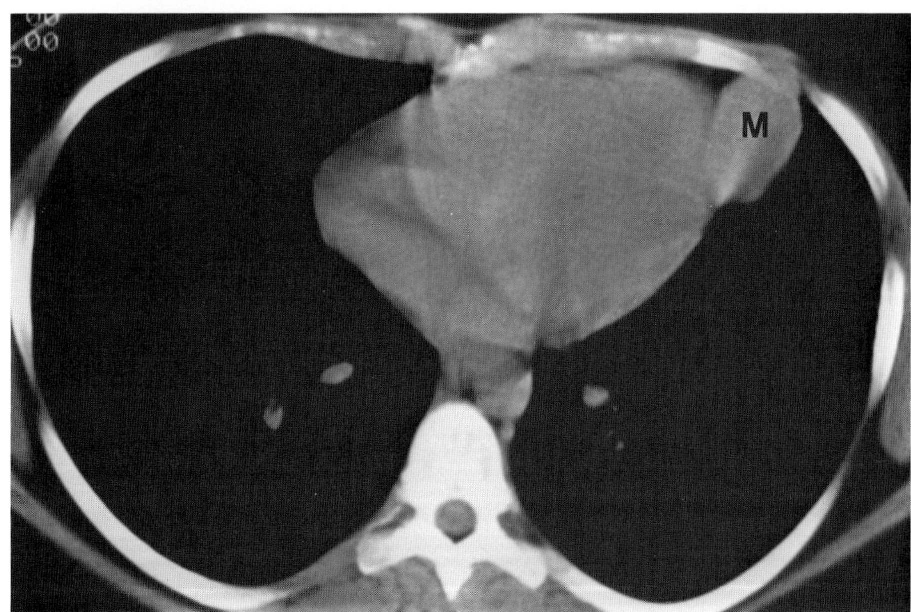

FIG. 20. (A) A pleural fibroma adjacent to the left heart border was detected incidentally on a routine chest radiograph in an asymptomatic 22-year-old woman. **(B)** On CT, the mass (*M*) is soft tissue attenuation, arising from the visceral pleura in the right anterior hemithorax. Diagnosis was established at thoracotomy.

any age, although the peak incidence is in the sixth and seventh decades. Treatment is adequate surgical excision, which provides a complete cure in the majority of patients. Histologic examination may reveal malignant features, however, which are associated with a poorer prognosis (62,63). If malignant features are present, 55 percent of patients will succumb as a result of tumor invasion, recurrence, or metastases (59).

Pleural lipomas are rare tumors, which may be discovered on routine chest radiographs in asymptomatic individuals on routine chest radiographs. They can be contained within the thorax, or can extend in a transmural fashion into the chest wall. Pleural lipomas can be accurately diagnosed preoperatively by their characteristic appearance on CT (Fig. 21). The tumors are well-defined and are of homogeneous fat density, with attenuation values of -50 to -150 H (64). If soft tissue components are present within the mass, or if the mass enhances after contrast administration, the diagnosis of liposarcoma should be considered (65).

Malignant Pleural Tumors

Mesothelioma and Asbestos-Related Disease

Malignant pleural mesothelioma is a rare tumor, but its incidence is increasing along with the increasing use of asbestos. Approximately 70 percent of patients with mesothelioma can provide a history of exposure to asbestos. Exposure is usually on an occupational basis, from work in shipbuilding, insulation and building construction, or the asbestos industry itself (66). The interval between first exposure to asbestos and the diagnosis

of pleural mesothelioma ranges from 20 to 50 years (average = 35 years). Patients usually present with dyspnea and chest pain. The chest radiographs typically show irregular pleural thickening and a loculated pleural effusion. On CT, nodular pleural thickening may extend into the interlobar fissures (67) (Fig. 22). Mesothelioma is usually unilateral, but the tumor can extend into the chest wall, the mediastinum, or abdomen. Associated changes of asbestosis and calcified pleural plaques support the diagnosis of mesothelioma, but are only present in 20 percent of patients. Pleural fluid cytology and needle biopsy can be misleading. Open thoracotomy is necessary to obtain an adequate specimen for diagnosis.

Asbestos exposure can produce benign pleural reactions as well. The most common pleural reaction is a circumscribed parietal pleural hyaline plaque. On chest radiographs, plaques are often seen *en face* and produce a faint opacity with an irregular contour. Oblique radiographs often help to demonstrate the plaques in profile, where they are seen as discrete plateau-like structures paralleling the inner margin of the lateral thoracic wall. They rarely extend over more than four intercostal spaces, and spare the lateral costophrenic angles and apices. On CT, both calcified and noncalcified pleural plaques are readily apparent, and can be easily distinguished from subcostal fat by their higher attenuation values.

Diffuse pleural thickening occurs less commonly and may be due to confluence of pleural plaques. Diffuse pleural thickening involving both the visceral and parietal pleura can also occur as a consequence of benign asbestos pleural effusion (68). This diffuse pleural thickening may resolve, or can cause imprisonment of the lung, requiring surgical decortication.

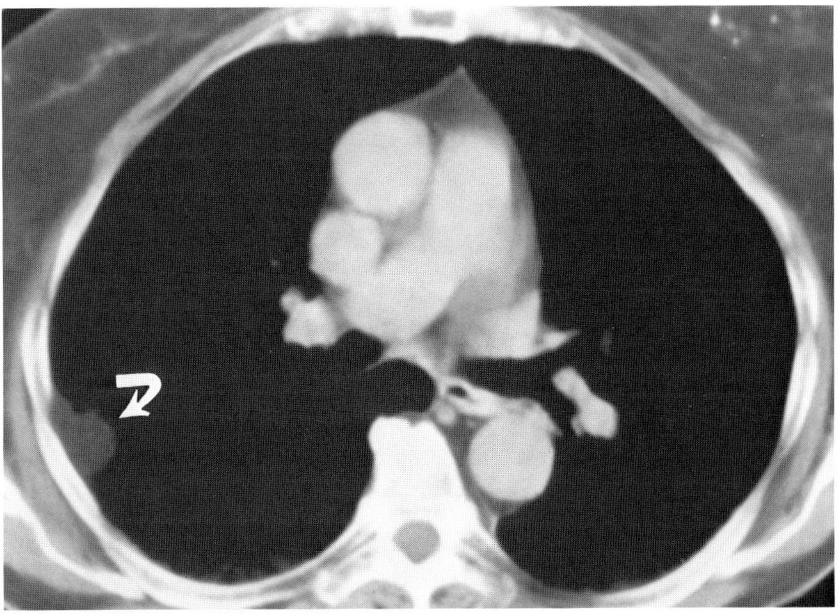

FIG. 21. A pleural lipoma (*arrow*) can be recognized by its fat attenuation on CT.

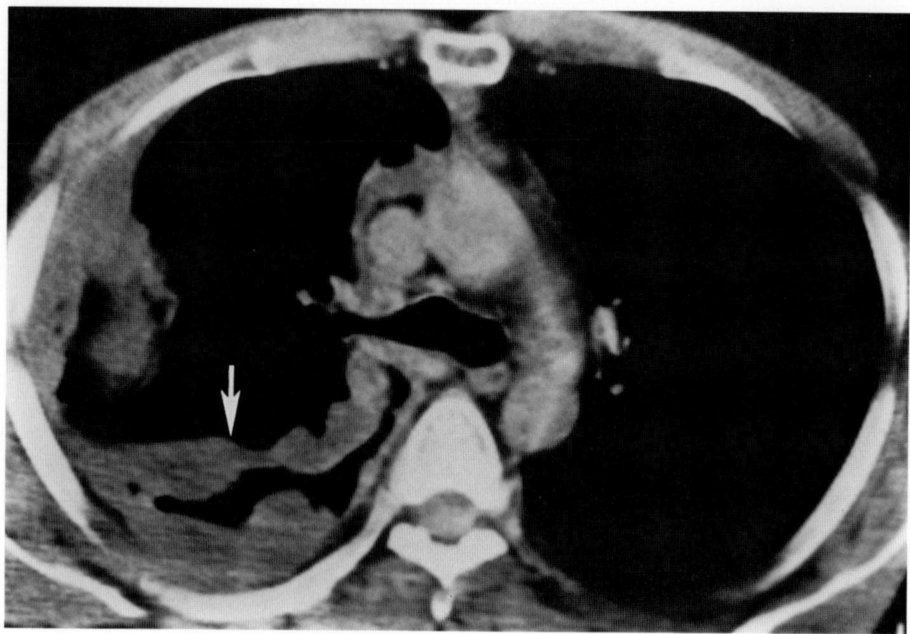

FIG. 22. A mesothelioma produces nodular thickening of the pleura, often extending into the interlobar fissures (*arrow*).

Patients with pleural disease as a result of asbestos exposure are also at risk for developing focal lung masses, which may represent either bronchogenic carcinoma or rounded atelectasis (69). Rounded atelectasis occurs when an abnormally thickened pleural surface causes infolding of a collapsed area of pulmonary parenchyma. Because of the spiraling nature of the abnormal pleural, the bronchi and vessels appear to converge into the mass in a comet-tail appearance. The diagnosis is suspected when there is a combination of volume loss, a typical comet-tail, and contiguity with pleural thickening. The lesion mimics bronchogenic carcinoma. The goal remains to exclude bronchogenic carcinoma, which is increased in the asbestos-exposed population. Close follow-up and a low threshold for biopsy have been recommended to avoid mistaking one lesion for the other.

Metastatic Disease to the Pleura

The most common manifestation of pleural metastatic disease is pleural effusion. Pleural effusions may result from either metastatic deposits on the visceral and parietal pleura, or neoplastic infiltration of mediastinal lymph nodes with subsequent obstruction of small vessels and lymphatics (70). The primary tumor is breast carcinoma in 25 to 50 percent of all malignant effusions (71). Other primary tumors that account for a significant percentage of malignant pleural effusions are bronchogenic carcinoma, ovarian carcinoma, and lymphoma. Malignant pleural effusions can cause significant de-

bilitation due to lung compression and the resulting loss of pulmonary function. Some malignant pleural effusions are responsive to chemotherapy or radiation therapy. Obliteration of the pleural space may be necessary to prevent reaccumulation of malignant pleural effusions. This may be achieved by either pleurectomy, or pleural sclerosis, with talc or tetracycline introduced into the pleural space to produce adhesion of the visceral and parietal pleural surfaces. Pleuroperitoneal shunting provides an alternative approach to management of pleural effusion (72).

On CT, pleural metastases are visible as nodules or plaques involving the visceral or parietal pleura (Fig. 23). Because diffuse pleural disease can be caused by both benign and malignant processes, the following criteria may help to diagnose pleural tumor: pleural nodularity, circumferential pleural involvement (pleural rind), pleural thickening greater than 1 cm, and involvement of the mediastinal pleura (73).

Accumulation of technetium-99m methylene diphosphonate may occasionally be seen in patients undergoing bone scanning to look for skeletal metastases (74,75). Although this accumulation was originally felt to be pathognomonic of a malignant pleural effusion, it has also been reported in inflammatory pleural effusions (76,77).

Pleural lymphoma occurs in three forms: pleural effusion, subpleural nodules, and subpleural plaques. The most common manifestation of pleural involvement in a patient with lymphoma is pleural effusion, which does not necessarily reflect intrinsic involvement of the pleura, but may occur as a result of obstruction of hilar and mediastinal lymphatics and veins by enlarged

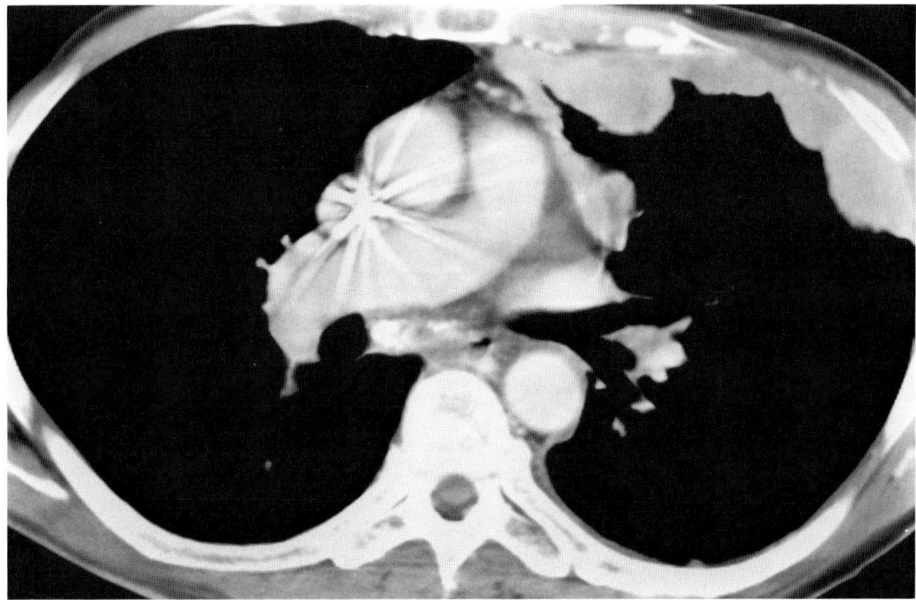

FIG. 23. Nodular pleural thickening in the left hemithorax represented pleural metastases.

lymph nodes (78). Pleural effusion occurs in 7–13 percent of patients with lymphoma, either Hodgkin disease or non-Hodgkin lymphoma (78).

Solid pleural manifestations of lymphoma include subpleural nodules of lymphoid tissue, and subpleural plaque formation, representing spread of lymphoma along the subvisceral pleural plane (79). Pleural effusions and pleural or subpleural masses are rarely the sole initial manifestation of lymphoma, but are occasionally the only site of recurrent disease (79).

Pleural effusions have been reported as the initial presentation of B-cell lymphoma in patients with acquired immune deficiency syndrome (AIDS) (80). In a patient at risk for AIDS or with known infection with human immunodeficiency virus, the presence of pleural effusion should prompt consideration of three diagnoses: pleural involvement by Kaposi sarcoma, lymphoma, and infection with mycobacterium tuberculosis.

Trauma

The radiographic hallmark of pneumothorax is displacement of the visceral pleura from the parietal pleura by air in the pleural space. The visceral pleura is visible as a thin, white line, outlined by air in the pleural space laterally and air within the lung medially. In the upright patient, pneumothorax collects over the apex of the lung. A chest radiograph obtained in expiration or in a lateral decubitus position may facilitate recognition of a small pneumothorax.

In the supine patient, air in the pleural space rises to the highest point of the thorax—the anterior costophrenic sulcus. On a chest radiograph, pneumothorax in a supine patient produces hyperlucency over the abdomen, sharply outlining the diaphragm. The lateral costophrenic angle appears deeper and more lucent than normal, which has been termed the deep sulcus sign (81–84).

Tension pneumothorax is generally recognized clinically, but may be suspected radiographically when pneumothorax causes shift of the mediastinum to the contralateral side, inversion of the diaphragm, and flattening of the cardiac contour. The ipsilateral lung is typically collapsed due to the increased pressure in the pleural space. The radiographic signs of tension pneumothorax may be present without any of the clinical criteria of tension pneumothorax.

Pneumothorax in the hospitalized patient is often due to iatrogenic causes, such as thoracentesis or central venous catheter placement. Pneumothorax may also occur as a result of trauma, with laceration of the lung by a fractured rib, producing an air leak into the pleural space.

Pneumothorax can also result from the rupture of a congenital apical bleb or an emphysematous bulla, which lies immediately beneath the visceral pleura. The development of spontaneous pneumothorax in these patients may be related to sudden pressure changes, which can occur when a scuba diver ascends too rapidly or when the flight crew of an airplane experience sudden loss of cabin pressure. There is also a relationship between spontaneous pneumothorax and unusual changes in the ambient atmospheric pressure in individuals on land (85). The collapsed lung surrounded by pneumothorax provides the radiologist with an opportunity to detect apical blebs and bullae. A variety of chronic lung diseases, including sarcoidosis, eosinophilic granuloma, and lymphangioleiomyomatosis, are also associated with spontaneous pneumothoraces.

The Postoperative Pleural Space

Pleural effusion is commonly present after thoracic or abdominal surgery. In a review of 128 patients with recent upper abdominal surgery, pleural effusions were seen in 89, and were not indicative of surgical complications (86).

After pneumonectomy, the pleural space gradually fills with fluid, and an air-fluid level can be seen at successively higher levels within the hemithorax on postoperative films. Complete opacification of the postpneumonectomy space requires weeks to months (Figure 24A). A drop in the air-fluid level on serial radiographs suggests bronchopleural fistula, usually heralded clinically by the onset of a cough productive of copious amounts of fluid.

After lobectomy, segmental or wedge resection, a postoperative pneumothorax is usually present on the initial

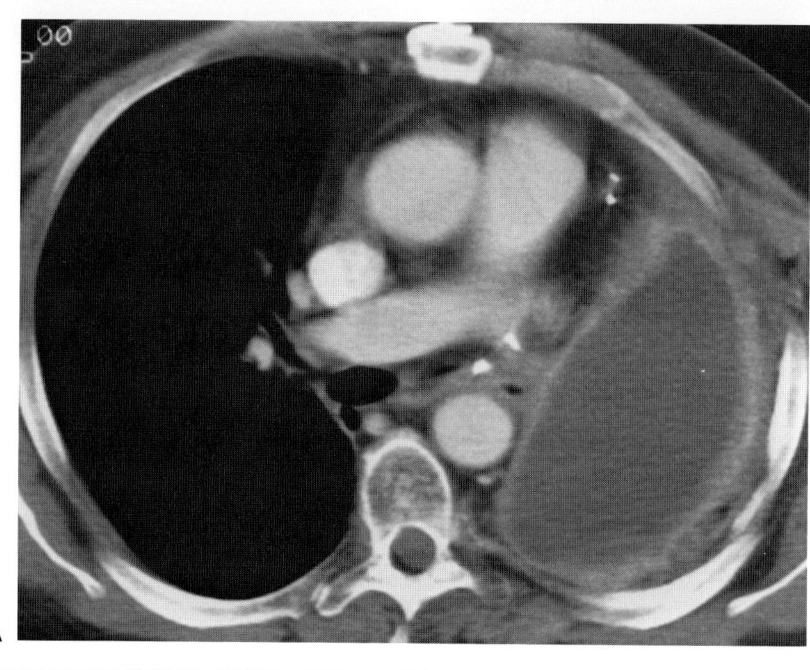

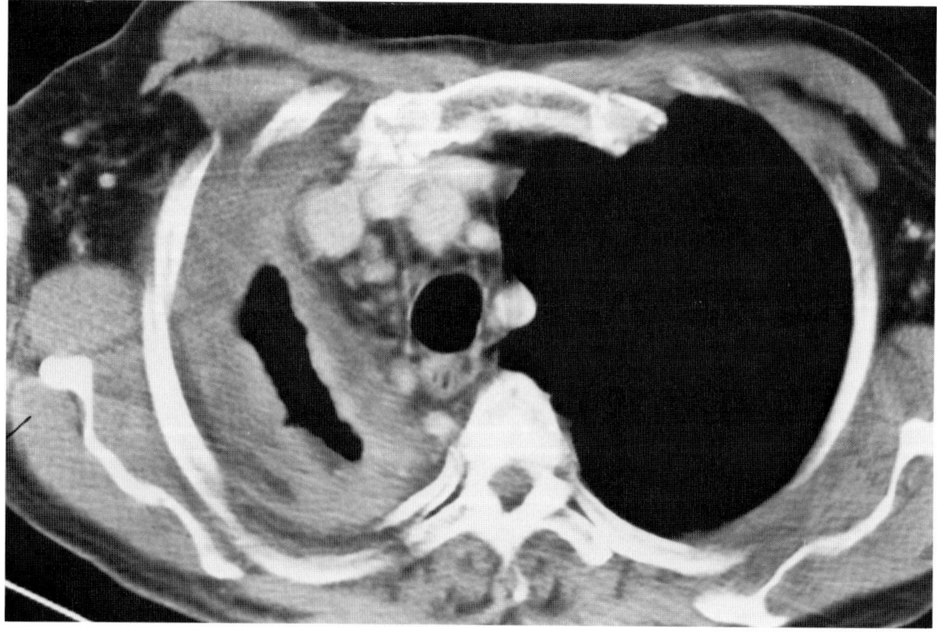

FIG. 24. (**A**) Normal postpneumonectomy space. The pleural space fills with fluid over a period of weeks to months after surgery. (**B**) Empyema developing after partial pulmonary resection from the right lung produces thickened visceral and parietal pleura.

postoperative radiographs. A small postoperative pleural air collection persists beyond the first several days in 10 to 20 percent of lobectomies, and in a higher percentage of segmental and wedge resections (87). A benign pleural space typically closes over the next several weeks. Empyema or bronchopleural fistula can occur, producing a thickened, irregular pleura, and prolonged drainage or purulent fluid from the thoracostomy tube (Fig. 24B).

Infection in the Pleural Space

An empyema is, by definition, pus in the pleural space. Most empyemas develop in association with pneumonia. A focus of infection contiguous to the pleura causes increased permeability of the visceral pleura. The small amount of sterile fluid that accumulates is exudative, characterized by primarily polymorphonuclear leukocytes, a normal glucose level, and a normal pH (88). At this point, the pleural fluid can be considered a parapneumonic effusion.

As the parapneumonic effusion becomes infected with bacteria, it becomes an empyema. Fibrin is deposited as a continuous sheet over the visceral and parietal pleura, which causes loculation of the fluid collection.

If the empyema is left untreated, a pleural peel develops, encasing the lung. Fluid may drain spontaneously through the chest wall (empyema necessitatis), or into the lung, producing a bronchopleural fistula. Peripheral lung necrosis in the infected lung creates a communication between a peripheral airway and the pleural space. A bronchopleural fistula may also develop as a consequence of pleural infection extending into the lung.

The therapeutic approach to empyema is external drainage, usually by tube thoracostomy. Lung abscesses, on the other hand, are treated with antibiotic therapy and postural drainage. It is important to distinguish accurately empyema from lung abscess, so that appropriate therapy is initiated.

On chest radiographs, the key to the distinction of empyemas from abscesses is based on their three-dimensional shapes (89). Empyemas conform to the adjacent chest wall and are therefore lenticular in shape, whereas a lung abscess is spherical. The appearance of the air-fluid level within the abscess or empyema on two orthogonal projections, such as the posteroanterior and lateral radiographs, can therefore provide significant diagnostic information. In an empyema, the air-fluid level is short in one projection and long in the other projection. The air-fluid level extends to the chest wall. Within the spherical lung abscess, however, the air-fluid level is of the same length in any projection. The lung abscess is surrounded by the pneumonia in which it developed, and therefore the air-fluid level does not extend to the chest wall.

The most reliable sign of empyema on CT has been termed the split-pleura sign (90). The thickened visceral and parietal pleural surfaces are separated by fluid and air in the pleural space. The hypervascular pleural surfaces enhance after intravenous administration of contrast material, and the split-pleura sign is seen to better advantage on contrasted images. As with all pleural lesions, the angle that an empyema forms with the chest wall is obtuse, in contrast to the acute angle formed by a lung abscess.

The mass effect of an empyema causes compression of adjacent lung, and the bronchi and pulmonary vessels may appear distorted. A lung abscess within the lung parenchyma replaces, rather than compresses, the lung. The bronchi and pulmonary vessels maintain a normal course, but terminate abruptly at the advancing wall of the abscess (90).

Wall characteristics further help to distinguish the two entities. The wall of an empyema is thin and uniform, and the inner surface is smooth. There is a sharply defined border between the empyema and adjacent lung. The wall of a lung abscess is thicker and irregular in width. The inner luminal margin is irregular, and there is no discrete boundary between the abscess and lung.

An entity that can mimic an empyema is accumulation of fluid within a preexisting bulla or lung cyst (Fig. 25) (91). In a manner analogous to the development of a parapneumonic pleural effusion, fluid develops within the bulla due to increased permeability of the wall of the bulla in response to adjacent pneumonitis (92).

The presence of adjacent pneumonitis may cause confusion with lung abscess and empyema. The bulla is usually larger than most lung abscesses, however, and has a sharp inner wall (93). The lenticular shape and smooth, uniform inner wall is similar to the appearance of an empyema. The wall of the bulla may enhance after the administration of intravenous contrast material, simulating the split-pleura sign of empyema. Two criteria help to distinguish this entity from empyema. One is its presence in the upper lobes, an unusual location for empyema. The second is the presence of a bulla on previous radiographs. A large, coexisting effusion is typically absent.

The fluid-filled bulla responds to conservative therapy with antibiotics. Attempts to externally drain a peripherally located lesion may result in empyema or bronchopleural fistula (92). Resolution of the fluid is slow, occurring in 6 weeks to 6 months.

Interventional Procedures of the Pleural Space

Chest fluoroscopy, ultrasonography, and CT may be used to guide pleural biopsy, thoracentesis, and percutaneous drainage of pleural fluid collections.

Large pleural fluid collections have traditionally been treated with chest tube drainage. Percutaneous drainage may be used as the primary diagnostic or therapeutic procedure, or it may be used for drainage of pleural fluid

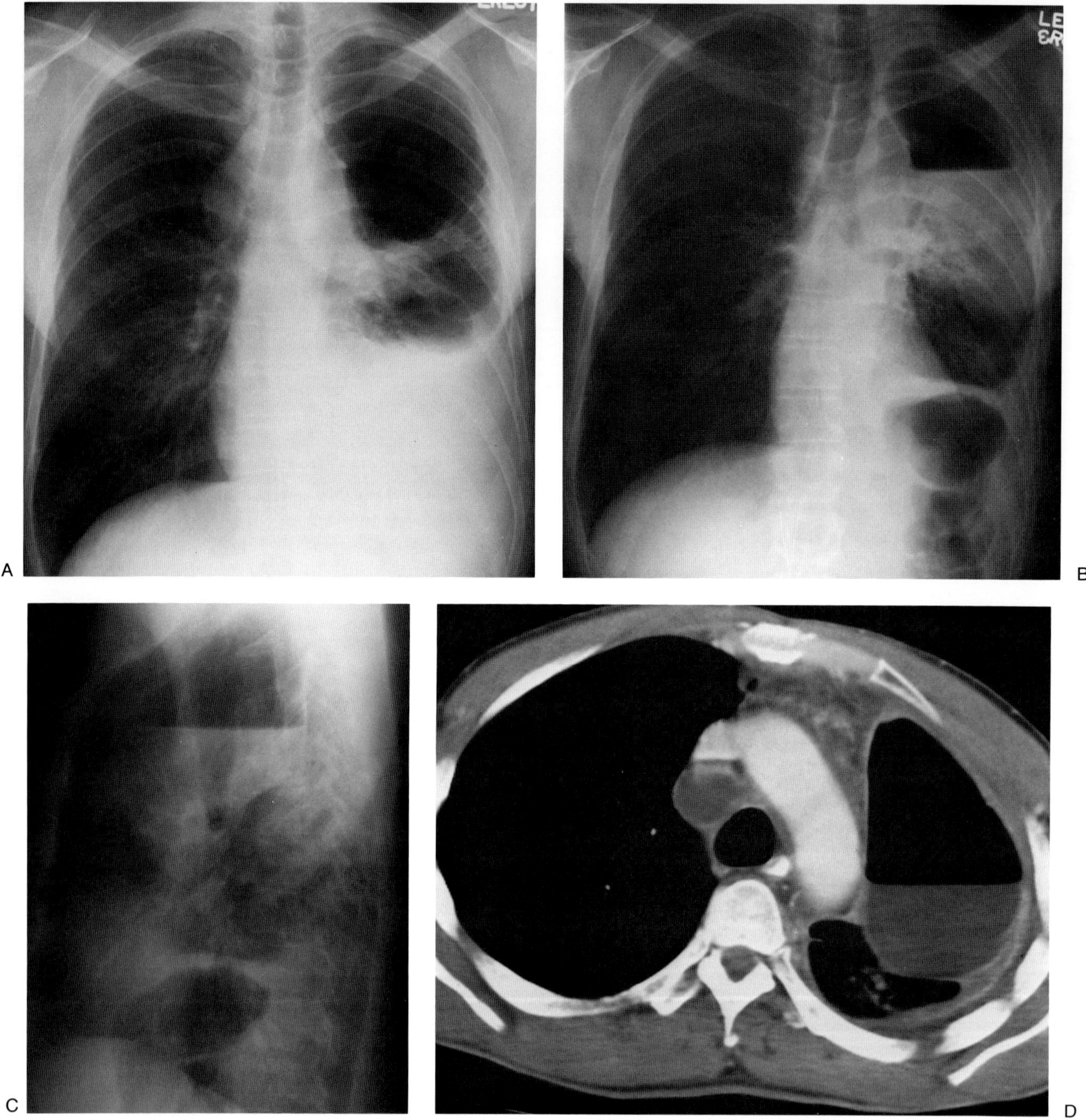

FIG. 25. Fluid within a preexisting bulla mimicking empyema. **(A)** A large left upper lobe bulla is present in a patient with metastatic bronchogenic carcinoma (malignant left pleural effusion, mediastinal adenopathy). **(B)** Three months later, an air-fluid level is present in the left upper hemithorax. Air bronchograms are noted in adjacent lung. **(C)** On the lateral radiograph, the air-fluid level is of a different length than on the frontal examination. **(D)** On CT, the air-fluid level within the bulla mimics empyema. Its location within the upper lobe and the existence of a large bulla on a previous chest radiograph help in the diagnosis of a parapneumonic effusion in this patient with clinical and radiographic evidence of pneumonia.

collections incompletely drained by chest tubes (94,95). The smaller caliber percutaneous catheters provide less patient discomfort than conventional chest tubes. A 6–7 Fr catheter is used to drain simple pleural effusions; a 10–14 Fr catheter is used for viscous empyemas (95–98). Instillation of urokinase via the percutaneous catheter into loculated hemorrhagic or fibrinous nonhemorrhagic pleural fluid collections may facilitate drainage (99). A contraindication to percutaneous catheter drainage, however, is the multilocular pleural fluid collection, which is likely to require thoracotomy (100).

REFERENCES

1. Clemente CD. *Anatomy: a regional atlas of the human body.* Philadelphia: Lea & Febiger, 1975.
2. Warwick R, Williams PL. *Gray's anatomy,* 35th British ed. Philadelphia: WB Saunders Co., 1973.
3. Snell RS. *Clinical anatomy for medical students.* Boston: Little, Brown & Co., 1981.
4. Gilmartin D. The serratus anterior muscle on chest radiographs. *Radiology* 1979;131:629–635.
5. Hölbert BL, Holbert JM, Libshitz HI. CT of interpectoral lymph nodes. *Am J Roentgenol* 1987;149:687–688.
6. Chiles C. Lesions of the chest wall. *Contemp Diagn Radiol* 1988;11:1–5.
7. King RM, Pairolero PC, Trastek VF, Piehler JM, Payne WS, Bernatz PE. Primary chest wall tumors: factors affecting survival. *Ann Thor Surg* 1986;41:597–601.
8. Weiss SW, Enzinger FM. Malignant fibrous histiocytoma: an analysis of 200 cases. *Cancer* 1978;41:2250–2266.
9. McAfee MK, Pairolero PC, Bergstralh EJ, Piehler JM, Unni KK, McLeod RA, Bernatz PE, Payne WS. Chondrosarcoma of the chest wall: factors affecting survival. *Ann Thor Surg* 1985;40:535–541.
10. Stelzer P, Gay WA Jr. Tumors of the chest wall. *Surg Clin North Am* 1980;60:779–791.
11. Barnes R, Catto M. Chondrosarcoma of bone. *J Bone Joint Surg* 1966;48:729.
12. Chiles C, Chen JTT, Elson CE, Roggli V. Anterior chest wall mass in an elderly male. *Invest Radiol* 1985;20:355–359.
13. Aoki J, Moser Jr RP, Kransdorf MJ. Chondrosarcoma of the sternum: CT features. *J Comput Assist Tomogr* 1989;13:806–810.
14. Lindfors KK, Meyer JE, Busse PM, Kopans DB, Munzenrider JE, Sawicka JM. CT evaluation of local and regional breast cancer recurrence. *Am J Roentgenol* 1985;145:833–837.
15. Shea WJ Jr, de Geer G, Webb WR. Chest wall after mastectomy. Part II. CT appearance of tumor recurrence. *Radiology* 1987;162:162–164.
16. Glazer HS, Duncan-Meyer J, Aronberg DJ, Moran JF, Levitt RG, Sagel SS. Pleural and chest wall invasion in bronchogenic carcinoma: CT evaluation. *Radiology* 1985;157:191–194.
17. Pennes DR, Glazer GM, Wimbish KJ, Gross BH, Long RW, Orringer MB. Chest wall invasion by lung cancer: Limitations of CT evaluation. *Am J Roentgenol* 1985;144:507–511.
18. Pearlberg JL, Sandler MA, Beute GH, Lewis Jr JW, Madrazo BL. Limitations of CT in evaluation of neoplasms involving chest wall. *J Comput Assist Tomogr* 1987;11:290–293.
19. Haggar AM, Pearlberg JL, Froelich JW, Hearshen DO, Beute GH, Lewis Jr JW, Schkudor GW, Wood C, Gniewek P. Chest-wall invasion by carcinoma of the lung: detection by MR imaging. *Am J Roentgenol* 1987;148:1075–1078.
20. Press GA, Glazer HS, Wasserman TH, Aronberg DJ, Lee JKT, Sagel SS. Thoracic wall involvement by Hodgkin disease and nonHodgkin lymphoma: CT evaluation. *Radiology* 1985;157:195–198.
21. Cho CS, Blank N, Castellino RA. Computerized tomography evaluation of chest wall involvement in lymphoma. *Cancer* 1985;55:1892–1894.
22. Patten RM, Shuman WP, Teefey S. Subcutaneous metastases from malignant melanoma: prevalence and findings on CT. *Am J Roentgenol* 1989;152:1009–1012.
23. Hidalgo H, Korobkin M, Breiman RS, Heaston DK, Moore AV, Ram PC. CT demonstration of subcutaneous venous collaterals. *J Comput Assist Tomogr* 1982;6:514–518.
24. Fernandez GG, Coblentz CL, Cooper C, Sallee DS. Hickman nodule: a mimic of metastatic disease. *Radiology* 1989;171:401–402.
25. Harley DP, Mena I. Cardiac and vascular sequelae of sternal fractures. *J Trauma* 1986;26:553–555.
26. De Luca SA, Rhea JT, O'Malley T. Radiographic evaluation of rib fractures. *Am J Roentgenol* 1982;138:91–92.
27. Richardson JD, McElvein RB, Trinkle JK. First rib fracture: a hallmark of severe trauma. *Ann Surg* 1975;181:251–254.
28. Woodring JH, Fried AM, Hatfield DR, Stevens RK, Todd EP. Fractures of first and second ribs: predictive value for arterial and bronchial injury. *Am J Roentgenol* 1982;138:211–215.
29. Fisher RG, Ward RE, Ben-Menachem Y, Mattox KL, Flynn TC. Arteriography and the fractured first rib: too much for too little? *Am J Roentgenol* 1982;138:1059–1062.
30. Livoni JP, Barcia TC. Fracture of the first and second rib: incidence of vascular injury relative to type of fracture. *Radiology* 1982;145:31–33.
31. Shea WJ Jr, de Geer G, Webb WR. Chest wall after mastectomy. Part I: CT appearance of normal postoperative anatomy, postirradiation changes and optimal scanning techniques. *Radiology* 1987;162:157–161.
32. Ziter Jr FMH. Major thoracic dehiscence: radiographic considerations. *Radiology* 1977;122:587–590.
33. Carter D, Otis CN. Three types of spindle cell tumors of the pleura: fibroma, sarcoma, and sarcomatoid mesothelioma. *Am J Surg Pathol* 1988;12:747–753.
34. Berkow AE, Demos TC. The midsternal stripe and its relationship to postoperative sternal dehiscence. *Radiology* 1976;121:525.
35. Goodman LR, Kay HR, Teplick SK, Mundth ED. Complications of median sternotomy: computed tomographic evaluation. *Am J Roentgenol* 1983;141:225–230.
36. Flynn MW, Felson B. The roentgen manifestations of thoracic actinomycosis. *Am J Roentgenol* 1970;110:707–716.
37. Webb WR, Sagel SS. Actinomycosis involving the chest wall: CT findings. *Am J Roentgenol* 1982;139:1007–1009.
38. Bilbey JH, Muller NL, Connell DG, Luoma AA, Nelams B. Thoracic outlet syndrome: evaluation with CT. *Radiology* 1989;171:381–384.
39. Roos DB. Congenital anomalies associated with thoracic outlet syndrome: anatomy, symptoms, diagnosis, and treatment. *Am J Surg* 1976;132:771–778.
40. Kellman GM, Kneeland JB, Middleton WD, Cates JD, Pech P, Grist TM, Foley WD, Jesmanowicz A, Froncisz W, Hyde JS. MR imaging of the supraclavicular region: normal anatomy. *Am J Roentgenol* 1987;148:77–82.
41. Stark P, Jamarillo D. CT of the sternum. *Am J Roentgenol* 1986;147:72–77.
42. Stark P. Midline sternal foramen: CT demonstration. *J Comput Assist Tomogr* 1985;9:489–490.
43. Goodman LR, Teplick SK, Kay H. Computed tomography of the normal sternum. *Am J Roentgenol* 1983;141:219–223.
44. Stark P, Watkins GE, Hildebrandt-Stark HE, Dunbar RD. Episternal ossicles. *Radiology* 1987;165:143–144.
45. Henschke CI, Davis SD, Romano PM, Yankelevitz DF. Pleural effusions: pathogenesis, radiologic evaluation, and therapy. *J Thor Imag* 1989;41:49–60.
46. Black LF. The pleural space and pleural fluid. *Mayo Clin Proc* 1972;47:493–506.
47. Im J, Webb WR, Rosen A, Gamsu G. Costal pleura: appearances at high-resolution CT. *Radiology* 1989;171:125–131.
48. Moskowitz H, Platt RT, Schachar R, Mellins H. Roentgen visualization of minute pleural effusion. *Radiology* 1973;109:33–35.
49. Alexander ES, Proto AV, Clark RA. CT differentiation of

subphrenic abscess and pleural effusion. *Am J Roentgenol* 1983;140:47–51.

50. Federle MP, Mark AS, Guillaumin ES. CT of subpulmonic pleural effusions and atelectasis; criteria for differentiation from subphrenic fluid. *Am J Roentgenol* 1986;146:685–689.

51. Dwyer A. The displaced crus: a sign for distinguishing between pleural fluid and ascites on computed tomography. *J Comput Assist Tomogr* 1978;2:598–599.

52. Silverman PM, Baker ME, Mahony B. Atelectasis and subpulmonic fluid: a CT pitfall in distinguishing pleural from peritoneal fluid. *J Comput Assist Tomogr* 1985;9:763–766.

53. Teplick JG, Teplick SK, Goodman L, Haskin ME. The interface sign: a computed tomographic sign for distinguishing pleural from intra-abdominal fluid. *Radiology* 1982;144:359–362.

54. Naidich DP, Megibow AJ, Hilton S, Hulnick DH, Siegelman SS. Computed tomography of the diaphragm: peridiaphragmatic fluid localization. *J Comput Assist Tomogr* 1983;7:641–649.

55. Hirsh JH, Rogers JV, Mack LA. Real-time sonography of pleural opacities. *Am J Roentgenol* 1981;136:297–301.

56. Dorne HL. Differentiation of pulmonary parenchymal consolidation from pleural disease using the sonographic fluid bronchogram. *Radiology* 1986;158:41–42.

57. Tscholakoff D, Sechtem U, deGeer G, Schmidt H, Higgins CB. Evaluation of pleural and pericardial effusions by magnetic resonance imaging. *Eur J Radiol* 1987;7:169–174.

58. Watts DM, Jones GP, Bowman GA, Olsen JD. Giant benign mesothelioma. *Ann Thor Surg* 1989;48:590–591.

59. England DM, Hochholzer L, McCarthy MJ. Localized benign and malignant fibrous tumors of the pleura: a clinicopathologic review of 223 cases. *Am J Surg Pathol* 1989;13:640–658.

60. Weisbrod GL, Yee AC. Computed tomographic diagnosis of a pedunculated fibrous mesothelioma. *J Canad Assoc Radiol* 1983;34:147–148.

61. Dedrick CG, McLoud TC, Shepard JO, Shipley RT. Computed tomography of localized pleural mesothelioma. *Am J Roentgenol* 1985;144:275–280.

62. Okike N, Bernatz PE, Woolner LB. Localized mesothelioma of the pleura: benign and malignant variants. *J Thorac Cardiovasc Surg* 1978;75:363–372.

63. Carter DC, Otis CN. Three types of spindle cell tumors of the pleura: fibroma, sarcoma, and sarcomatoid mesothelioma. *Am J Surg Path* 1988;12:747–753.

64. Buxton RC, Tan CS, Khine NM, Cuasay NS, Shor MJ, Spigos DG. Atypical transmural thoracic lipoma: CT diagnosis. *J Comput Assist Tomogr* 1988;12:196–198.

65. Munk PL, Muller NL. Pleural liposarcoma: CT diagnosis. *J Comput Assist Tomogr* 1988;12:709–710.

66. Chahinian AP, Pajak TF, Holland JF, Norton L, Ambinder RM, Mandel EM. Diffuse malignant mesothelioma: prospective evaluation of 69 patients. *Ann Intern Med* 1982;96:746–755.

67. Alexander E, Clark RA, Colley DP, Mitchell SE. CT of malignant pleural mesothelioma. *Am J Roentgenol* 1981;137:287–291.

68. McLoud TC, Woods BO, Carrington CB, Epler GR, Gaensler EA. Diffuse pleural thickening in an asbestos-exposed population: prevalence and causes. *Am J Roentgenol* 1985;144:9–18.

69. Lynch DA, Gamsu G, Ray CS, Aberle DR. Asbestos-related focal lung masses: manifestations on conventional and high-resolution CT scans. *Radiology* 1988;169:603–607.

70. Meyer PC. Metastatic carcinoma of the pleura. *Thorax* 1966;21:437–443.

71. Leff A, Hopewell PC, Costello J. Pleural effusion from malignancy. *Ann Intern Med* 1978;88:532–537.

72. Little AG, Kadowaki MH, Ferguson MK, Staszek VM, Skinner DB. Pleuro-peritoneal shunting. *Ann Surg* 1988;208:443–450.

73. Leung AN, Muller NL, Miller RR. CT in differential diagnosis of diffuse pleural disease. *Am J Roentgenol* 1990;154:487–492.

74. Lamki L, Cohen P, Driedger A. Malignant pleural effusion and Tc-99m MDP accumulation. *Clin Nucl Med* 1982;7:331–333.

75. Siegel ME, Walker Jr WJ, Campbell III JL. Accumulation of 99m Tc-diphosphonate in malignant pleural effusions: detection and verification. *J Nucl Med* 1975;16:883–885.

76. Babbell RW, Jackson DE, Conte FA. Technetium-99m MDP accumulation in a nonmalignant pleural effusion. *Clin Nucl Med* 1982;7:298–299.

77. Goldstein HA, Gefter WB. Detection of unsuspected malignant pleural effusion by bone scan. *Clin Nucl Med* 1984;9:556.

78. Castellino RA, Blank N, Hoppe RT, Cho C. Hodgkin disease: contributions of chest CT in the initial staging evaluation. *Radiology* 1986;160:603–605.

79. Shuman LS, Libshitz HI. Solid pleural manifestations of lymphoma. *Am J Roentgenol* 1984;142:269–273.

80. Sider L, Horton ES. Pleural effusion as a presentation of AIDS-related lymphoma. *Invest Radiol* 1989;24:150–153.

81. Rhea JT, van Sonnenberg E, McLoud TC. Basilar pneumothorax in supine adult. *Radiology* 1979;133:593–595.

82. Gordon R. The deep sulcus sign. *Radiology* 1980;136:25–27.

83. Tocino IM, Miller MH, Fairfax WR. Distribution of pneumothorax in the supine and semirecumbent critically ill adult. *Am J Roentgenol* 1985;144:901–905.

84. Chiles C, Ravin CE. Radiographic recognition of pneumothorax in the intensive care unit. *Crit Care Med* 1986;14:677–680.

85. Scott GC, Berger R, McKean HE. The role of atmospheric pressure variation in the development of spontaneous pneumothoraces. *Am Rev Respir Dis* 1989;139:659–662.

86. Nielsen PH, Jepsen SB, Olsen AD. Postoperative pleural effusion following upper abdominal surgery. *Chest* 1989;96:1133–1135.

87. Goodman LR. Postoperative chest radiograph. II. Alterations after major intrathoracic surgery. *Am J Roentgenol* 1980;134:803–813.

88. Light RW. Parapneumonic effusions and empyema. *Clin Chest Med* 1985;6:55–62.

89. Friedman PJ, Hellekant CAG. Radiologic recognition of bronchopleural fistula. *Radiology* 1977;124:289–295.

90. Stark DD, Federle MP, Goodman PC, Podrasky AE, Webb WR. Differentiating lung abscess and empyema: radiography and computed tomography. *Am J Roentgenol* 1983;141:163–167.

91. Bersack SR. Fluid collection in emphysematous bullae. *Am J Roentgenol* 1960;83:283–292.

92. Zinn WL, Naidich DP, Whelan CA, Litt AW, McCauley DI, Ettener NA. Fluid within preexisting pulmonary air-spaces: a potential pitfall in the CT differentiation of pleural from parenchymal disease. *J Comput Assist Tomogr* 1987;11:441–448.

93. Stark P, Gadziala N, Greene R. Fluid accumulation in preexisting pulmonary air spaces. *Am J Roentgenol* 1980;134:701–706.

94. Silverman SG, Mueller PR, Saini S, Hahn PF, et al. Thoracic empyema: management with image-guided catheter drainage. *Radiology* 1988;169:5–9.

95. Westcott JL. Percutaneous catheter drainage of pleural effusion and empyema. *Am J Roentgenol* 1985;144:1189–1193.

96. Reinhold C, Illescas FF, Atri M, Bret PM. Treatment of pleural effusions and pneumothorax with catheters placed percutaneously under imaging guidance. *Am J Roentgenol* 1989;152:1189–1191.

97. van Sonnenberg E, Nakamoto SK, Mueller PR, Casola G, et al. CT- and ultrasound-guided catheter drainage of empyemas after chest-tube failure. *Radiology* 1984;151:349–353.

98. O'Moore PV, Mueller PR, Simeone JF, Saini S, et al. Sonographic guidance in diagnostic and therapeutic interventions in the pleural space. *Am J Roentgenol* 1987;149:1–5.

99. Moulton JS, Moore PT, Menchini RA. Treatment of loculated pleural effusions with transcatheter intracavitary urokinase. *Am J Roentgenol* 1989;153:941–945.

100. Merriam MA, Cronan JJ, Dorfman GS, Lambiase RE, Haas RA. Radiographically guided percutaneous catheter drainage of pleural fluid collections. *Am J Roentgenol* 1988;151:1113–1116.

Thoracic Radiology, edited by
J.D. Newell, Jr., and R.D. Tarver,
Raven Press, Ltd., New York © 1993.

CHAPTER 8

Thoracic Aortic Imaging*

Imaging Strategies for Diagnosis

Janette D. Durham

Noninvasive imaging tests have taken on an increasingly important role in the evaluation of acquired disorders of the thoracic aorta, frequently obviating the need for aortography. The variety of diagnostic imaging tests now available have surprisingly confused rather than simplified the work-up of thoracic aortic disease. This stems from the lack of prospective comparison studies that demonstrate the strength of each new exam as it is promoted for a new indication. These studies are particularly difficult in this critically ill patient population. With time the best role of each imaging test will become obvious, and cost-effective screening tests that allow a reduction in aortography will be found. Currently it is important to look at the strengths and weaknesses of each test as suggested by the existing literature, so that an efficient diagnostic algorithm can be followed. A haphazard approach results in prohibitive time, cost, and risk to the patient.

The following is a discussion of the diagnostic evaluation of thoracic aortic aneurysm (TAA), traumatic aortic rupture (TAR), aortic dissection (AD), and aortic occlusive disease (AOD) of the thoracic aorta. It has been organized to define the important questions that must be answered in order to direct therapy and to assess the success of imaging tests in providing answers.

THORACIC AORTIC ANEURYSMS

A bulge in the wall of a blood vessel, whether localized or diffuse, is an aneurysm. True aneurysms histologi-cally have all three layers of vessel wall, including intima, media, and adventitia. Enlargement occurs symmetrically as a result of weakening of the media, and is either fusiform or cylindrical. Common causes of true aneurysms are atherosclerosis and cystic medial necrosis. False aneurysms have an incomplete wall due to penetration. They tend to be localized, enlarge asymmetrically, and are described as saccular. Common causes of false aneurysms are trauma and infection. Dissecting aneurysm is a misnomer. AD occurs when blood obtains access to the medial layer of a blood vessel and dissects the media, resulting in two parallel vascular channels. Aneurysms and dissection occur in different patient populations and have different causes.

Aortic aneurysms are found at autopsy in 2–4 percent of the population (1). The most common etiology for acquired TAA is atherosclerosis or medial degeneration of unknown etiology with superimposed atherosclerosis (2). Trauma is the second most common etiology and is discussed separately. Medial cystic degeneration, infection, syphilis, and aortitis are less common. Both the configuration and the location of thoracic aneurysms help predict etiology (3).

Aneurysms of the aortic sinus and tubular ascending aorta are usually the result of cystic medial necrosis either genetic (associated with Marfan or Ehlers–Danlos syndrome) or idiopathic. Typically there is fusiform enlargement of the ascending aorta, sparing the arch. These true aneurysms have little calcification, involve the sinuses of Valsalva symmetrically, result in aortic insufficiency, and are frequently complicated by dissection.

Infectious aneurysms occur when injured intima secondary to atherosclerosis, trauma, surgery, or catheterization is exposed to bacteria. Patients who are immunocompromised, use intravenous drugs, or who have bacterial endocarditis are at risk. Infection occurs by em-

J. D. Durham: Department of Radiology, University of Colorado Health Sciences Center, Denver, Colorado 80262.

* Figure 3 and parts of this chapter have been adapted from a chapter entitled, "Imaging of Acquired Thoracic and Abdominal Aortic Diseases," by J. D. Durham and J. A. Kaufman. In: Strandness D. E., Jr., van Breda A., eds. *Vascular Diseases, Surgical and Interventional Surgery.* 1993 (in preparation).

bolization, contiguous spread from an extra or intravascular source, or lymphangitic spread. The infection eventually destroys the elastic lamella, media, and adventitia. Infectious aneurysms are false, saccular aneurysms, most commonly located in the ascending aorta in proximity to an infected heart valve. Presentation may be insidious with uncontrolled sepsis and rupture.

Aortitis, aortic insufficiency, and aortic aneurysm are the cardiovascular complications of untreated syphilis. Syphilitic aneurysms are uncommon inflammatory aneurysms that develop 10–30 years after infection. They are thick-walled true aneurysms resulting from chronic inflammation that destroys the media. They tend to be asymmetric, saccular aneurysms with pencil-thin wall calcification, and perianeurysmal fibrosis. The ascending aorta, arch, and proximal descending aorta are involved in equal frequency. The aortic sinuses are typically spared.

Atherosclerotic aneurysms occur when intimal lesions cause the underlying media to atrophy and undergo fibrosis. Degeneration leads to dilation. Ultimately the vessel wall is reduced to a thin acellular, avascular connective tissue layer prone to rupture. Early changes in atherosclerosis may be limited to aortic ectasia, diffuse enlargement of the aortic lumen, and tortuosity. Progression leads to localized dilation or aneurysm. Atherosclerotic aneurysms involve the descending aorta distal to the left subclavian artery, most often in elderly males. Associated abdominal aneurysms are common. Thoracic aneurysms tend to be fusiform although a saccular appearance may occur.

Penetrating thoracic ulcer is a recently recognized complication of an atherosclerotic ulcer that ruptures into the media. Hemorrhage in the media mimics AD. Elderly, hypertensive males are at risk, and the propensity for rupture necessitates repair (4,5).

Discovery of a focal aneurysm of the proximal descending aorta at the aortic isthmus is suspicious for a previously undetected traumatic aneurysm. Two percent of patients that survive aortic rupture develop chronic aneurysms. These false aneurysms develop secondary atherosclerosis, resulting in smooth intimal calcification. The saccular, localized appearance and the location at the aortic isthmus help identify the etiology (6).

Indications for Imaging

Imaging nontraumatic TAAs is performed for four indications: diagnosis and surveillance of asymptomatic aneurysms, preoperative evaluation of asymptomatic aneurysms prior to elective repair, preoperative evaluation of symptomatic aneurysms prior to urgent or emergent repair, and follow-up after surgery for postoperative complications.

Diagnosis and Surveillance

Most patients with aortic aneurysms are either asymptomatic and diagnosis is made following plain radiography performed for other indications or have mild symptoms secondary to aneurysmal compression of adjacent structures. Plain radiographic diagnosis is confirmed by axial imaging with ultrasound (US), computed tomography (CT), or magnetic resonance imaging (MRI) in order to obtain an accurate aortic diameter; to define the configuration, location, and extent; and to assess for complications, including rupture. Surveillance is performed to determine aneurysmal enlargement or complications that would prompt repair.

Chest Radiographs

Aneurysms of the thoracic aorta produce masses in the mediastinum resulting in mediastinal widening. An ascending aortic aneurysm causes a convex contour to the right superior mediastinum on frontal radiographs and fills the retrosternal space on lateral radiographs. Involvement of the aortic root is hidden. An arch aneurysm may result in an aorticopulmonary window mass on a frontal projection that can be localized in the anterior-posterior dimension on the lateral. A descending aortic aneurysm produces a mass to the left of the spine on frontal radiographs, widening and displacing the left paraspinal line to the left. Intimal calcification can be seen in the majority of atherosclerotic aneurysms and helps identify the aortic wall. On the lateral radiograph both borders of the descending aorta may be surrounded by lung allowing visualization and measurement of aortic diameter. Left ventricle enlargement from aortic insufficiency, tracheal compression, and bone erosion are complications of the aneurysm (7,8).

Ultrasound

Aneurysms of the ascending aorta can be visualized in most patients by transthoracic echocardiography (TTE) (9). In addition the aortic valve can be studied for vegetations or dilation, aortic insufficiency confirmed, and pericardial fluid detected. Successful use of TTE depends on an appropriate ultrasonic window to study the ascending aorta within the thorax. This window is obscured by abnormal chest wall configuration, narrow intercostal spaces, obesity, pulmonary emphysema, and mechanical ventilation. Unfortunately the aortic arch and descending aorta are visualized infrequently, limiting the usefulness of this technology in the majority of patients with aneurysms (9).

The recent addition of transesophageal echocardiography (TEE) to TTE has improved the sensitivity of US for aortic pathology, with most of the present experience being confined to the diagnosis of AD. TEE allows evaluation of the ascending and descending thoracic aorta, except for a small segment of the aortic arch that is obscured by the trachea and proximal left bronchus. The abdominal aorta cannot be visualized. The exam has the advantage of being performed at the bedside in approximately 15 minutes. Cardiac arrhythmias account for minimal morbidity. A combination of TEE and TTE should improve the usefulness of US in diagnosis of TAA, but to date experience is limited.

Computerized Tomography

CT allows differentiation of aneurysms from nonvascular mediastinal or lung masses causing mediastinal widening. Measurement of aneurysmal size, detection of subtle calcification, evaluation of aortic wall thickness, and examination of the periaortic space are also accomplished. Dynamic incremental scanning of the entire thorax and abdomen with contiguous 10 mm scan collimation is performed. One hundred and fifty milliliters of ionic or nonionic contrast are mechanically injected with a short scan delay. Apparatus exterior to the chest, including chest leads, nasogastric tube, and respiratory equipment, need to be removed, and the arms positioned above the head to avoid artifacts. In addition, patient movement must be minimized. Early experience with helical scanning suggests that rapid scan times allow better vascular enhancement and decreased motion artifact. The tradeoff for speed is a loss in resolution (10).

Aneurysms are identified on CT images by focal or diffuse aortic dilation extending over a variable length. Thrombus is usually crescentic and circumferential, and may be separated from the aortic lumen after contrast administration. Measurement of correct aneurysmal size is important in determining a patient's prognosis and risk of rupture. CT allows accurate aortic measurement by revealing both the patent aortic lumen and intravascular thrombus. Aortography can only visualize the patent lumen, and aneurysm size is frequently underestimated, unless the aortic wall can be identified by calcification.

Normal aortic measurements by CT are 3.6 cm at the valve ring, 3.5 cm in the tubular ascending aorta, 2.6 cm in the proximal descending aorta, and 2.4 cm in the distal descending aorta (11). A simplistic approach to the diagnoses of aortic aneurysm is the recognition that the aorta should decrease in size as it proceeds distally, and any enlargement is pathologic. CT measurement of aortic diameter may be factitious when aortic tortuosity results in the measured segment obliquely traversing the scan plane. Narrow slice thickness and long axis reconstructions can help overcome this limitation (6).

Seventy-five percent of aneurysms have intimal calcification helping to identify the aortic wall. Localization of calcification peripherally helps exclude the diagnosis of AD. Displacement of calcification centrally suggests AD. Punctuate calcification within aneurysm thrombus can confuse this distinction, and other signs of AD must be used to support the diagnosis (12).

Magnetic Resonance Imaging

Axial spin echo image acquisition is used most frequently to diagnosis TAA. Cardiac gating is used to eliminate phase-encoding artifacts from cardiac motion and breathing. Gradient echo image acquisition can be used to enhance flow velocities and help distinguish slow flow from thrombus. Examination time with MRI is dependent on the number of acquisitions obtained, but 30 minutes appears to be the minimum. Acquisition of gradient echo and multiplanar images extends the exam. Pacemakers, intracranial aneurysm clips, intraocular metallic fragments, and a dependence on metallic monitoring equipment are absolute contraindications to MRI. Patient motion, inability to cooperate, and cardiac arrhythmias detract from the exam. Acutely ill, unstable patients are therefore not suitable candidates (13).

Imaging in oblique sagittal and coronal planes allows large field of view imaging with better examination of the aortic root and proximal descending aorta, difficult areas for CT (Fig. 1A,B). Small aneurysms that may be missed by axial CT images are more accurately demonstrated by sagittal MRI images (14). Preliminary experience with a combination of magnetic resonance angiography with MRI suggests moderate success at visualizing the origins of branch vessels. The disadvantages of MRI include the loss of signal secondary to calcification, and the exam cost compared with CT. No large comparative studies are yet available to demonstrate an advantage of MRI over CT in surveillance of TAA.

Elective Operative Repair

Operative repair is recommended when an ascending aortic aneurysm becomes greater than 6 cm in size, twice the size of the adjacent aorta, or when there is a rapid increase in size. Additional indications include symptomatic aortic insufficiency, tracheal or esophageal compression, bone erosion, infection, or emboli (15). Preoperative imaging is performed to ensure successful treatment with low morbidity and mortality. In order to plan the time of operation, the surgical approach, and the method of reconstruction, the following questions must be answered: What is the cranial and caudal extent? What is the location in respect to the great vessels and coronary arteries? What is the status of the aortic valve? What is the size and the extent of mural thrombus? What is the status of downstream vessels? What is the wall integrity? Is there fluid or fibrosis in the perivascular space? And, what other conditions or anatomic anomalies are present that might complicate surgery? A

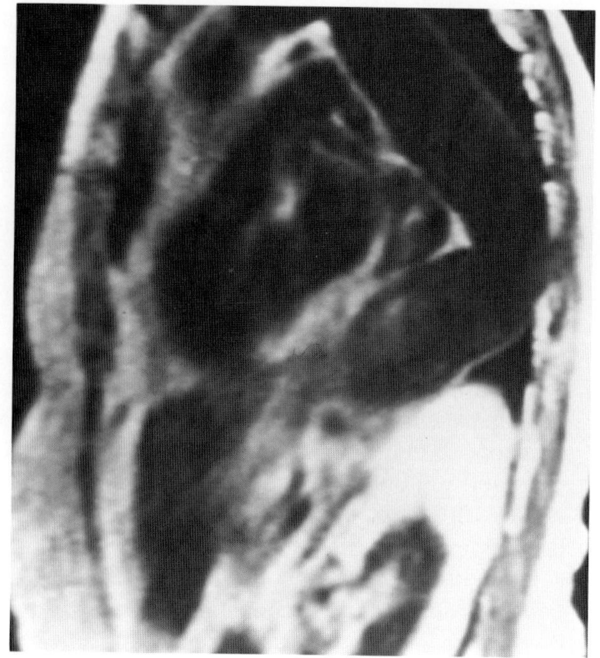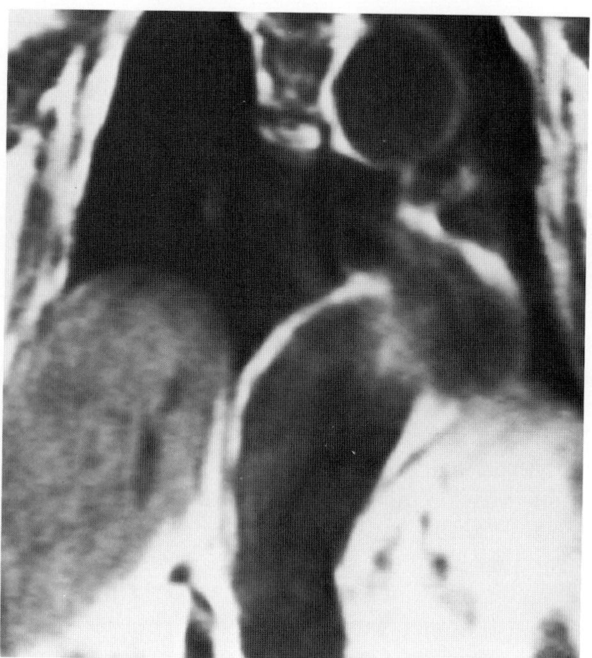

FIG. 1. *Technique:* Spine echo T1-weighted MRI images of the chest and abdomen [TR 365/TE 20 sagittal image of the chest and upper abdomen **(A)**; TR 375/TE 15 coronal image of the chest and upper abdomen **(B)**]. *Discussion:* The descending and abdominal aorta is enlarged from the left subclavian artery to the iliac bifurcation. The large field of view in both sagittal and coronal planes depicts the aneurysm course, allowing an accurate measurement of aneurysm size that might be overestimated on an axial image because of the striking elongation and tortuosity. *Diagnosis:* Atherosclerotic thoracoabdominal aneurysm. Courtesy of E. Kent Yucel, M.D., Massachusetts General Hospital, Boston.

combination of axial imaging with CT and aortography provides these answers. CT evaluates the aneurysm size and amount of thrombus, and the periaortic space for complications and anatomic anomalies. CT directs the surgical approach and the timing of operation. Aortography directs the type of surgical reconstruction performed by demonstrating the extent of the lesion, the status of the aortic valve, the involvement of branch vessels, and the downstream vasculature (16,17).

Thoracic Aortography

Conventional thoracic aortography is performed most often from a femoral approach using 6 or 7 Fr. catheters. Two views are routinely obtained, 45° right posterior oblique and straight anterior-posterior or 10° left posterior oblique projections, following injection of 60–70 ml of ionic or nonionic contrast. Intraarterial digital aortography in some authors' experience has proved adequate, replacing conventional filming, reducing the required catheter size to 5 Fr., and reducing contrast volume to 30–50 ml (18). Intravenous digital aortography has been abandoned due to insufficient resolution. Catheterization complications, even in the hands of radiologists in-training, are surprisingly minimal. Contrast-induced renal failure is the most common serious adverse outcome.

An aneurysm is demonstrated by aortography as a widened aortic lumen, either fusiform, cylindrical, or saccular. Aortic plaque and thrombus result in irregularity of the vessel wall. The size of the aneurysm portrayed is misleading, because the patent lumen is demonstrated, and thrombus masks the true aneurysm size. Identification of calcification or the soft tissue of the aortic wall suggests the true size. Aortography provides a road map of the aorta, precisely displaying the extent and location of the aneurysm. The origins of the coronary arteries and great vessels are evaluated to exclude involvement. Absence of branch vessels, even when the lumen is normal in size, suggests aneurysm. Thoracic aneurysms are frequently associated with abdominal aneurysms, and complete aortic evaluation of the downstream vessel is necessary to determine the extent of aorta requiring replacement.

Urgent or Emergent Repair of Symptomatic Aneurysms

Symptomatic aneurysm implies complications or expansion heralding imminent or existent rupture. Rupture occurs in 90 percent of patients with TAA by 5 years if untreated (2). Complications of ascending aortic aneurysms include cardiac ischemia, aortic insufficiency, and rupture into the pericardium. Descending aortic aneurysms rupture into the pleural space.

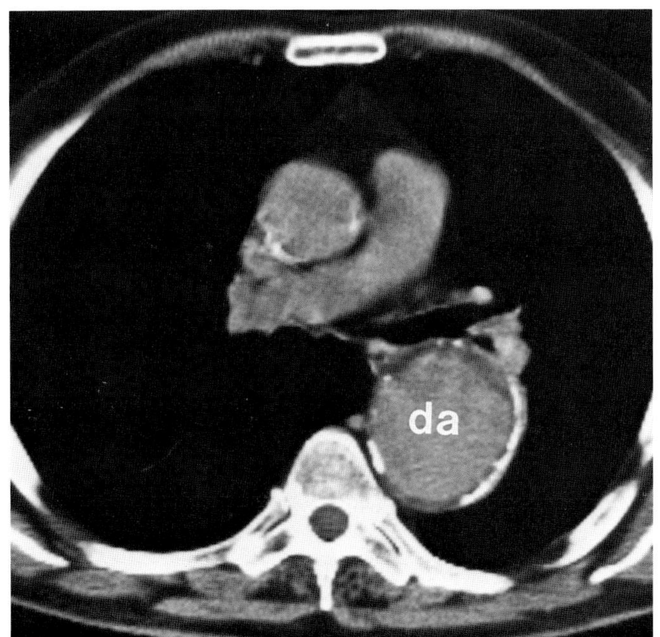

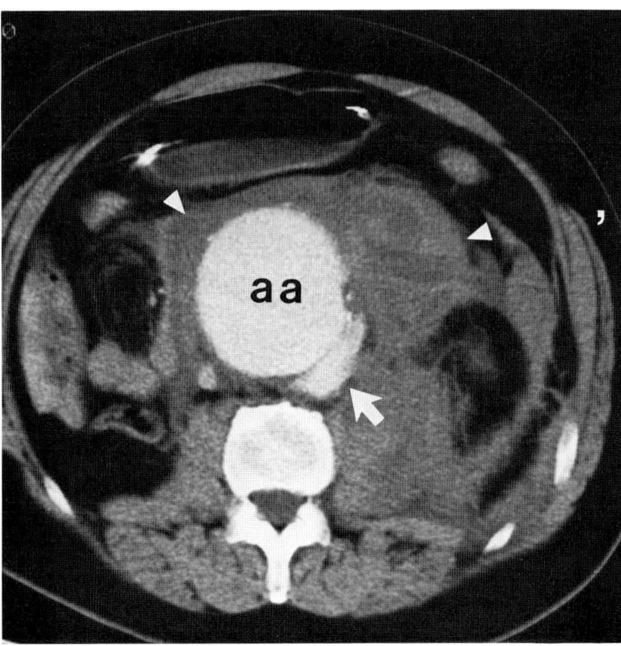

FIG. 2. *Technique:* Contrast-enhanced axial CT images though the descending aorta (**A**) and abdomen (**B**). *Discussion:* The descending aorta (*da*) is aneurysmal with peripheral calcification. There is minimal thrombus. The abdominal aorta (*aa*) is similarly enlarged. Besides contrast in the lumen of the vessel, there is a collection of contrast outside the lumen (*arrow*). In addition there is a large amount of perivascular fluid (*arrowheads*) diagnostic of rupture. *Diagnosis:* Thoracoabdominal aneurysm with rupture.

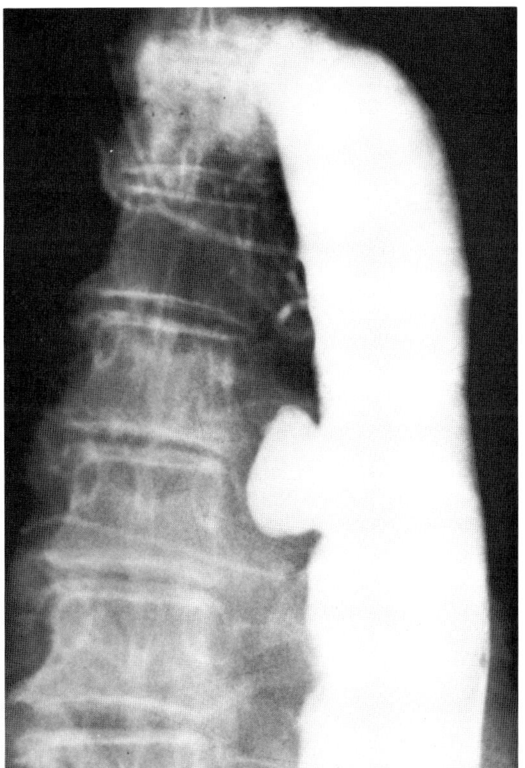

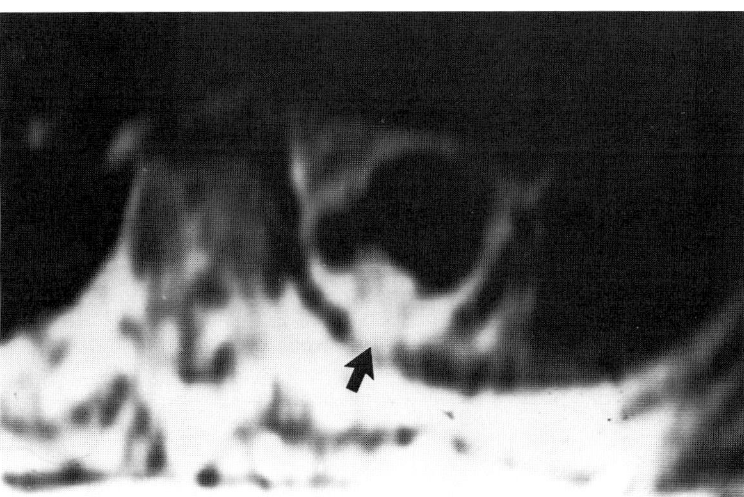

FIG. 3. *Technique:* Antero-posterior aortogram (**A**). T2-weighted spin echo axial MRI (TR 2000/TE48) through the descending aorta (**B**). *Discussion:* There is diffuse irregularity of the aortic wall suggesting atherosclerosis. A medial saccular outpouching from the aortic lumen is worrisome for a false aneurysm. The T2-weighted MRI image shows the outpouching in an axial plane. High signal in the aortic wall is consistent with hemorrhage (*arrow*). *Diagnosis:* Penetrating thoracic aortic ulcer. Courtesy of E. Kent Yucel, M.D., Massachusetts General Hospital, Boston.

The mortality associated with rupture necessitates an expeditious evaluation that contributes to operative survival but does not unjustifiably delay treatment. The ready availability of CT and its ability to assess the pericardial and periaortic spaces for blood permit its use prior to operative repair to confirm the clinical impression of rupture prior to operation (Fig. 2A,B) (19). In the abdominal aorta clinical misdiagnosis of rupture may be as high as 50 percent, resulting in unnecessary emergent surgery that is fraught with increased morbidity (20). The utility of CT for this indication is dependent on an imaging environment that can provide CT evaluation in 15 to 30 minutes. If time permits and the patient is hemodynamically stable, aortography can be performed to supply more detailed information prior to reconstruction. An unusual presentation of aortic rupture and a difficult diagnosis without MRI is penetrating thoracic aortic ulcer demonstrated in Fig. 3A,B.

Postoperative Complications

Postoperative complications include infection, false aneurysm formation, and rupture. These processes affect the periaortic tissues and are best detected by axial imaging with CT or MRI. Perigraft gas and fluid 6 weeks postoperatively suggest infection (21,22). A false aneurysm is detected by focal dilation, commonly at an anastomosis. Pericardial, pleural, or perivascular fluid is diagnostic of rupture. Angiography, except for demonstration of a pseudoaneurysm, contributes little to the diagnosis, but may be required for preoperative planning.

RECOMMENDATIONS FOR IMAGING TAA

Summary

Diagnosis and Surveillance
   chest radiography and CT
Preoperative Imaging of Asymptomatic Aneurysms
   CT and aortography
Preoperative Imaging of Symptomatic Aneurysm
   CT (and aortography, if time permits)
Postoperative Complications
   CT or MRI

TRAUMATIC AORTIC RUPTURE

A small fraction (15 percent) of patients who sustain blunt chest trauma from sudden deceleration will survive TAR and present for medical evaluation (23,24). Although autopsy specimens reveal isthmic tears to ac-

count for only 50 percent of injuries, 95 percent of patients who survive to undergo aortography will have tears that occur at the aortic isthmus, between the left subclavian artery and the ligamentum arteriosum (25–27). Rupture of the ascending aorta above the aortic valve, the descending aorta, or one of the proximal great vessels is rare.

The exact mechanism for aortic rupture is unknown. Rapid deceleration of the mobile ascending and descending aorta relative to a fixed aortic isthmus produces sheering of the aortic wall at the level of the isthmus (28). A recent hypothesis explains that compression of the bony thorax results in an osseous pinch of the aorta that causes laceration (29). Whatever the mechanism, the outcome is complete disruption of the intima, the intima and media, or all layers of the aortic wall, with the surrounding mediastinal tissues containing the rupture. Mediastinal hemorrhage is the result of simultaneous rupture of small arteries and veins in the mediastinum.

Clinical findings in patients with TAR are frequently absent, subtle, or unreliable. The suspicion of aortic injury is raised by the mechanism of injury suffered and confirmed by aortography. Surgical repair or replacement of the injured aorta is necessary for survival, with only 5 percent of untreated patients surviving 4 months (23). Imaging is performed for diagnosis and preoperative planning. The information that must be obtained prior to surgical repair includes the presence of aortic rupture, the location of the tear, and the presence of associated injury of the great vessels, coronary arteries, and aortic valve.

Chest Radiographs

In patients who have undergone a deceleration injury, the presence of mediastinal hematoma suggests severe chest trauma and raises the possibility of TAR. A chest radiograph that demonstrates a widened mediastinum with loss of the aortic contour is the most sensitive predictor of TAR, and the most frequent indication for aortography (30–34). The sensitivity of a widened mediastinum for TAR is 92–100 percent, but the specificity is only 10–67 percent (31,32,34). In older patients the mediastinum is more difficult to evaluate because of aortic ectasia and tortuosity, and is less useful in predicting TAR. Numerous accessory radiographic findings have been described to predict aortic injury, including loss of the aorticopulmonary window, rightward deviation of the trachea, left bronchus depression, rightward deviation of the nasogastric tube, widened left paraspinous stripe, apical cap, hemothorax, rib and clavicle fractures, and pulmonary contusion (25). Unfortunately most of these findings are prevalent in trauma populations without aortic injury and are useful only to support a suspicion of significant chest trauma.

The incidence of a normal chest radiograph in a patient with TAR is unknown but felt by most authors to be rare (35). In a recent investigation, TAR was found in 2 of 199 (1 percent) patients with negative chest radiographs (36). In a literature review by Woodring (37), 48 of 656 (7.3 percent) patients were found who had vascular injury and a radiographically normal mediastinum (37).

Computed Tomography

The possibility of false-negative chest radiographs has liberalized the indication for aortography to mechanism of injury alone without chest radiograph abnormality, and has increased the utilization of aortography so that TAR is found in my own experience in only 5 percent of patients studied. In order to decrease this seemingly overutilization of aortography, investigators have sought more specific screening tests. CT has undergone the most extensive evaluation and is discussed herein. MRI might be superior to CT in demonstrating TAR, but at present logistics make MRI inappropriate in critically ill patients who require close observation and monitoring.

Dynamic incremental contrast-enhanced scanning protocols to evaluate for aortic rupture have been described using contiguous 5 or 10 mm scan collimation through the upper mediastinum and aortic arch, with mechanical injection of 1 ml/second of contrast following a short scan delay. Technically inadequate or equivocal scans can be expected in 10 percent of patients (38).

Criteria for diagnosis of TAR, originally described by Heiberg et al. (39), has been used in subsequent publications. Direct signs of injury include false aneurysm; an intimal tear, a linear lucency within the opacified aortic lumen resulting from the torn edge of the aorta; and marginal irregularity of the opacified aortic lumen. Indirect signs include intramural or periaortic hematoma. Most authors have broadened these criteria to include any mediastinal hematoma, intraluminal, periaortic, or remote (Fig. 4, A–D) (40–43).

The superiority in resolution and speed of modern scanners strongly influences the success and feasibility of CT in diagnosing subtle aortic pathology. Table 1 shows the results of the most recent prospective series (36,38,40,44,45). In these studies unstable patients and patients felt at high risk for TAR were excluded, and all patients underwent subsequent abdominal CT to evaluate abdominal injuries. Selection criteria varied between reports in respect to chest radiograph findings and therefore the likelihood of injury varied from low probability of injury in patients who had normal chest radiographs to moderate probability of injury in patients who had equivocal or positive x-rays. Sensitivity and specificity

calculated from a combination of this data are 82 and 85 percent, respectively. Miller et al. (40) reported the only false-negative exams, including two cases of missed TAR and three cases of great vessel injury. None of the great vessel injuries required repair. One missed TAR was an error in diagnosis where mediastinal hematoma was missed, and the other case was technically inadequate. Raptopoulos et al. (36) evaluated all patients undergoing abdominal CT despite chest x-ray findings. They found CT to have a sensitivity of 100 percent and a specificity of 86 percent for TAR, compared with 80 and 62 percent, respectively, for chest radiography. Two patients with normal chest radiographs had abnormal CT studies and subsequent positive aortography.

Several authors have attempted to address the impact of CT on aortography, although no cost studies have been completed. Morgan et al. (45) evaluated 28 patients with abnormal chest x-rays, in addition to the group cited previously, who were felt to be at low risk for aortic injury. They were able to exclude mediastinal hemorrhage in 22 (78 percent) patients, and 19 (68 percent) were treated without aortography. Richardson et al. (38), who selected patients with equivocal or technically inadequate chest x-rays, found no hematoma in 77 percent of patients who were treated without aortography. Raptopoulos et al. (36) found that when CT was used as an adjunct to chest radiography to screen patients prior to aortography, utilization of aortography fell by 56 percent.

Several questions remain unanswered. Can CT be normal in the presence of aortic laceration or great vessel injury? Is there a role for CT screening in high-risk patients? And, can CT direct patients to surgery without aortography? Obviously large numbers of patients with TAR will need to be studied to find the true incidence of false-negative exams or the sensitivity of CT in detecting rare great vessel injuries. No investigator has attempted to study patients at high risk for TAR who have mediastinal hemorrhage evident on chest radiographs. The number of positive CT studies that have been found to date is therefore small, making the false-negative rate more difficult to evaluate and leaving the role of CT in high-risk patients unknown. All authors recommend aortography prior to surgical exploration, because most positive CT exams reflect the presence of mediastinal hematoma. The false-positive rate for CT calculated from Table 4 is 84% (positive predictive value 16%) (Fig. 5) (36,38,40,44,45).

The administration of additional contrast to trauma patients who may require subsequent aortography is the major medical risk of performing CT. Fortunately the contrast requirement can be reduced if the exam is limited to the ascending and proximal descending aorta, the area of interest. The investment of time to obtain a scan is the second concern. Obviously no patient who is hemo-

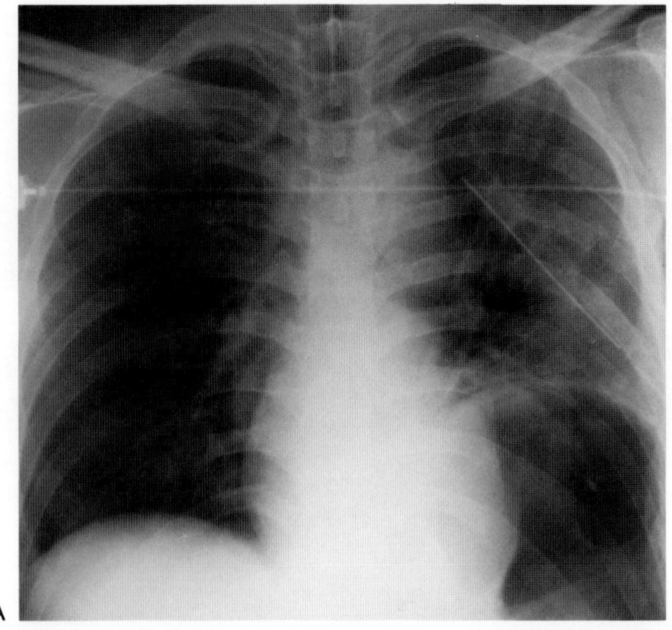

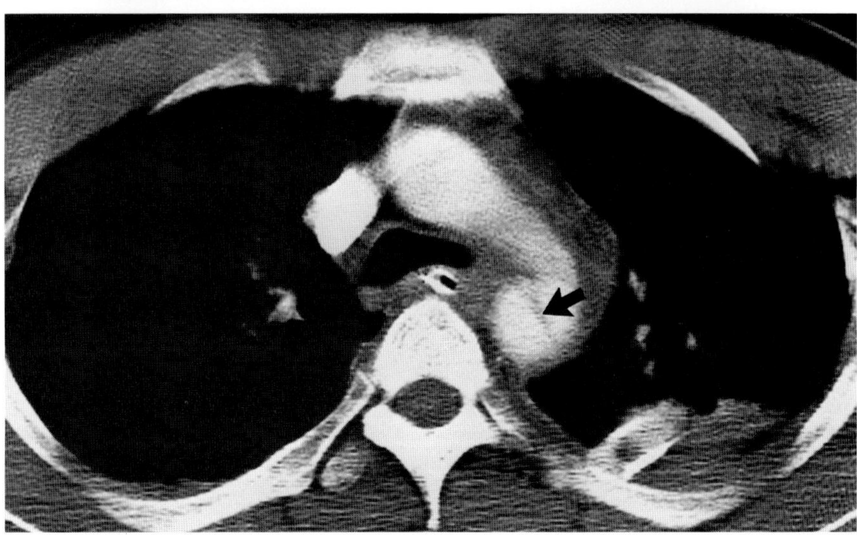

FIG. 4. *Technique:* Supine frontal chest radiograph (**A**). Contrast-enhanced 10 mm axial CT images through the aortic arch (**B**) and descending aorta (**C**). Right posterior oblique aortogram (**D**). *Discussion:* The antero-posterior chest film demonstrates a left chest tube and endotracheal (ET) tube. There is elevation of the left diaphragm with left lung base atelectasis. The aortic arch is indistinct and the aorticopulmonary window is full. CT images reveal mediastinal fluid surrounding the aortic arch and descending aorta. The proximal descending aorta is enlarged, and there is a filling defect (intimal flap) traversing the lumen (*arrow*). These findings are direct evidence for aortic rupture. Aortography confirms the presence of a false aneurysm in the typical location at the aortic isthmus. *Diagnosis:* Traumatic aortic rupture and diaphragmatic hernia. Courtesy of Marsha J. Heinig, M.D., Ph.D., Denver General Hospital, Denver.

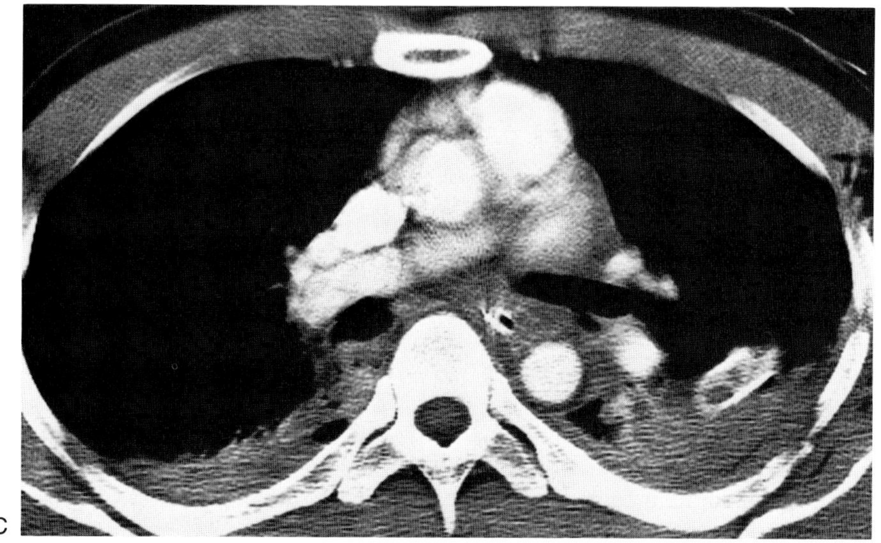

C

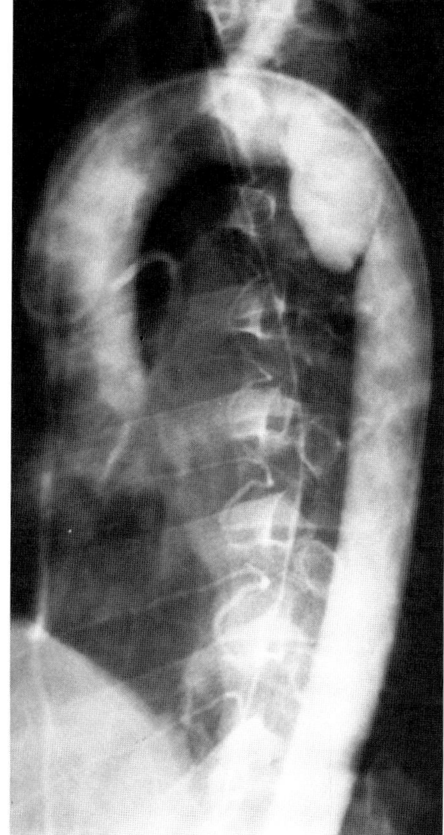

D

FIG. 4. *Continued.*

TABLE 1. *Results of CT in TAR*

Author	Patients	Chest x-ray	CT results vs. aortography/surgical/clinical follow-up			
			TP	FN	TN	FP
Miller, 1989	104	P	6	5	62	31
Maydayag, 1991	93	N	1	0	83	9
Richardson, 1991	90	E	4	0	63	23
Raptopoulos, 1992	326	P&N	10	0	272	44
Morgan, 1992	160	N	1	0	152	7
Total	773		22	5	632	114

P, positive; N, negative; E, equivocal; TP, true positive; FP, false positive; TN, true negative; FN, false negative.

dynamically unstable should undergo CT examination of any kind, and the addition of this step to the work-up of stable patients largely depends on an imaging department that is organized to investigate critically ill patients efficiently. CT examination of the aorta can easily be added to CT evaluation of the head or abdomen, requiring only 15–20 additional minutes (42).

Ultrasound

The use of TEE for screening patients with TAR has recently been suggested by Sparkes et al. (46), who studied a series of 11 patients with chest trauma, including six patients with arteriographic proof of TAR. They identified TAR in three patients, and excluded it in three patients with false-positive aortograms (one patient confirmed surgically and two patients confirmed clinically). This preliminary experience represents a selected group of patients likely to have injury, and investigators were aware of aortographic findings at the time of evaluation. The simplicity, low-cost, and quickness with which TEE can be performed makes this test worthy of future investigation.

Thoracic Aortography

Arteriographically, the torn edges of the intima can be seen as sharp, transverse linear defects. Intimal injuries may be multiple and discontinuous. Changes in the outer aortic wall may be absent, with intimal injury the evidence of laceration range from subtle irregularity of the aortic contour to a false aneurysm. Extravasation of contrast through the injured wall is rare. Injuries at the isthmus are associated with injuries of the great vessels in 5 percent of cases, including stenosis or thrombosis secondary to intimal injury, or rupture with false aneurysm (47). Tears of the ascending aorta may be associated with cardiac, coronary artery, and aortic valve injuries.

Conventional aortography has been reported to have a 100 percent sensitivity and 99 percent specificity for the diagnosis of TAR, with a positive predictive value of 97 percent and a negative predictive value of 100 percent (48). The 1–2 percent false-positive rate necessitates a rare negative exploration. The most common reason for an equivocal or false-positive aortogram is an atypical ductus bump. The ductus usually forms gentle obtuse angles at its junction with the aortic wall; however, a few

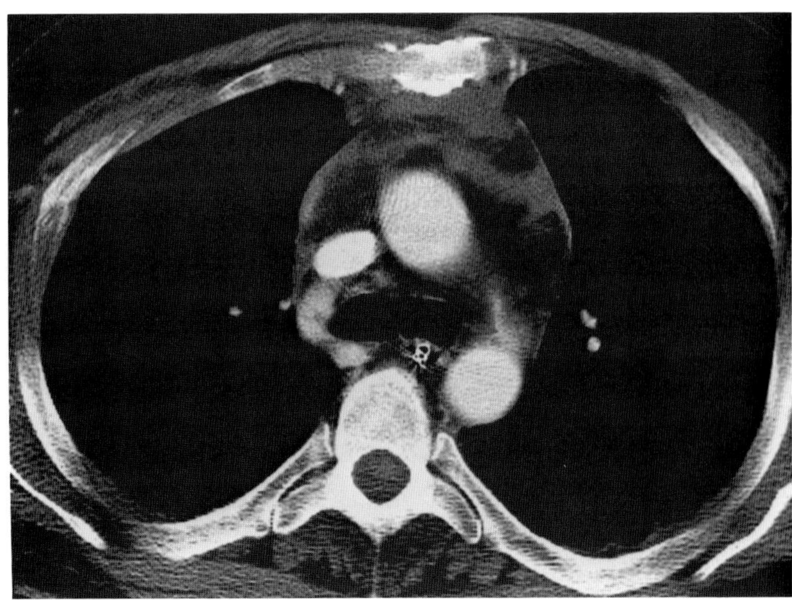

FIG. 5. *Technique:* Contrast-enhanced 10 mm axial CT just inferior to the aortic arch. *Discussion:* A large amount of anterior mediastinal fluid is present. This indirect evidence of aortic rupture requires further evaluation with aortography. Mediastinal hemorrhage will account for a 80–90 percent false-positive rate. *Diagnosis:* Mediastinal hemorrhage without aortic injury demonstrated by aortography. Courtesy of Marsha J. Heinig, M.D., Ph.D., Denver General Hospital, Denver.

patients will have an acute angle superiorly that can cause uncertainty. The absence of an intimal flap helps distinguish this normal variant (49).

A report of two patients with TAR who died during aortography underscores the importance of avoiding any catheter manipulation in the region of potentially injured aorta (50). Other reported complications have been rare, despite the critical patient population being studied. The administration of contrast to patients who have recently been treated for shock is the greatest concern. Aortography for this indication takes an average of 70 minutes, including 30 minutes of preparation and postangiography care. Digital imaging can reduce the time required for acquiring images from 40 to 20 minutes (18). Patients who are comatose or intoxicated may be difficult to study with digital acquisition.

RECOMMENDATIONS FOR IMAGING TAR

Despite its poor specificity, chest radiography remains the most widely used screening test for aortic injury. The use of CT to screen for TAR is still investigational, and appropriate only in institutions were CT can be provided in expeditious fashion and is indicated already for evaluation of abdominal trauma. Aortography remains the most direct and accurate diagnostic test for TAR with little patient risk, and is required in all patients undergoing operative repair. The cost and personnel requirement to provide emergency aortography to a group of patients who are going to have the suspected disease as infrequently as 10 percent provide the motivation for seeking a more specific screening exam.

The multiplicity of injuries resulting from high-speed injuries demands a rapid diagnostic plan. In unstable patients peritoneal lavage and emergent exploration to control major abdominal hemorrhage are performed. If chest radiography suggests aortic injury and the patient cannot be stabilized, thoracotomy is indicated without imaging tests of any kind. In hemodynamically stable patients who have suffered a deceleration injury and have chest radiographs that demonstrate mediastinal hemorrhage or suggest aortic injury, aortography should be performed immediately.

Patients who are felt to be at high risk because of the type of injury sustained and who have normal chest x-rays, and patients at low or moderate risk but who have equivocal or technically inadequate chest x-rays, can be screened with CT prior to abdominal CT. If the mediastinum is normal, the patient is observed and followed with serial chest radiography. If mediastinal hematoma or any direct evidence of TAR is present, the patient undergoes aortography. Even with the addition of chest CT to an already complex work-up, one can expect the majority of patients to be in the operating room within 4 hours of presentation (51).

Summary

  Diagnosis and Preoperative Planning
    Normal chest radiograph
      High risk: CT
      Low-moderate risk: observe
    Equivocal or inadequate chest radiograph
      Low-moderate risk: CT
    Abnormal chest radiograph
      Aortography

AORTIC DISSECTION

AD is most commonly thought to occur as a result of a structural defect in or degeneration of the aortic media. Blood gains entry to the media and dissects the aortic wall. Patients with AD who are younger than 40 frequently have genetic cystic medial necrosis (Marfan syndrome). Older patients have smooth muscle degeneration related to aging and hypertension (52). The recognition of medial dissections that occur in the absence of intimal injury supports a structural abnormality of the media as the etiologic factor. Although this presentation of disease has been reported in only 5 percent of surgical and autopsy series, recent recognition by MRI and CT suggests a higher incidence (53). Bleeding from the vasa vasorum into the media is suspected. An alternative theory for the cause of AD proposes intimal trauma as the initial injury that allows blood to enter the media even if the media is normal or near normal. This theory is supported by the common sites for intimal injury in dissection occurring at the same locations as TAR, the supravalvular ascending aorta and the aortic isthmus.

AD results in the development of two aortic channels, a native or true channel that is compressed by an abnormal medial or false channel. The two channels are separated by the intima. The false channel spirals around the true channel from the right, anterior ascending aorta, to the superior, posterior arch, to the left, posterior descending aorta. With time the false channel endothelializes and may calcify.

After gaining entry into the media, blood may reenter the true lumen, come to a halt, or rupture into the pericardium, pleural space, or periaortic tissues. Communications between the true and false channel can be multiple. Most often dissection occurs in an antegrade direction, but retrograde dissection from an intimal injury at the aortic isthmus also occurs. The arch and iliac arteries are involved in half, and renal arteries in one-fourth of autopsied patients, but less frequently in survivors (54).

Since prognosis and treatment depend on the segment of involved aorta, classification is based on location. Two classification schemes are commonly used. A Stanford A dissection involves the ascending aorta, and a B dissection involves the descending aorta beginning distal to the left subclavian artery (55). The DeBakey classification differentiates type A lesions into DeBakey I lesions that extend from the ascending aorta to involve the descending aorta and type II lesions that are confined to the ascending aorta. A DeBakey III lesion is similar to a Stanford B lesion (56). The incidence of DeBakey I, II, and III dissections is 51, 6, and 42 percent, respectively (57). Dissections that present within 2 weeks of the event are considered acute—the rest chronic.

Medical treatment is directed toward immediate and long-term control of hypertension and reduction of pulse pressure. This is the standard therapy for uncomplicated Stanford B dissections. Surgery for B dissections is necessary when complications develop, including rupture, vascular compromise, pain, extension of dissection, or aneurysmal enlargement of the false channel (52). Stanford A dissections require immediate surgery because of the tendency for rupture, coronary artery occlusion, and acute aortic insufficiency. The goal of surgical treatment is to prevent extension of the dissection to the aortic root and to prevent rupture. Therapy includes correction of aortic insufficiency, either by valve replacement or resuspension, replacement or less commonly repair of the ascending aorta, preventing communication of the false channel with the aortic root, and coronary artery reconstruction if needed (58,59). The persistence of the false channel following operative repair due to multiple persistent communications between the true and false channel argues that repair of the proximal intimal injury site may not be mandatory, as long as the injury is separated from the aortic valve by an aortic graft (60,61).

Large series of untreated patients with type A AD have a 75% mortality in the first 2 weeks, and 90 percent mortality by 3 months. Early survival following surgical repair of Stanford A dissections is greater than 80 percent. Five-year survival is 65 percent, and 10-year survival is 40 percent (52,58,59). Neurologic compromise is the most devastating morbidity and is as high as 28 percent after thoracoabdominal procedures (58).

Indications for Imaging

There are two indications for imaging patients with suspected or known AD, diagnosis and preoperative imaging of acute AD, and surveillance of postoperative and chronic AD.

Diagnosis and Preoperative Imaging of Acute AD

Imaging in the setting of suspected acute dissection is performed to confirm the diagnosis, and to localize the aortic injury to the ascending or descending aorta in order to direct therapy. Other important information includes the competency of the aortic valve, and the involvement of the coronary arteries, great vessels, and abdominal vessels when there is evidence of visceral or renal ischemia. Correctly identifying the site of intimal tear and other communications between the true and false channels (entry and reentry points) may not be important if the surgical approach used does not focus on correction of the intimal injury but instead on proximal reconstruction and valve replacement (40,52).

Chest Radiographs

Although routine chest radiographs tend to be abnormal with evidence of a widened mediastinum, this finding is nonspecific and common in a population of elderly males. Twenty-five percent of patients with acute AD will have normal chest radiographs (54). The finding of mediastinal widening is most helpful when previous radiographs reveal this finding is acute. Internal displacement of calcification from the peripheral wall of the aorta and disparity in the size of the ascending and descending aorta are other suspicious signs.

Ultrasound

TTE has been used to screen patients for AD, with a sensitivity ranging from 77–80 percent (62). The descending aorta is not well visualized in 30 percent of cases, making diagnosis of type B lesions difficult. TEE has improved the sensitivity of US, particularly for type B lesions. Diagnostic criteria include the identification of two lumens with a separating intimal flap, detection of a thrombosed lumen with displaced intimal calcification or separation of intimal layers by thrombus, and identification of intimal tears by disruption in the continuity of the flap, with fluttering of the ruptured intimal borders.

Hashimoto et al. (63) evaluated TEE in comparison with TTE and CT in a series of 22 patients with AD, 12 with surgical confirmation. TEE successfully made the diagnosis of AD and identified the involved aortic segment in all patients, and identified the site of intimal tear in 17. TTE failed to make the diagnosis in seven patients, failed to accurately localize the involved aortic segment in 11, and failed to diagnose the site of intimal tear in 17. CT, although as successful as TEE in identifying the intimal flap and localizing the involved aortic segment, was unable to diagnose the site of intimal tear in any patient. TTE and TEE were successful in identifying aortic regurgitation in 12 of the 17 patients confirmed by aortography.

A comparative study by Erbel et al. (62) determined the sensitivity and specificity of combined TTE and TEE compared with CT and aortography in 164 patients with suspected AD, 71 patients with autopsy or surgical proof of AD, and 82 patients with proof by two or more imaging tests. The sensitivity of TTE and TEE (98 percent) was superior to both CT (83 percent) and aortography (88 percent). False-positive exams with TEE occurred in two patients with aortic ectasia because of reverberation artifact in the ascending aorta, and false-negative exams in one patient with a small localized tear of the aortic root missed also by aortography and subsequently detected at surgery.

In 29 patients evaluated by TEE, 22 of which had subsequent aortography and 22 CT, Mügge et al. (64) found discrepancies in the diagnosis of seven patients. Aortography in one and CT in three patients failed to identify AD due to a large tear, with similar blood flow in both the true and false lumen. In addition CT was unable to diagnose AD in three patients with proximal AD due to a thrombosed false channel.

These data suggest that the presence and location of dissection and the site of intimal tear are diagnosed more frequently with TEE than with TTE, CT, and even the gold standard aortography, especially in the circumstance of a large tear with rapid flow through the false channel or the opposite extreme when the false channel is thrombosed. In addition, TEE allows the detection of complications of AD, including aortic regurgitation, pericardial effusion, left pleural effusion, abnormal cardiac wall motion, and compression of cardiac structures (57). TEE cannot evaluate the coronary arteries and great vessels. Angiography is still necessary prior to surgical repair.

Computed Tomography

CT is currently the most widely used screening test for AD because of its availability. Diagnosis depends on the demonstration of the true and false channels within the aortic lumen, separated by an intimal flap following administration of intravenous contrast media (65–68). Aortic wall thickening, widening of the aorta, clotted blood in the false lumen, inward displacement of intimal calcification, and compression of the true lumen support the diagnosis of AD. Pleural, mediastinal, and pericardial fluid suggest rupture and herald death.

Accurate diagnosis relies on high-quality exams with appropriately timed contrast media administration. Initial protocols utilized dynamic nonincremental scanning at three levels through the arch during the administration of contrast. Decreased scanning times now allow the entire ascending aorta to be imaged during mechanical contrast injection, with 5 to 10 mm scan collimation. Images must be reviewed at multiple window and level settings to avoid missing subtle differences in enhancement between the true and false channels, and to visualize the intimal flap.

Extensive experience with the use of CT for evaluation of acute AD exists. Three studies are presented in Table 2 (65,67,68). The sensitivity and specificity of CT using a combination of this data is 93 and 99 percent, respectively. False-negative studies have been reported when simultaneous or equal opacification of the true and false channels occurs, or when there is complete thrombosis of the false lumen, making differentiation from TAA difficult (64,69). The aortic root and the proximal descending aorta are difficult to evaluate because of artifact and volume averaging in these areas.

Although CT is sensitive for the presence of AD and can separate type A and B lesions, it does not evaluate the aortic valve, the coronary arteries, or the great vessels. The entry site is not established. Therefore, any patient requiring surgery, including patients with type A or symptomatic B lesions, must subsequently undergo aortography. CT is adequate for evaluation of patients with asymptomatic B lesions. The double dose of contrast that patients with acute AD require when CT is used prior to aortography is less than ideal.

Magnetic Resonance Imaging

The inherent contrast between flowing blood and soft tissue allows visualization of the intimal flap as a linear structure of medium signal intensity surrounded by signal void in the true and false channels on spin echo MRI (Fig. 6). Unlike CT, similar flow in the true and false channels does not mask the flap. MRI is valuable in the diagnosis of intramural hemorrhage without intimal tear secondary to vasa vasorum rupture within the wall. This results in medial hematoma demonstrated by high-signal intensity on T1 images. This finding is missed at aortography.

TABLE 2. *Results of CT in acute AD*

Author	Patients	CT results vs. aortography/surgical follow-up			
		TP	FP	TN	FN
Oudkerk, 1983	26	21	0	5	0
Thorsen, 1983	42	17	1	24	0
Vasile, 1986	137	54	0	76	7
Total	205	92	1	105	7

TP, true positive; FP, false positive; TN, true negative; FN, false negative.

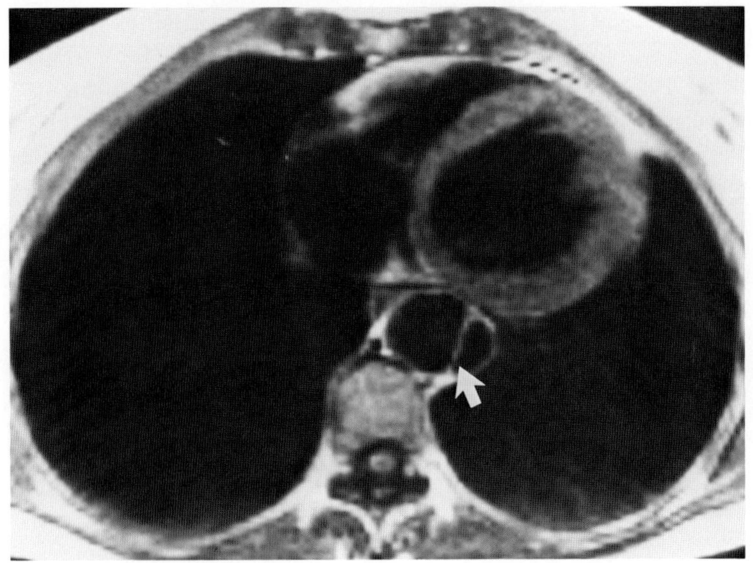

FIG. 6. *Technique:* T1-weighted axial MRI through the midchest. *Discussion:* Within the descending aorta, there is a linear line of intermediate signal intensity (*arrow*) separating the two channels. The medial channel is large and compresses the lateral channel, suggesting that the true aortic lumen is the lateral channel. The ascending aorta is not involved. *Diagnosis:* Type B aortic dissection. Courtesy of David A. Lynch, M.B., University of Colorado Health Sciences Center, Denver.

Spin echo image acquisition in the transverse plane is used most commonly. Gradient echo acquisition can be used to enhance flow velocities and identify entry sites, as well as distinguish slow flow in the false channel from thrombus.

Kerstin-Sommerhoff et al. (70) studied 54 patients, 23 with AD, to evaluate the effect of experience level on the sensitivity of MRI for acute AD. Readers with three levels of experience were studied. The most experienced reader had a sensitivity of 96 percent, with a 100 percent specificity; the least experienced reader had a sensitivity of 78 percent, with a 94 percent specificity. Fruehwald et al. (71) reported a comparison study of MRI with TTE, CT, and aortography that demonstrated a sensitivity of MRI for AD of 100 percent compared with 44 percent for TTE, 83 percent for CT, and 77 percent for aortography. Aortography results were compromised by the use of intravenous digital angiographic examination in 20 percent of the patients.

Frequent anatomic and artifactual findings that mimic AD include the left brachiocephalic vein, arch artery origins, superior pericardial recess, aortic plaque, apposition of the azygos vein and descending aorta, mediastinal fibrosis, subacute thrombus on gradient echo images, and motion induced phase encoding artifacts (72).

Just as with CT, the coronary arteries, great vessels, and aortic valve are not evaluated by MRI, therefore acute type A dissections and symptomatic B dissections will need subsequent aortography prior to surgery. MRI is sufficient for evaluation of acute type B dissections and has the advantage over CT of not requiring contrast, multiplanar imaging, better evaluation of the aortic root, and improved sensitivity. A decided disadvantage is the cost of the exam, which, in our institution, approaches aortography.

Thoracic Aortography

Visualization of the intimal flap separating the true and false channels is the hallmark of dissection on aortography. Other signs of AD include narrowing and compression of the true lumen by the nonopacified false lumen, an abnormal catheter position separated from the outer wall of the aorta, differential opacification of the two channels, occluded branch vessels, aortic wall thickening, and aortic insufficiency (Fig. 7A,B). Aortography is the only imaging method that is able to define the involvement of the coronary arteries and branch vessels, and assess the involvement and function of the aortic valve. The exact site of entry and reentry can be demonstrated in some but not all cases.

Pitfalls include failure to opacify a thrombosed false lumen, necessitating the radiographic recognition of aortic wall thickening to make the diagnosis, simultaneous opacification of both channels hiding the intimal flap, and missing small localized dissections near the aortic root. Aortography cannot diagnose dissection that occurs without intimal injury.

Because coronary arteriography may be necessary prior to surgical repair, cineangiography may be performed rather than conventional or digital arteriography. The ability to image at 30 frames/second makes cineangiography well suited to evaluate the dynamic action of the aortic valve, the motion of an intimal flap, and entry and reentry sites (73,74). The tradeoff for improved temporal imaging is a loss of spatial resolution when the descending aorta is panned as a bolus of contrast proceeds down the aorta. This hinders the diagnosis of dissection in subtle cases and limits the understanding of branch vessel involvement in the abdomen. Subsequent conventional angiography may be necessary.

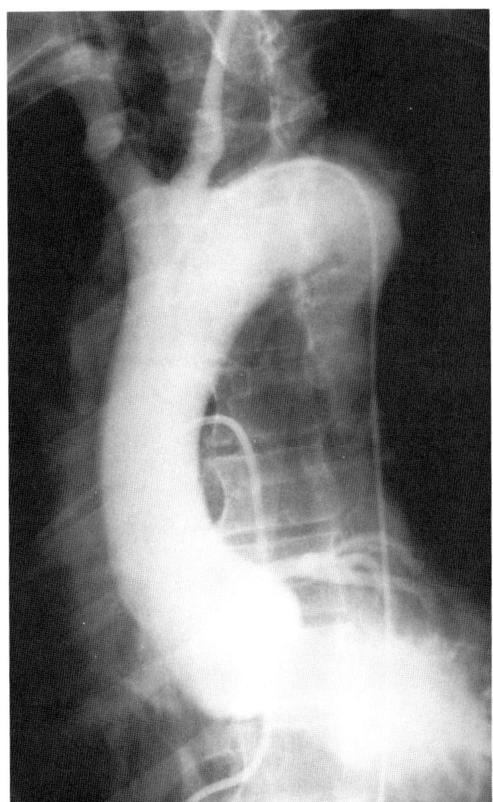
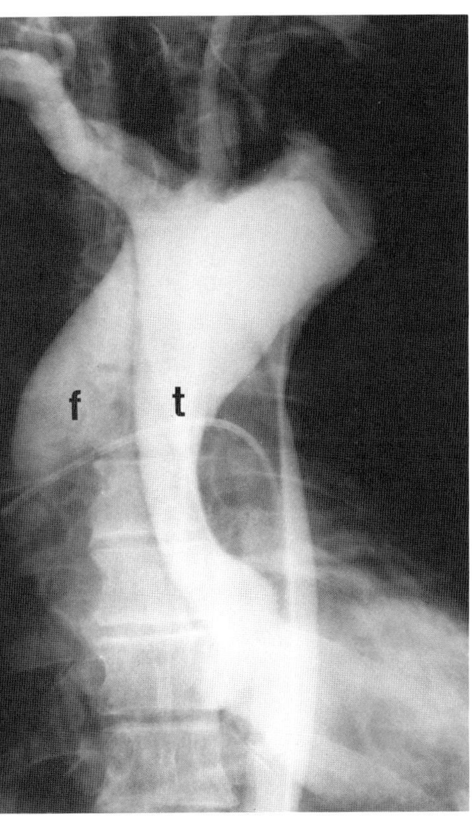

FIG. 7. *Technique:* Right posterior oblique (**A**) and antero-posterior (**B**) aortogram. *Discussion:* The ascending aorta is narrowed. The left coronary artery fills, but the right does not. A later film shows slow opacification of a second false channel (*f*) that is large and compresses the medial true channel (*t*). Both channels continue into the descending aorta. An intimal flap separates the two channels. The two channels extend into the innominate and left carotid. The left subclavian artery fills slowly. There is aortic insufficiency. *Diagnosis:* Type A aortic dissection with left coronary, right innominate, left carotid, and left subclavian artery involvement, and aortic valvular insufficiency.

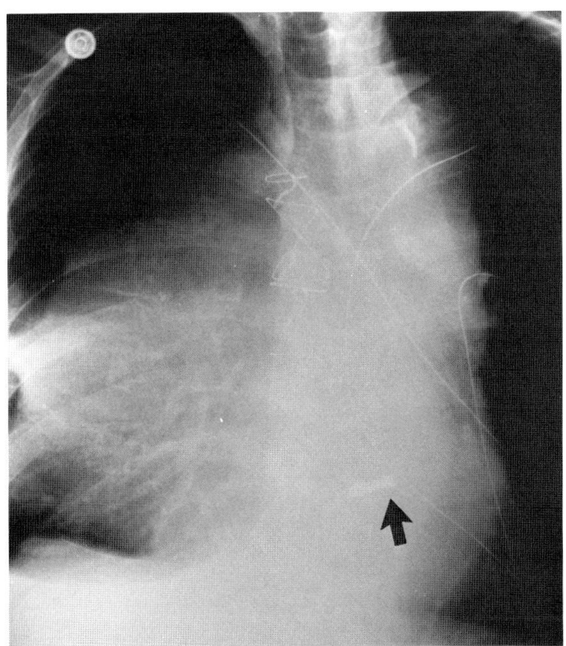
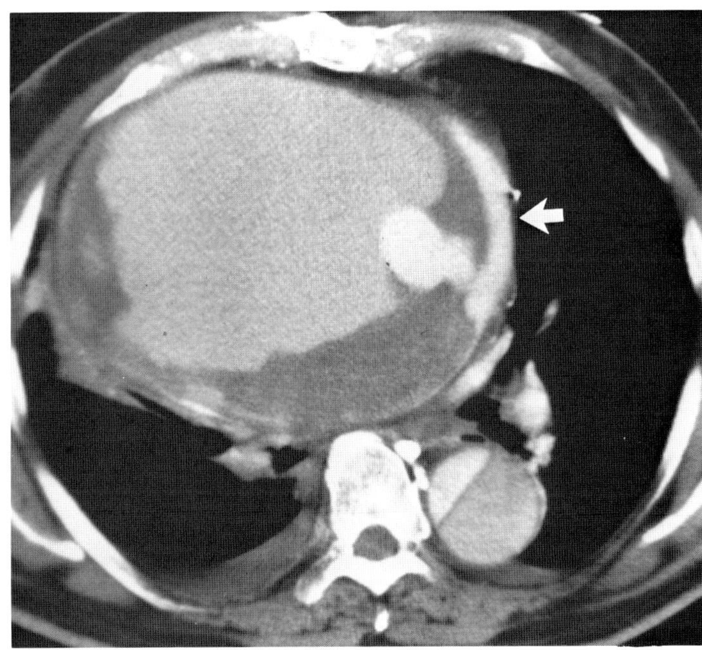

FIG. 8. *Technique:* Erect frontal chest radiograph (**A**). Contrast-enhanced 10 mm axial CT through the midaortic arch (**B**). *Discussion:* On the chest film a prosthetic aortic valve is evident as well as sternotomy wires. To the right of the spine there is a large mass that obliterates the right heart border and extends to obscure the right lung. CT demonstrates two channels in the descending aorta diagnostic of chronic aortic dissection. Contrast extravasates from the ascending aorta into a large thrombus filled mass that compresses the ascending aorta (*arrow*). *Diagnosis:* False aneurysm of the ascending aorta complicating aortic grafting and aortic valve replacement for type A aortic dissection.

Surveillance of Postoperative and Chronic AD

Following surgical therapy for type A dissection, 40 percent of patients may require repeat operation for complications (60). Indications for reoperation of type A AD or operative repair of type B AD include an enlarging thoracic false channel, pseudoaneurysm formation, redissection, extension of dissection, dilation of a sinus of Valsalva, persistence of mediastinal or pericardial fluid, and ischemia resulting from branch vessel involvement (Fig. 8A,B) (60,61).

Either CT or MRI can be used to survey patients with chronic or postoperative AD, and demonstrate subsequent changes in the true and false lumens, including size, patency, thrombosis, and calcification (60,75). CT surveillance has added to our understanding of the usual postoperative course, including the persistence of the false channel in 70–90 percent of patients due to multiple fenestrations between the true and false lumen that are not obliterated with surgery (60,76,77). The persistence of the false lumen in postoperative and chronic AD emphasizes the importance of the investigation of vital arteries threatened by ischemia (6,77).

RECOMMENDATIONS FOR IMAGING AD

Currently TEE appears to be the most appealing screening test for acute AD because it determines accurately which patients require aortography and surgery, with minimal morbidity. When it is not available CT may be used in its place; however, if there is a high suspicion for type A AD, immediate aortography is more expeditious, and avoids the large volume of contrast required to perform both CT and aortography. If a type A lesion is found by TEE or CT, aortography is pursued. Type B dissections found by TEE need to be further evaluated with CT or MRI to confirm the diagnosis and provide a baseline exam. CT or MRI are adequate for surveillance of chronic and postoperative dissections, reserving aortography for preoperative evaluation when complications develop.

Summary

Acute Dissection
  Positive TEE
    If type A: aortography
    If type B: MRI

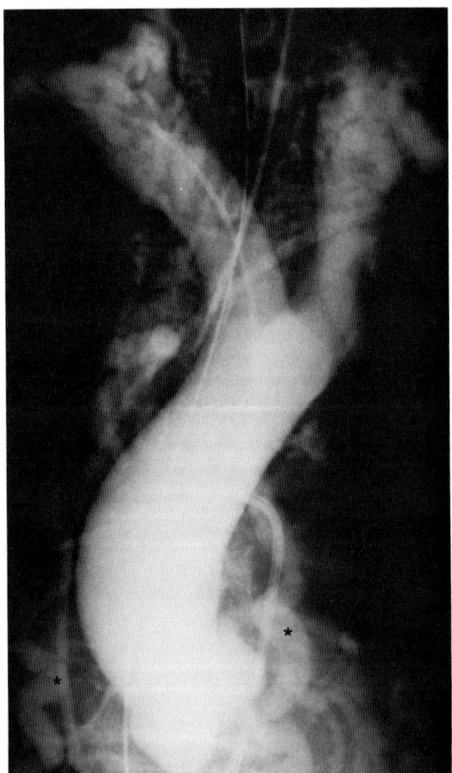
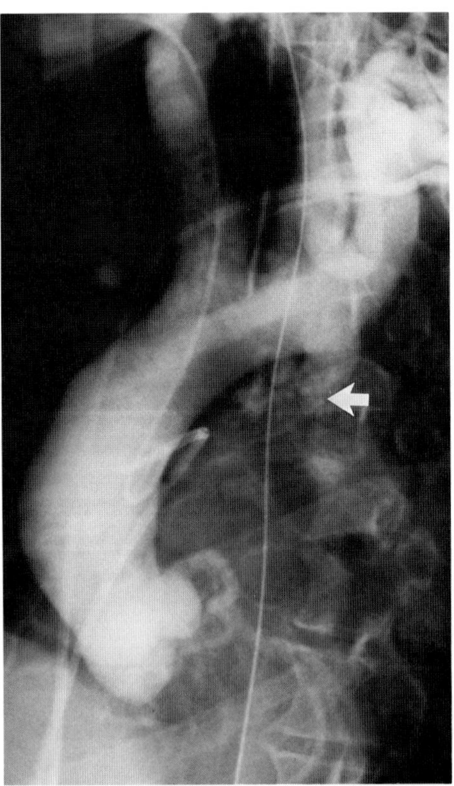

FIG. 9. *Technique:* Antero-posterior (**A**) and right posterior oblique (**B**) aortogram. *Discussion:* The ascending aorta and great vessels are mildly enlarged. Large tortuous collaterals overlie the great vessels, and the internal mammary arteries are enlarged (*asterisk*). The aortic lumen is occluded just past the left subclavian artery (*arrow*). *Diagnosis:* Adult coarctation.

Negative TEE
  Observe
Chronic Dissection or Postoperative Dissection
  CT or MRI

AORTIC OCCLUSIVE DISEASE

AOD, except in the carotid location, is best demonstrated by arteriography. US, CT, and MRI have had limited success at visualizing the disease adequately. Diagnostic algorithms for imaging occlusive disease of the thoracic aorta are straightforward. If clinical symptoms and noninvasive laboratory measurements suggest arterial occlusive disease and surgical therapy is contemplated, arteriography is performed prior to intervention.

Atherosclerotic occlusive disease may involve the branch vessels of the thoracic aorta, coronary, innominate, and carotid arteries. Atherosclerosis of the thoracic aorta does not result in occlusion, but rather aortic ulceration or aneurysmal disease as previously discussed. When aortic narrowing is discovered a different etiology must be suspected. Two rare conditions that result in aortic occlusion that are often confused with AD are included herein.

Adult coarctation of the aorta results from congenital obstruction of the aortic arch at or just past the ligamentum arteriosum produced by an internal diaphragm or ridge of tissue composed of intima and media. Unlike preductal infantile coarctation, this disease may not be detected until late childhood or early adulthood. Patients present with chest pain. Clinical findings include hypertension, lower extremity claudication, and heart failure. Chest radiography suggests the diagnosis by the combination of left ventricular hypertrophy, poststenotic dilation of the proximal descending aorta immediately beyond the coarctation, resulting in a figure 3 configuration of the left mediastinum, an indistinct aortic arch, and rib notching. Because patients have hypertension, asymmetric pulses and other clinical findings that mimic AD, aortography may be requested emergently for clarification. In less dramatic presentations, the chest radiograph diagnosis can be confirmed by demonstrating aortic narrowing and multiple arterial collaterals with MRI, reserving aortography for preoperative planning (Fig. 9A,B) (78).

Takayasu's arteritis, a granulomatis vasculitis, involves the thoracic and abdominal aorta and its large branch arteries (79). Thoracic aortic stenosis or occlusion may result. The disease targets 20- to 30-year-old females. Cardiovascular or nonspecific systemic symptoms and an elevated sedimentation rate may suggest the diagnosis, but depending on the presenting complaints asymmetric pulses may again suggest acute AD. Aortography reveals focal, smooth symmetric narrowing of the aorta and multiple arterial branch vessel stenosis or occlusions (Fig. 10).

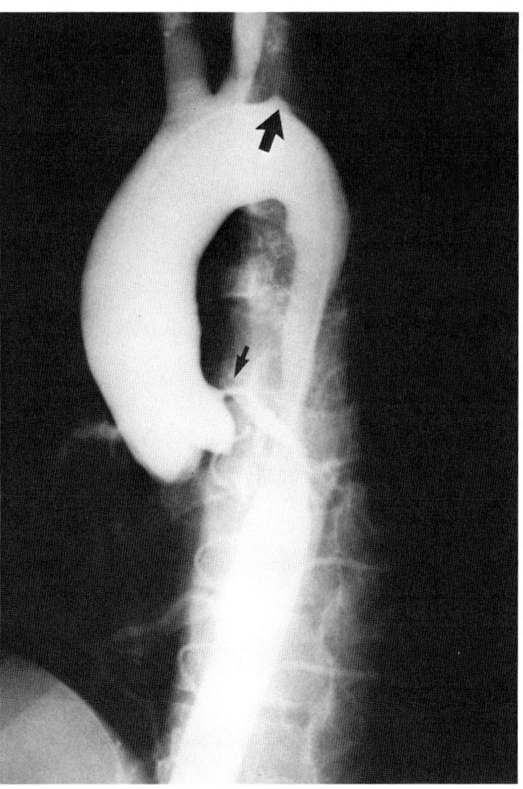

FIG. 10. *Technique:* Right posterior oblique aortogram. *Discussion:* There is smooth tapered narrowing of the descending aorta. The left coronary artery origin is narrowed (*small arrow*). The subclavian artery is occluded (*large arrow*). *Diagnosis:* Takayasu's arteritis.

Summary

Preoperative Planning of AOD
  Aortography

REFERENCES

1. Pasch AR, Ricotta JJ, May AG, Green RM, DeWeese JE. Abdominal aortic aneurysm—the case for elective resection. *Circulation* 1984;70(suppl I):I1–4.
2. Crawford ES. Replacement of the thoracic aorta. In: Grillo HC, Austen WG, Wilkins EW, Mathisen DJ, Vlahakes GJ, eds. *Current therapy in cardiothoracic surgery.* Philadelphia: BC Decker, Inc., 1989;336–340.
3. Posniak HV, Demos TC, Marsan RE. Computed tomography of the normal aorta and thoracic aneurysms. *Semin Roentgenol* 1989;24:7–21.
4. Cooke JP, Kazmier FJ, Orszulak TA. The penetrating aortic ulcer: pathologic manifestations, diagnosis and management. *Mayo Clin Proc* 1988;63:718–725.
5. Yucel EK, Steinberg FL, Egglin TK, Geller SC, Waltman AC, Athanasoulis CA. Penetration aortic ulcers: diagnosis with MR imaging. *Radiology* 1990;177:779–781.

6. Godwin JD. Conventional CT of the aorta. *J Thorac Imaging* 1990;5:18–31.

7. Guthaner DF. The plain chest film in assessing aneurysms and dissecting hematomas of the thoracic aorta. In: Taveras JM, Ferrucci J, Buonocore E, eds. *Radiology. Diagnosis-Imaging-Intervention,* 1990 ed., chap 33. Philadelphia: JB Lippincott Co., 1986.

8. Daves ML. Aortic "aneurysms." In: Daves ML, ed. *Cardiac roentgenology. Shadows of the heart.* Chicago: Year Book Medical Publishers, Inc., 1981;527–543.

9. Bruno L, Prandi M, Colombi P, La Vecchia L. Diagnostic and surgical management of patients with aneurysms of the thoracic aorta with various causes. Echocardiography and contrast enhanced computed tomography in prophylactic replacement of the ascending aorta. *Br Heart J* 1986;55:81–91.

10. Stanford W, Rooholamini SA, Galvin JR. Ultrafast computed tomography in the diagnosis of aortic aneurysms and dissections. *J Thorac Imaging* 1990;5:32–39.

11. Aronberg DJ, Glazer HS, Madsen K, Sagel SS. Normal thoracic aortic diameters by computed tomography. *J Comput Assist Tomogr* 1984;8:247–250.

12. Torres WE, Maurer DE, Steinberg HV, Robbins S, Bernardino ME. CT of aortic aneurysms: the distinction between mural and thrombus calcification. *Am J Roentgenol* 1988;150:1317–1319.

13. Link KM, Lesko NM. The role of MR imaging in the evaluation of acquired diseases of the thoracic aorta. *Am J Roentgenol* 1992;158:1115–1125.

14. Dinsmore RE, Liberthson RR, Wismer GL, et al. Magnetic resonance imaging of thoracic aortic aneurysms: comparison with other imaging methods. *Am J Roentgenol* 1986;146:309–314.

15. Akins CW. Composite aortic valve and aortic root replacement in aneurysmal disease. In: Grillo HC, Austen WG, Wilkins EW, Mathisen DJ, Vlahakes GJ, eds. *Current therapy in cardiothoracic surgery.* Philadelphia: BC Decker, Inc., 1989;381–383.

16. Todd GJ, Nowygrod R, Benvenisty A, Buda J, Reemtsma K. The accuracy of CT scanning in the diagnosis of abdominal and thoracoabdominal aortic aneurysms. *J Vasc Surg* 1991;13:302–310.

17. Williams LR, Flinn WR, Yao JST, et al. Extended use of computed tomography in the management of complex aortic problems: a learning experience. *J Vasc Surg* 1986;4:264–271.

18. Pozzato C, Fedriga E, Donatelli F, Gattoni F. Acute posttraumatic rupture of the thoracic aorta: the role of angiography in a 7-year review. *Cardiovasc Intervent Radiol* 1991;14:338–341.

19. Kucich VA, Vogelzang RL, Hartz RS, LoCicero J, Dalton D. Ruptured thoracic aneurysm: unusual manifestation and early diagnosis using CT. *Radiology* 1986;160:87–89.

20. Zarnke MD, Gould HR, Goldman MH. Computed tomography in the evaluation of the patient with symptomatic abdominal aortic aneurysm. *Surgery* 1988;103:638–642.

21. Auffermann W, Olofsson PA, Rabahie GN, Tavares NJ, Stoney RJ, Higgins CB. Incorporation versus infection of retroperitoneal aortic grafts: MR imaging features. *Radiology* 1989;172:359–362.

22. O'Hara PJ, Borkowski GP, Hertzer NR, O'Donovan PB, Brigham SL, Beven EG. Natural history of periprosthetic air on computerized axial tomographic examination of the abdomen following abdominal aortic aneurysm repair. *J Vasc Surg* 1984;1:429–433.

23. Parmley LF, Mattingly TW, Manion WC, Jahnke EJ. Nonpenetrating traumatic injury of the aorta. *Circulation* 1958;17:1086–1101.

24. Greendyke RM. Traumatic rupture of aorta. *JAMA* 1966;195:119–122.

25. Fisher RG, Hadlock F, Ben-Menachem Y. Laceration of the thoracic aorta and brachiocephalic arteries by blunt trauma: report of 54 cases and review of the literature. *Radiol Clin North Am* 1981;19:91–110.

26. Fishbone G, Robbins DI, Osborn DJ, Grnja V. Trauma to the thoracic aorta and great vessels. *Radiol Clin North Am* 1973;11:543–554.

27. Daniels DL, Maddison FE. Ascending aortic injury: an angiographic diagnosis. *Am J Roentgenol* 1981;136:812–813.

28. Lundevall J. The mechanism of traumatic rupture of the aorta. *Acta Pathol Microbiol Scand* 1964;62:34–46.

29. Crass JR, Cohen AM, Motta AO, Tomashefski JF, Wiesen EJ. A proposed new mechanism of traumatic aortic rupture: the osseous pinch. *Radiology* 1990;176:645–649.

30. Clark DE, Zeiger MA, Wallace KL, Packard AB, Nowicki ER. Blunt aortic trauma: signs of high risk. *J Trauma* 1990;30:701–705.

31. Barcia TC, Livoni JP. Indications for angiography in blunt thoracic trauma. *Radiology* 1983;147:15–19.

32. Gundry SR, Williams S, Burney RE, MacKenzie JR, Cho KJ. Indications for aortography. Radiography after blunt chest trauma: a reassessment of the radiographic findings associated with traumatic rupture of the aorta. *Invest Radiol* 1983;18:230–237.

33. Sefczek DM, Sefczek RJ, Deeb ZL. Radiographic signs of acute traumatic rupture of the thoracic aorta. *Am J Roentgenol* 1983;141:1259–1262.

34. Kram HB, Appel PL, Wohlmuth DA, Shoemaker WC. Diagnosis of traumatic thoracic aortic rupture: a 10-year retrospective analysis. *Ann Thorac Surg* 1989;47:282–286.

35. Ayella RJ, Hankins JR, Turney SZ, Crowley RA. Ruptured thoracic aorta due to blunt trauma. *J Trauma* 1977;17:199–205.

36. Raptopoulos V, Sheiman RG, Phillips DA, Davidoff A, Silva WE. Traumatic aortic tear: screening with chest CT. *Radiology* 1992;182:667–673.

37. Woodring JH. The normal mediastinum in blunt traumatic ruptures of the thoracic aorta and brachiocephalic arteries. *J Emerg Med* 1990;8:467–476.

38. Richardson P, Mirvis SE, Scorpio R, Dunham CM. Value of CT in determining the need for angiography when findings of mediastinal hemorrhage on chest radiographs are equivocal. *Am J Roentgenol* 1991;156:273–279.

39. Heiberg E, Wolverson MK, Sundaram M, Shields JB. CT in aortic trauma. *Am J Roentgenol* 1983;140:1119–1124.

40. Miller FB, Richardson JD, Thomas HA, Cryer HM, Willing SJ. Role of CT in diagnosis of major arterial injury after blunt thoracic trauma. *Surgery* 1989;106:596–603.

41. Mirvis SE, Kostrubiak I, Whitley NO, Goldstein LD, Rodriquez A. Role of CT in excluding major arterial injury after blunt thoracic trauma. *Am J Roentgenol* 1987;149:601–605.

42. Fenner MN, Fisher KS, Sergel NL, Porter DB, Metzmaker CO. Evaluation of possible traumatic thoracic aortic injury using aortography and CT. *Am Surg* 1990;56:497–499.

43. Ishikawa T, Nakajima Y, Kaji T. The role of CT in traumatic rupture of the thoracic aorta and its proximal branches. *Semin Roentgenol* 1989;24:38–46.

44. Maydayag MA, Kirshenbaum KJ, Nadimpalli SR, Fantus RJ, Cavallino RP, Crystal GJ. Thoracic aortic trauma: role of dynamic CT. *Radiology* 1991;179:853–855.

45. Morgan PW, Goodman LR, Aprahamian C, Foley WD, Lipchik EO. Evaluation of traumatic aortic injury: does dynamic contrast-enhanced CT play a role? *Radiology* 1992;182:661–666.

46. Sparkes MB, Burchard KW, Marrin CAS, Bean CHG, Nugent WC, Plehn JF. Transesophageal echocardiography. Preliminary results in patients with traumatic aortic rupture. *Arch Surg* 1991;126:711–714.

47. Magilligan DJ Jr, Davila JC. Innominate artery disruption due to blunt trauma. *Arch Surg* 1979;114:307–309.

48. Sturm JT, Hankins DG, Young G. Thoracic aortography following blunt chest trauma. *Am J Emerg Med* 1990;8:92–96.

49. Morse SS, Glickman MG, Greenwood LH, et al. Traumatic aortic rupture: false-positive aortographic diagnosis due to atypical ductus diverticulum. *Am J Roentgenol* 1988;150:793–796.

50. LaBerge JM, Jeffrey RB. Aortic lacerations: fatal complications of thoracic aortography. *Radiology* 1987;165:367–369.

51. Richardson JD, Wilson ME, Miller FB. The widened mediastinum. Diagnostic and therapeutic priorities. *Ann Surg* 1990;211:731–736.

52. DeSanctis RW, Doroghazi RM, Austen WG, Buckley MJ. Aortic dissection. *N Engl J Med* 1987;317:1060–1067.

53. Yamada T, Tada S, Harada J. Aortic dissection without intimal rupture: diagnosis with MR imaging and CT. *Radiology* 1988;168:347–352.

54. Demos TC, Posniak HV, Marsan RE. CT of aortic dissection. *Semin Roentgenol* 1989;24:22–37.

55. Daily PO, Trueblood HW, Stinson EB, Wuerflein RD, Shumway NE. Management of acute aortic dissection. *Ann Thorac Surg* 1970;10:237–247.
56. DeBakey ME, Henly WS, Cooley DA, et al. Surgical management of dissecting aneurysms of the aorta. *J Thorac Cardiovasc Surg* 1965;49:130–149.
57. Wechsler RJ, Kotler MN, Steiner RM. Multimodality approach to thoracic aortic dissection. *Cardiovasc Clin* 1986;17:385–408.
58. Crawford ES, Svensson LG, Coselli JS, Safi HJ, Hess KR. Aortic dissection and dissecting aortic aneurysm. *Ann Surg* 1988;208:254–272.
59. Wolfe WG, Oldham HN, Rankin JS, Moran JF. Surgical treatment of acute ascending aortic dissection. *Ann Surg* 1983;197:738–742.
60. Yamaguchi T, Guthaner DF, Wexler L. Natural history of the false channel of type A aortic dissection after surgical repair: CT study. *Radiology* 1989;170:743–747.
61. Guthaner DF, Miller DC, Silverman JF, Stinson EB, Wexler L. Fate of the false lumen following surgical repair of aortic dissections: an angiographic study. *Radiology* 1979;133:1–8.
62. Erbel R, Daniel W, Visser C, Engberding R, Roelandt J, Rennollet H. Echocardiography in diagnosis of aortic dissection. *Lancet* 1989;March 4:457–460.
63. Hashimoto S, Kumada T, Osakada G, et al. Assessment of transesophageal Doppler echography in dissecting aortic aneurysm. *J Am Coll Cardiol* 1989;14:1253–1262.
64. Mügge A, Daniel WG, Laas J, Grote R, Lichtlen PR. False-negative diagnosis of proximal aortic dissection by computed tomography or angiography and possible explanations based on transesophageal echocardiographic findings. *Am J Cardiol* 1990;65:527–529.
65. Thorsen MK, San Dretto MA, Lawson TL, Foley WD, Smith DF, Berland LL. Dissecting aortic aneurysms: accuracy of computed tomographic diagnosis. *Radiology* 1983;148:773–777.
66. Landtman M, Kivisaari L, Standertskjöld-Nordenstam C-G, Taavitsainen M. Computed tomography in pre- and postoperative evaluation of aortic dissection. *Acta Radiol Diag* 1986;27:273–278.
67. Vasile N, Mathieu D, Keita K, Lellouche D, Block G, Cachera JP. Computed tomography of thoracic aortic dissection: accuracy and pitfalls. *J Comp Assist Tomogr* 1986;10:211–215.
68. Oudkerk M, Overbosch E, Dee P. CT recognition of acute aortic dissection. *Am J Roentgenol* 1983:141:671–676.
69. St. Amour TE, Gutierrez FR, Levitt RG, McKnight RC. CT diagnosis of type A aortic dissections not demonstrated by aortography. *J Comp Assist Tomogr* 1988;12:963–967.
70. Kersting-Sommerhoff BA, Higgins CB, White RD, Sommerhoff CP, Lipton MJ. Aortic dissection: sensitivity and specificity of MR imaging. *Radiology* 1988;166:651–655.
71. Fruehwald FXJ, Neuhold A, Fezoulidis J, et al. Cine-MR in dissection of the thoracic aorta. *Eur J Radiol* 1989;9:37–41.
72. Solomon SL, Brown JJ, Glazer HS, Mirowitz SA, Lee JKT. Thoracic aortic dissection: pitfalls and artifacts in MR imaging. *Radiology* 1990;177:223–228.
73. Archiniegas JG, Soto B, Little WC, Papapietro SE. Cineangiography in the diagnosis of aortic dissection. *Am J Cardiol* 1981;47:890–894.
74. Gutierrez FR, Gowda S, Ludbrook PA, McKnight RC. Cineangiography in the diagnosis and evaluation of aortic dissection. *Radiology* 1980;135:759–761.
75. White RD, Ullyot DJ, Higgins CB. MR imaging of the aorta after surgery for aortic dissection. *Am J Roentgenol* 1988;150:87–92.
76. Mathieu D, Keita K, Loisance D, Cachera JP, Rousseau M, Vasile N. Postoperative CT follow-up of aortic dissection. *J Comp Assist Tomogr* 1986;10:216–218.
77. Hendrickx P, Rieder P, Prokop M, Milbradt H, Karck M, Laas J. Intravenous DSA and dynamic computed tomography for postoperative follow-up of type A aortic dissections. *Eur J Radiol* 1989;9:158–162.
78. Gomes AS, Lois JF, George B, Alpan G, Williams RG. Congenital abnormalities of the aortic arch: MR imaging. *Radiology* 1987;165:691–695.
79. Procter CD, Hollier LH. Takayasu's arteritis and temporal arteritis. *Ann Vasc Surg* 1992;6:195–197.

Thoracic Radiology, edited by
J.D. Newell, Jr., and R.D. Tarver,
Raven Press, Ltd., New York © 1993.

CHAPTER 9

Intensive Care Unit Chest Radiology

Robert D. Tarver

In a busy hospital-based practice, portable chest radiographs may comprise almost 50 percent of the total volume of radiographs taken in a department. The portable chest films are usually of very ill patients in the intensive care units (ICUs). The films are an important tool used by the clinicians when making decisions. The morning portable films are used extensively, much as lab values are used in assessing the clinical status of the patients. The extent of the patient's pulmonary disease, the noisy ICU environment, and the inability of the patient to co-operate make physical examination of the patient's cardiopulmonary status less reliable. Therefore, the intensivist often relies heavily on the portable chest radiograph to assess the patient's cardiopulmonary status. In addition, a number of tubes, lines, and catheters must be in a certain position to function properly, all of which can easily be inadvertently moved and only checked with a portable film. In summary, the portable chest radiograph is a common, important examination used extensively to assess the cardiopulmonary status of patients in the ICU (1,2).

PORTABLE CHEST RADIOGRAPHY

Chest radiology can be difficult even with an excellent postero-anterior (PA) and lateral chest radiograph. The ability to make radiographic diagnoses depends on the radiologist's experience in reading portable chest radiographs and his or her ability to obtain a high-quality radiograph. Correctly identifying pathological changes often depends on subtle radiographic changes. A radiologist's ability to see the radiographic abnormalities is dependent on high-quality radiographs. Despite the radiol-

ogist's experience, the portable radiograph is more difficult to interpret, is more difficult to obtain, and is less reliable than a PA and lateral chest radiograph. Abnormalities are easier to see and interpret on standard PA and lateral radiographs from a dedicated chest unit than from a portable unit. Several factors combine to make portable chest radiographs of inferior quality. Technical, geometric, and patient factors all detract from the ability to obtain excellent portable radiographs.

Technical Factors

Most portable chest radiographs are taken without grids that are used to reduce scatter. The grids are not used because cutoff will occur if they are not perpendicular to the x-ray beam and aligned with the center of the central beam of the x-ray. Grid cutoff prevents some of the x-ray beam from reaching the patient and produces underexposed films. The technologist cannot reliably align the portable cassette with the x-ray beam to prevent grid cutoff and, therefore, grids are not used. Films taken without grids have more scatter that adds an overall grayness to the images. Several techniques, developed to properly align the x-ray beam and the grid, have not achieved wide usage (3,4). They involve either a direct mechanical or electronic connection between the film cassette and the x-ray tube. Portable chest radiographs are not phototimed; PA and lateral films are. Phototimers turn off the x-ray beam after the proper exposure has been obtained. Portable film exposure is chosen by the technologist and is based on the individual's experience in taking a film on similar sized patients. An experienced technologist can take diagnostic quality radiographs over 90 percent of the time. However, intrathoracic pathology, unknown to the technologist, may require more or less exposure for a diagnostic radiograph and may result in the need to repeat the film. PA and lateral radiographs are usually obtained with a 140

R. D. Tarver: Department of Radiology, Indiana University Medical Center, and Wishard Memorial Hospital, Indianapolis, Indiana 46202.

kv beam. Portable chest radiographic machines usually do not go above 100 kv, and most portable chest radiographs are taken at about 80 kv. The 80 kv setting is used to decrease the scatter and, therefore, will increase contrast. One of the disadvantages of an 80 kv beam versus a 140 kv beam is that the lower energy beam has less penetrating ability and, in order to get an adequate exposure, a greater dose must be used. To obtain a greater dose the time of exposure must be increased (15–20 msec), creating more cardiac and respiratory motion artifact than that of a dedicated chest unit (2–4 msec). Longer exposures are also needed because the portable machines have lower mA settings available than standard chest radiographic units, and the time must be lengthened to get the required mA's. All of these technical factors contribute to the overall difficulty in obtaining high-quality portable chest radiographs.

Geometric Factors

Several geometric factors combine to degrade the diagnostic ability of portable radiographs. Standard chest films are taken at a tube-to-film distance of 6 feet, the patient's anterior chest against the film, and the patient standing upright. This positioning minimizes cardiac magnification and allows gravity to aid the diaphragm in moving the abdominal contents downward, thus ensuring a deep inspiration. Portable chest radiographs are taken with the patient sitting or supine. The tube to film distance varies from 40 to 60 inches, and the beam passes through the patient from anterior to posterior (AP), with the patient's back against the film. These factors cause the heart to appear enlarged, the diaphragms to be elevated, and the lung volume to be smaller when compared with a standard PA radiograph (Fig. 1). Patient rotation is difficult to judge at the bedside and, because of the shorter tube to film distance, small degrees of rotation are more noticeable than on standard radiographs. All of these factors must be considered when reading portable chest radiographs and comparing them with standard PA radiographs.

Patient Factors

Patient factors can also contribute to the overall poorer quality of portable chest radiographs. Because of their illness the patients often cannot cooperate with the technologist either to maintain proper positioning or to hold their breath. In addition pain from abdominal or thoracic trauma or surgery often prevents the patients from taking a maximal inspiration. The technologist may have difficulty coordinating maximum inspiration with the x-ray exposure in patients on high ventilatory rates or on patients with very shallow respirations (Fig. 2).

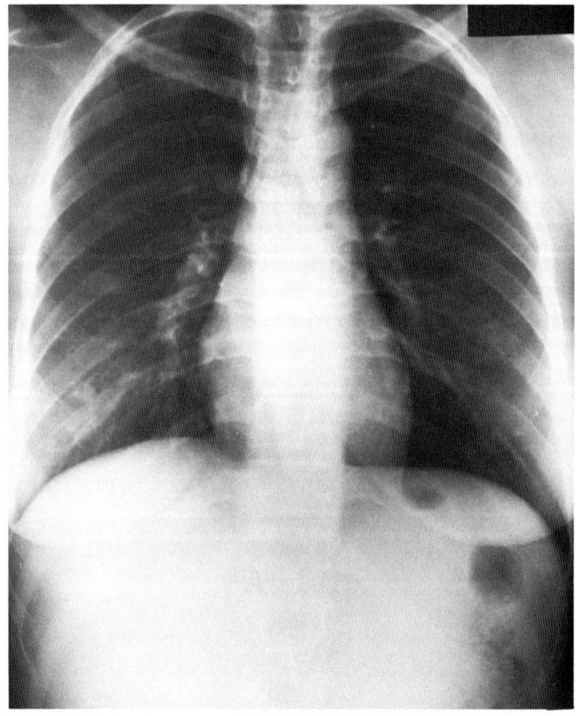
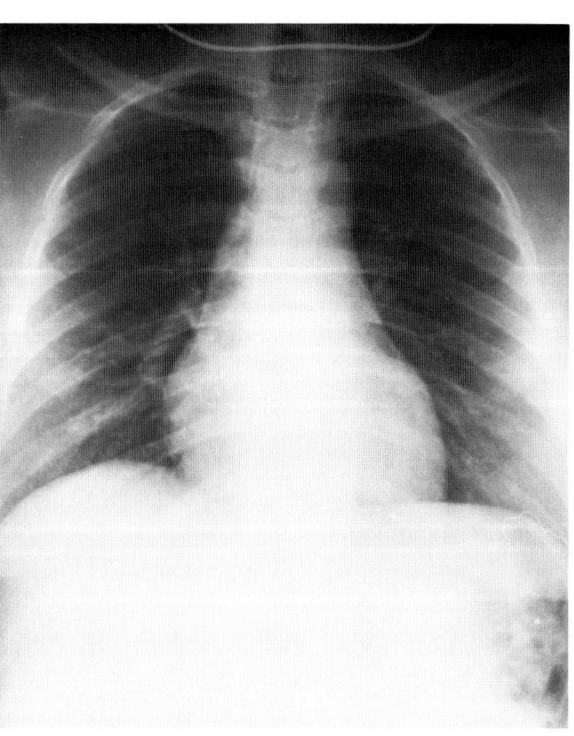

FIG. 1. **(A)** PA upright chest radiograph. **(B)** AP upright portable chest radiograph of the same patient 1 hour later. Notice the apparent increase in heart size due to positioning alone.

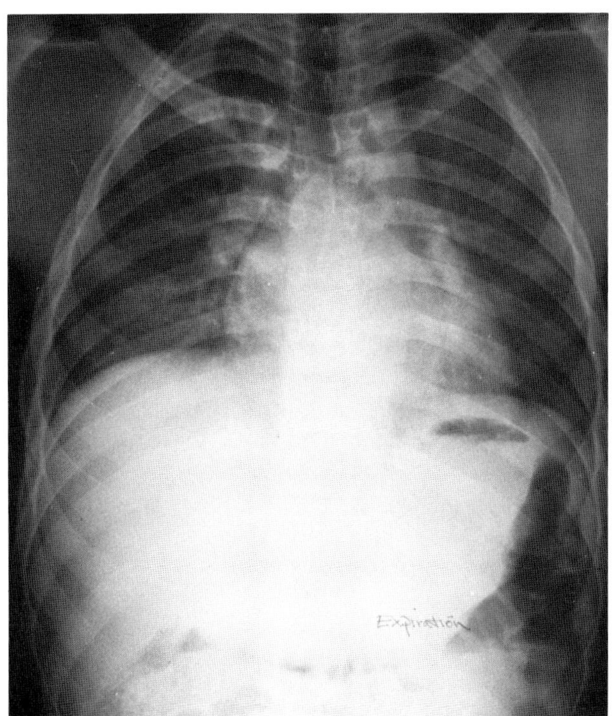
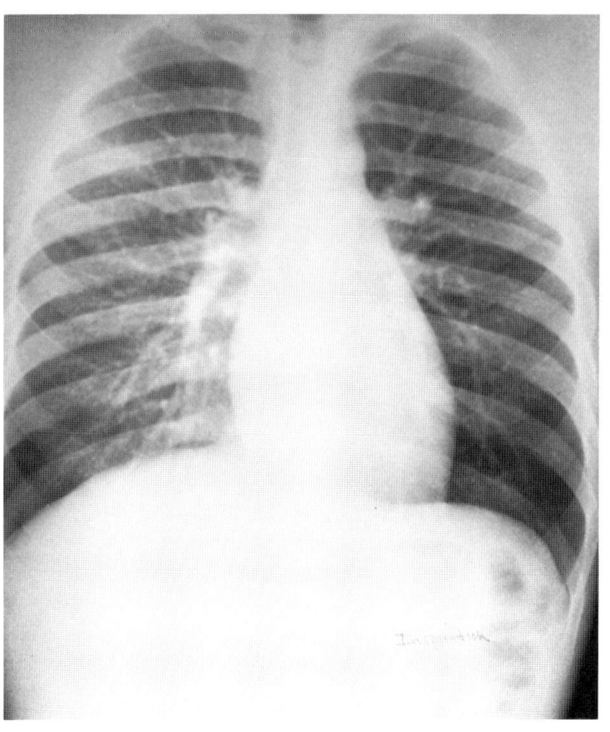

A

B

FIG. 2. **(A)** AP portable chest radiograph taken at low lung volumes shows diffuse pulmonary infiltrates and cardiomegaly. **(B)** Same patient a few minutes later with a better inspiratory effort shows normal heart size and clear lungs.

THE PORTABLE CHEST FILM TECHNOLOGIST

A technologist experienced in portable chest film technique is invaluable. The portable film technologist and the radiologist form a team that is responsible for obtaining and reading a chest film that may have an important impact on the patient's care. A little encouragement and occasional compliment from the radiologist will make the technologist realize what an important link he or she is in the patient's care. Ideally two technologists should perform the portable chest rounds. Moving and correctly positioning ill, intubated, often uncooperative patients is difficult with only one technologist, especially if he or she is slight of build. Also, the portable chest radiographic unit is a bulky, often unwieldy, machine that must be carefully positioned in small ICU rooms. Two technologists working as a team can often get the job done in less than half the time a solo technologist can. A technologist routinely performing portable chest radiographs has a better estimation of the proper technique for each patient, because this individual has critiqued his or her own films from previous films (Table 1). If different technologists do the films each day, it is helpful to chart the techniques that have been successfully used on each patient. Each technologist should review his or her own films so that minor adjustments in technique can be made the next time a film is taken on a particular patient. The portable film technologist should be experienced. A strong case can be made that the portable technologist should be a position of experience and seniority, because portable films (unlike many examinations) are more dependent on the technologist's particular knowledge and skills.

DIGITAL PORTABLE CHEST RADIOGRAPHS

The computed radiography system uses standard portable radiography equipment to make the exposure. The imaging receptor consists of a plate coated with a photostimulable phosphor (europium-activated barium fluorobromide) that functions as a large area detector instead

TABLE 1. *Portable film selections and techniques*

Company	Film	Screen	kv	mA's
Kodak	TMG-1	Lanex regular	100	0.64–2
Agfa	STG-2	Regular	75	1–2.5
Dupont	Cronex 41	Quanta Fast Detail	75	1.5–2
Fugi	Super HRG	GH-1	75	1–2

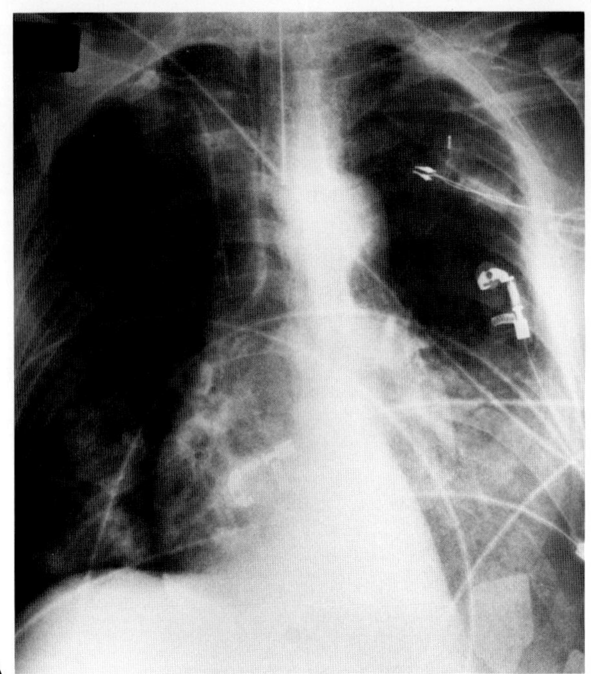

A

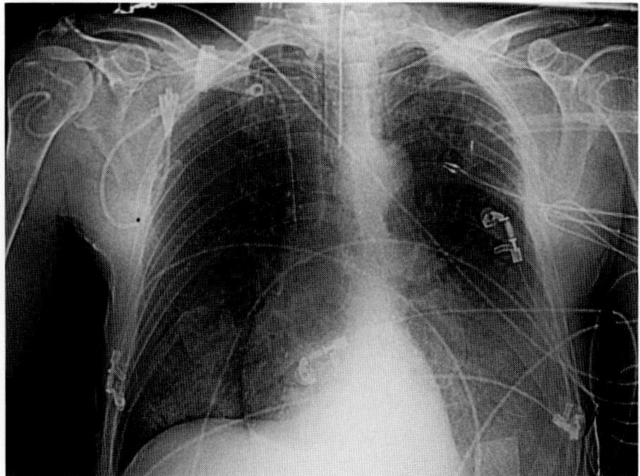

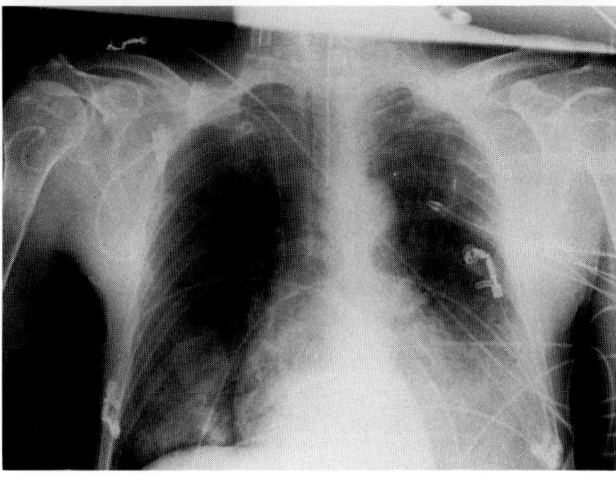

B

FIG. 3. **(A)** Conventional portable radiograph taken with film and screens. **(B)** Digital portable radiograph of the same patient taken with a Phillips digital imaging system. Two films are produced for each exposure. The *top image* is processed with edge enhancement to improve the visualization of tubes and lines. The *bottom image* is processed to appear like the conventional image.

of the conventional film-screen combination. When the phosphor is exposed to x-rays, a latent image is formed that is later converted to light image by a laser beam. The light image is detected by a photomultiplier, digitized, and an image is created on film. The computed radiography system has an extremely wide dynamic range. Its linear photoluminescence and dose response of 1:10,000 are far greater than the nonlinear 1:100 range of film-screen combinations. The systems of Fugi Photo (Japan) and Phillips Medical Systems (Shelton, CT) generate a hard-copy image pair from a single exposure. One image is processed to resemble a standard radiograph and the second is processed with a wider latitude and some spatial frequency enhancement. The resultant image has a spatial resolution of about 2.5 line pairs/mm, about half the resolution available with conventional film-screen systems (5,6) (Fig. 3).

The advantage of the computed chest radiography is that the images are of uniform density and excellent quality. Despite the smaller format and decreased spatial resolution, the advantages of a uniform density film (despite patient, technical, and technologist variations) makes

this system ideal for portable chest radiography. Computed chest radiography has reduced repeats to below 1 percent. Positioning errors are the most common reason for repeats. Comparison studies between computed and conventional radiography show computed radiography as the best choice for portable chest radiography (7,8).

ABNORMALITIES

Pleural Effusions

On a conventional PA and lateral chest radiograph, the lateral and posterior costophrenic sulci appear as sharp lucent angles of lung parenchyma against the diaphragm. Several milliliters of pleural fluid in the normal pleural space are not visible on radiographs. Blunting of the angles is manifested as a density that fills the normally sharp angle and has a meniscus-shaped upper surface. The fluid is first noticeable in the posterior costophrenic angles as blunting of the normally sharp angle and, as the fluid increases, the lateral costophrenic angles also become blunted. As more fluid accumulates the blunting becomes more pronounced, and the fluid is visible lateral to the lung as well. In cadaver studies, 175 ml of pleural fluid is required to blunt the lateral costophrenic angle (9). Large effusions displace the lung cephalad and the hemidiaphragms caudad. Decubitus chest radiographs allow for a more accurate estimation of the amount of pleural effusions. Decubitus views also demonstrate whether or not the effusion is loculated. Opposite decubitus views and prone cross-table lateral films are helpful in visualizing lung parenchyma that may be obscured by pleural effusions. On upright radiographs, subpulmonic effusions may be difficult to detect, because the costophrenic angles may be sharp. A tell-tale lateral displacement of the apparent apex of the diaphragm and lack of visualization of lung markings below the hemidiaphragm may be the only available radiographic evidence of an effusion.

Pleural effusions on upright portable films share many of the radiographic appearances of effusions of standard PA and lateral films. Most upright portable chest radiographs are not taken with the patient's thorax perpendicular to the floor, as in a standard PA radiograph. Most of the time an upright portable chest radiograph is taken with the patient in a slight recumbent position at an incline of between 70° and 50° in relationship to the horizontal. As a result a pleural effusion does not collect entirely inferiorly between the lung and hemidiaphragm. Instead, the effusion tracts upward, posterior to the lower lung to a varying degree. The effusion tracking behind the lower lobes adds radiographic density to the lower lobes and can simulate alveolar infiltrate. The posterior effusion can be identified because it produces an overall grayness to the lower lobes that increases inferiorly (Fig. 4). Breast shadows can also produce an artifact that simulates these posterior effusions. The posterior effusion often obscures the sharp border of the hemidiaphragm. The lack of visualization of a hemidiaphragm, without signs of a lower lobe alveolar infiltrate or atelectasis, can indicate that a pleural effusion is present.

Pleural effusions in supine patients can be difficult to detect and properly identify. A pleural effusion layers posteriorly, behind the lung in a supine patient. The caudad portions of the pleural space in supine patients are more dependent than the cephalad portions, causing a gradient of pleural fluid thickness, which is greatest in the caudad portions of the pleural space. Several anatomic factors contribute to this phenomena. The shoulder girdle serves to elevate the upper chest in the supine patient, and the weight of the abdomen forces the lower portion of the chest into the bed, making it more dependent than the upper portion of the chest. The radiographic appearance of a pleural effusion in a supine patient is an overall increased density of the hemithorax, which is greater toward the bases of the lungs. Differen-

tiating diffuse alveolar infiltrates from pleural effusions on a supine film is usually not difficult. Air bronchogram, the hallmark of alveolar infiltrates, is not seen in patients with only pleural effusions. Another helpful sign in differentiating effusions from diffuse alveolar infiltrates is the ability to see the pulmonary vessels. Despite the increased density of the hemithorax, caused by the posteriorly layering pleural effusion, the pulmonary vessels are visible because they are surrounded by normally aerated lung. If any doubt exists in differentiating a posterior effusion from an alveolar infiltrate, bilateral decubitus films are helpful. When the side in question is in the dependent position, the presence and amount of fluid can be visualized. When the side in question is in the nondependent position, the effusion layers against the mediastinum and the lung have a chance to expand, and any alveolar infiltrates can be seen free of the underlying effusion. Large pleural effusions are easy to identify in supine patients, because in addition to collecting posteriorly to the lung they tract around the lateral border of the lung producing a characteristic fluid density between the ribs and the lung.

Portable decubitus films can be difficult to obtain. However, there are several techniques that can improve diagnostic capability. Placing the patient on a backboard, while taking the decubitus film, keeps the dependent area of interest from being obscured as it sinks down into the bed. Small effusions are often not seen on portable decubitus films, because the beam is centered on the patient's midline. Due to geometric constraints of a short tube to film distance, the small effusion is projected over the dependent chest wall and ribs instead of being projected adjacent to the ribs. By centering the beam closer to the backboard or dependent portion of the patient's chest, small effusions can be detected.

Pneumothorax

Identifying a pneumothorax on an upright PA chest radiograph is a relatively easy task. A lucent collection of air lateral and superior to the thin white line of the pleura is easy to detect and identify as a pneumothorax. Ancillary signs, such as lack of lung markings in the apex and a relative lucency of the involved hemithorax, are occasionally helpful. The clinical history of acute chest pain, chest trauma, or central venous catheter placement may suggest the diagnosis of a pneumothorax. If a pneumothorax is suspected, but not detected, on standard PA and lateral radiographs, other views may be helpful. Expiratory films and lateral decubitus films, with the suspected side up, are occasionally helpful in detecting small pneumothoraces.

Identification of a pneumothorax on portable chest radiographs can be more difficult than on a standard PA chest radiograph. If the portable film can be taken in the

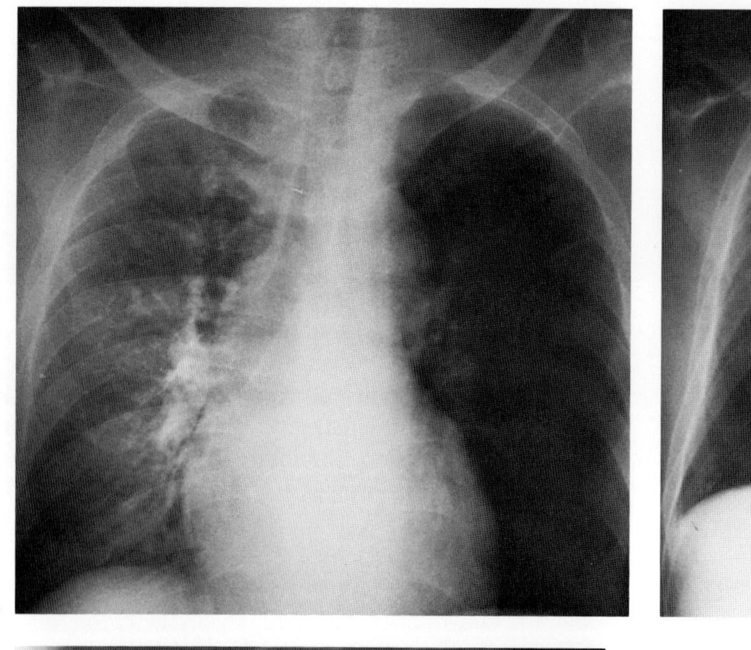

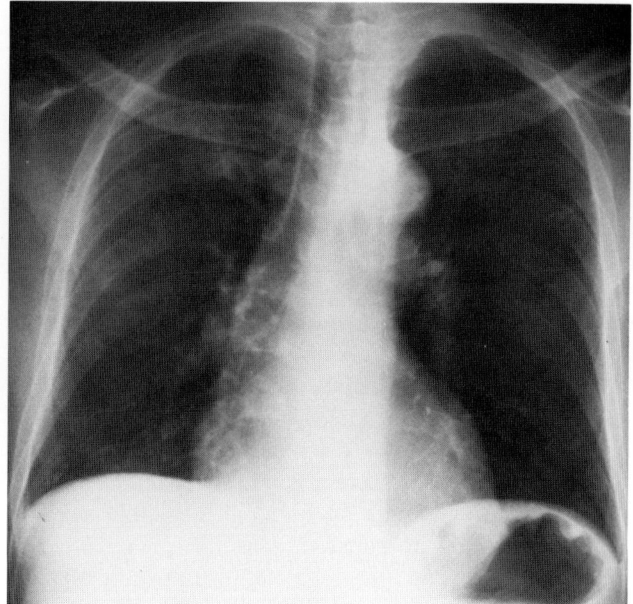

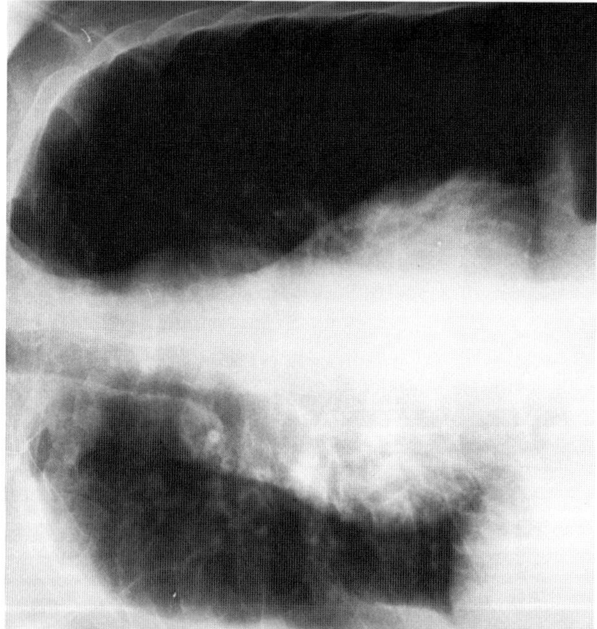

FIG. 4. **(A)** Supine portable chest radiograph showing an increased density throughout the right hemithorax due to a right pleural effusion layering posteriorly. Notice how the vessels can be seen and there are no air bronchograms. **(B)** Upright portable radiograph of the same patient at the same time showing the right lung to be clear. The effusion is collecting in a subpulmonic location and is difficult to detect. **(C)** Portable right lateral decubitus radiograph of the same patient showing a large, layering right pleural effusion.

upright position, the identification of a pneumothorax is relatively easy by using the same diagnostic signs that are found on a standard PA radiograph. The lucent crescent of air is still found over the superior and lateral aspects of the hemithorax. If the patient is supine, identifying a pneumothorax can be more difficult (Fig. 5). In a supine patient, the most superior aspect of the hemithorax is the anterio-lateral costophrenic sulcus. This anatomic fact is important, because radiologists usually look for pneumothoraces over the apex of the lung. However, on a supine radiograph, the bases of the lungs must be checked. The appearance of a pneumothorax on a supine film often gives rise to a lucency in the lateral costophrenic sulcus. This is termed the deep sulcus sign. The lateral costophrenic sulcus appears deep, lucent, and more pronounced, because the negative pleural pressure, which kept the diaphragm up and the chest wall in, is absent (Fig. 6). If a pneumothorax is suspected but not confirmed on a supine chest radiograph, additional views may be needed. Often the patient can be positioned for an upright view. However, if the patient cannot tolerate the upright position, a lateral decubitus view can be obtained. An overexposed film is one of the most common reasons for missing a pneumothorax on a portable chest radiograph. Often all that is needed to detect a pneumothorax is to repeat the portable chest radiograph with an improved technique.

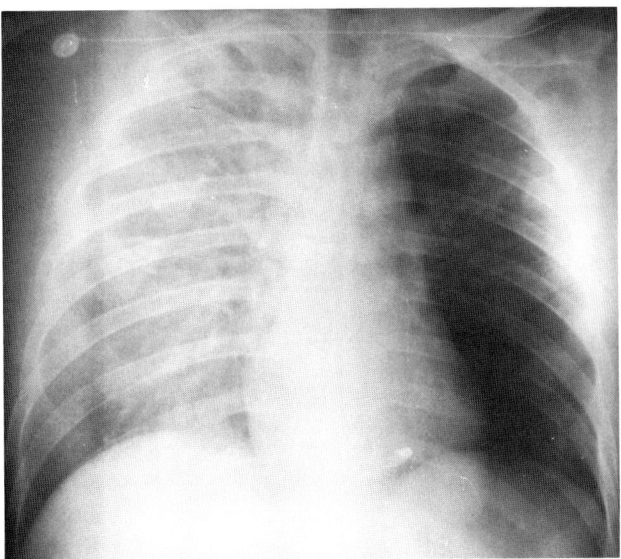

FIG. 5. Portable chest radiograph showing a partially opacified right hemithorax and a lucent left hemithorax. It is occasionally difficult to determine which side is abnormal. Is the denser side normal or is the more lucent side? In this trauma case both sides were abnormal. The right side was abnormally dense because of a large hemothorax, and the left side was abnormally lucent because of a large pneumothorax.

Pneumomediastinum

Pneumomediastinum is an abnormal collection of air within the mediastinum. The most common cause of pneumomediastinum (seen in the ICU setting) is ventilator-induced barotrauma. Using high positive end-expiratory pressure to ventilate patients can cause rupture of alveoli adjacent to small airways. The air then dissects back along the airways into the mediastinal fascial planes. Traumatic interruption of the tracheobronchial tree will produce a pneumomediastinum. The interruption may be in the upper trachea or larynx from one of the following: blunt trauma, penetrating injuries, traumatic intubation, or it may be in the lower airways due to traumatic rupture of a mainstem bronchi. Spontaneous pneumomediastinum, caused by raised intrathoracic pressures, can occur in asthmatics and patients with severe coughing or vomiting. Esophageal rupture caused by instrumentation or severe retching (Boerhaave's syndrome) also may cause pneumomediastinum. Occasionally patients with a pneumoperitoneum can develop a pneumomediastinum as the air dissects through the diaphragm and into the mediastinum.

The radiographic appearance of pneumomediastinum on portable chest radiographs is similar to that seen on standard PA radiographs. A lucent paramediastinal collection of air is usually seen on both sides of the mediastinum. Occasionally it is more apparent on one side than the other (Fig. 7). When the pneumomediastinum is seen unilaterally it can easily be confused with a medial pneumothorax. Decubitus films will easily distinguish between these two conditions, because the lucency of a medial pneumothorax will migrate to the nondependent side of the thorax, and the pneumomediastinum will remain fixed along the mediastinum. A normal lucency, termed the mach effect, is perceived next to the mediastinum and should not be confused with a pneumomediastinum. The mach effect is caused by a complex physiological response of the optic system when it sees a sharp difference in radiographic density. The air collections of a pneumomediastinum often extend into the paratracheal region where the pneumomediastinum produces a linear lucency paralleling the trachea. The linear lucencies may extend into the neck as well. The pneumomediastinum can also produce a lucency inferior to the heart—between the anterior pericardium and the diaphragm. This sign of pneumomediastinum is termed the continuous diaphragm sign. A pneumomediastinum can usually be differentiated from a pneumopericardium because the latter is found just around the heart and does not extend into the superior mediastinum.

Pneumomediastinum is usually a benign condition itself. However, it can result in more serious complications. Pneumopericardium is a common complication of pneumomediastinum in newborns on respirators. In

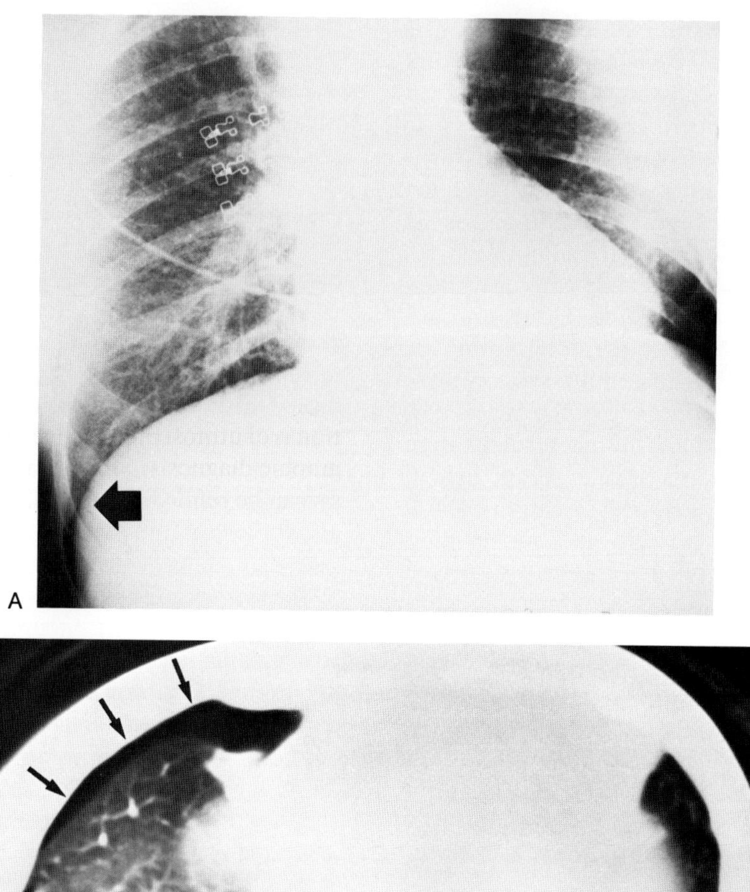

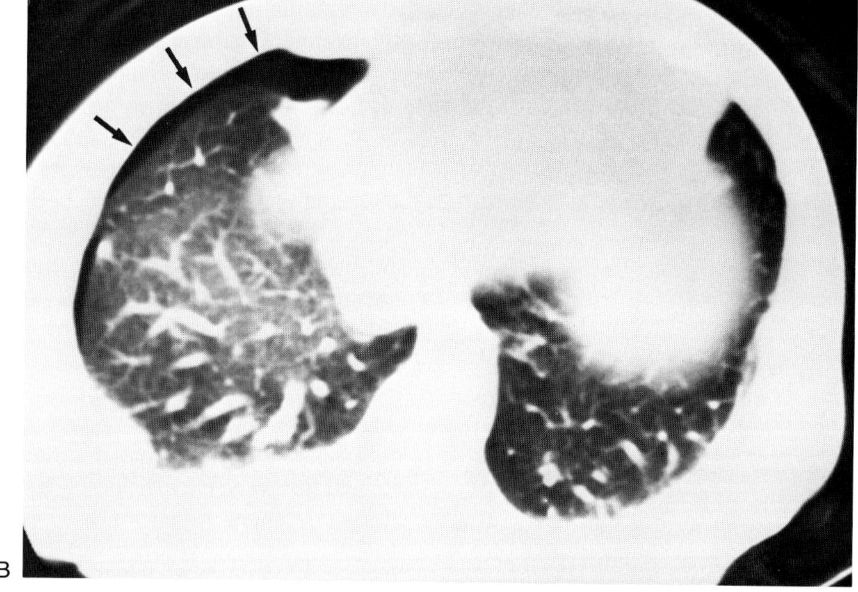

FIG. 6. (A) Supine portable chest radiograph of a trauma patient. The patient has several fractured right ribs. Notice the unusual lucency and depth of the right lateral costophrenic sulcus (*arrow*). This is the deep sulcus sign of a pneumothorax on a supine radiograph. **(B)** Chest CT demonstrating the deep sulcus sign. The pneumothorax (*arrows*) collects in the highest point of the supine hemithorax, which is the anterolateral costophrenic sulcus.

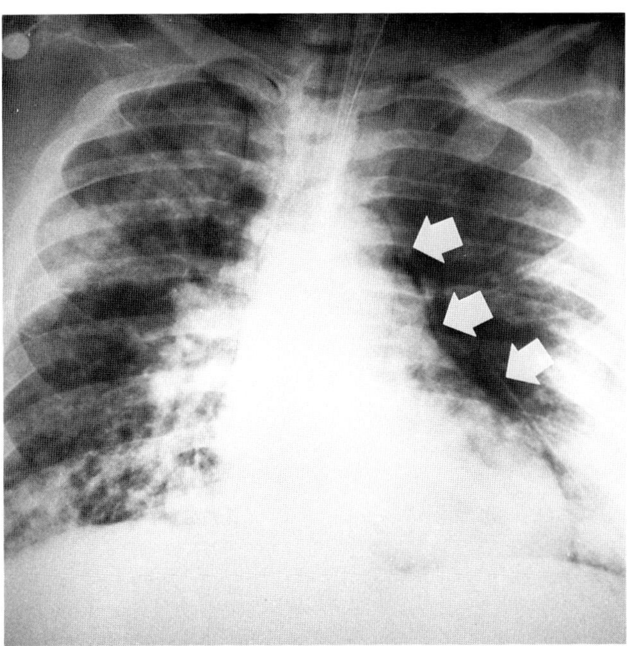

FIG. 7. Portable chest radiograph demonstrating a pneumomediastinum. The air is surrounding the aortic arch and extends along the left heart border (*arrows*).

newborns, pneumopericardium can cause cardiac tamponade and, therefore, is often drained. In adults, pneumopericardium is an uncommon complication of pneumomomediastinum. Rarely, a pneumomediastinum may rupture into the pleural space and cause a pneumothorax. Pneumomediastinum can dissect into the retroperitoneum and give rise to a pneumoperitoneum.

FOCAL PARENCHYMAL ABNORMALITIES

Focal parenchymal densities seen on portable chest radiographs can have numerous etiologies. The abnormalities are the same as seen on standard PA and lateral radiographs. However, in portable chest radiography a lateral view is not usually obtained, and the AP film is of lesser quality than a standard PA radiograph. The lack of a lateral film takes away important clues about the three-dimensional location and the appearance of abnormalities commonly seen on a standard PA and lateral radiograph. As less information can be obtained from a portable radiograph, greater use must be made of the patient's history, physical findings, and laboratory results. In addition, previous films and follow-up films are helpful in making and confirming a specific diagnosis.

Common causes of focal parenchymal densities seen on portable radiographs are atelectasis, pneumonia, aspiration, hemorrhage, and contusion. All of these abnormalities can produce a unique radiographic picture, but often they produce similar radiographic findings. If the patient's history, physical findings, and laboratory tests all point to a specific diagnosis, the nonspecific radiographic abnormality can be assumed to represent the specific diagnosis. However, many cases occur in which the clinical picture is no clearer or no more specific than the radiographic findings.

Lobar pneumonia is easy to diagnose on portable films, if there is a clear lobar parenchymal density and if the patient has a fever, a cough, and an elevated white blood cell count (Fig. 8). Lobar abnormalities can also be caused by partial lobar atelectasis, aspiration, or hemorrhage that involves only one lobe. Therefore, the value of follow-up films and close attention to the clinical situation is of utmost importance in making the correct radiographic diagnosis. Many times the radiographic diagnosis can be refined as the clinical picture becomes clearer and follow-up films are obtained.

Atelectasis is one of the most common radiographic abnormalities found on portable radiographs. Patients who are intubated, sedated, comatose, or in pain do not clear secretions normally. These same patients often do not breathe deeply. When these two factors combine, the lung is prone to develop areas of atelectasis. Atelectasis usually has an easily recognizable pattern of segmental, lobar, or whole lung opacity with evidence of volume loss (Fig. 9). Air bronchograms can be seen in atelectasis and usually indicate the atelectasis is peripheral and not the result of a central obstruction. Some patients have multiple areas of scattered atelectasis that can simulate patchy alveolar infiltrates of widespread pneumonia.

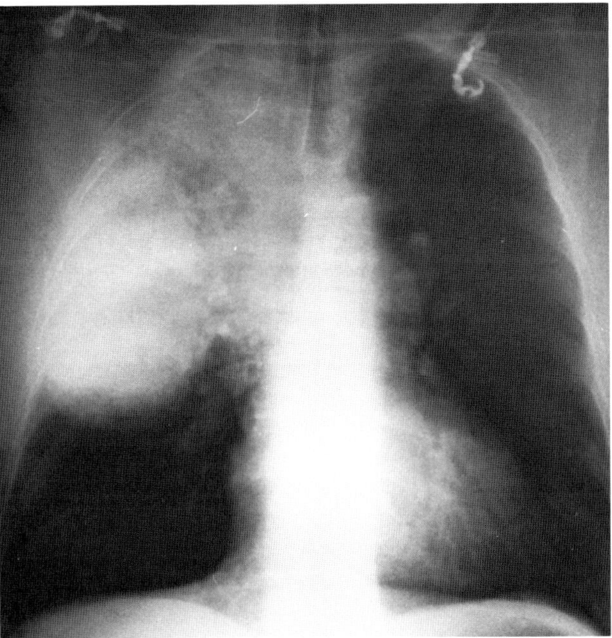

FIG. 8. Portable chest radiograph showing a patient with right upper lobe alveolar infiltrate. Despite having only one view, the appearance of right upper lobe consolidation is classic enough that it can be recognized on the AP view only.

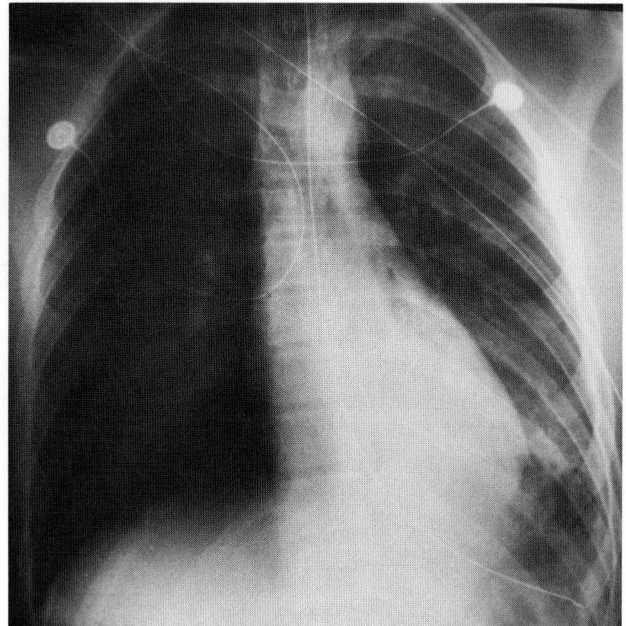
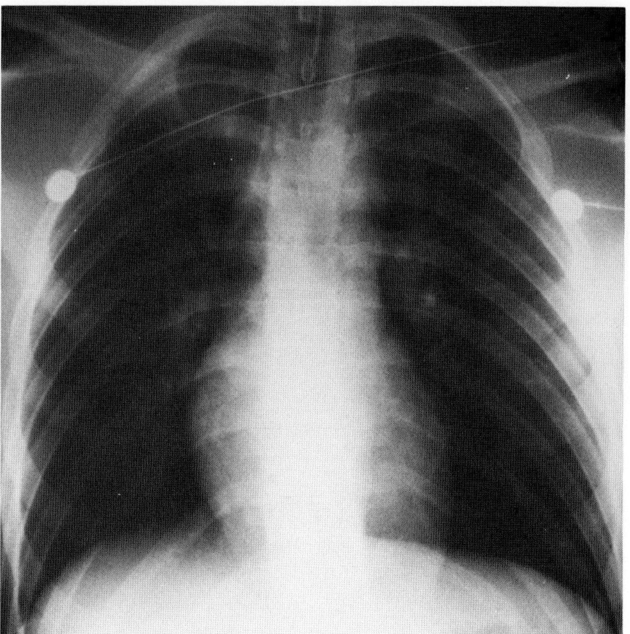

FIG. 9. (A) Portable chest radiograph of a young male immediately status-post appendectomy. The radiograph shows a retrocardiac density with lack of visualization of the descending aorta and the left hemidiaphragm. There is also shift of the mediastinum to the left. These are the findings of left lower lobe collapse most likely due to retained secretions. **(B)** Follow-up portable chest radiograph obtained 2 hours later. There has been reaeration of the left lower lobe.

Aspiration occurs commonly in ICU patients and has a varied radiographic appearance that can vary from the classic lower lobe parenchymal opacity to diffuse bilateral opacities. A clinical history of a witnessed aspiration, loss of consciousness, or seizure combined with an appropriate parenchymal opacity in a dependent location can be diagnostic of aspiration on a portable radiograph. Typical locations of aspiration are in the dependent portions of the lungs: the posterior segments of the upper and lower lobes and the superior segments of both lower lobes. Atypical aspirations may occur if the patient is in a position other than supine at the time of aspiration. Usually the clinical history is not forthcoming, and the radiographic diagnosis of aspiration is just one of the differential diagnostic choices.

Hemorrhage in the lung may produce a segmental, lobar, or diffuse parenchymal density depending on how much bleeding occurred and the location of the bleeding site. Without a history of hemoptysis or blood loss, the diagnosis of hemorrhage cannot be specifically made. Blood does clear rapidly, which may indicate the etiology of a parenchymal density as it is followed over a few days time.

Lung contusion is usually seen in the clinical situation of major trauma. Contusion can be thought of as a bruise within the lung parenchyma, with edema and hemorrhage causing the parenchymal opacity. A contusion is usually present on the initial radiographs or becomes manifest within 6 hours. The distribution of contusions are usually peripheral and may be associated with overlying rib fractures. Contusions may be extensive and may extend into the more central regions of the lung and mimic patchy areas of pneumonia.

DIFFUSE PARENCHYMAL DENSITIES

A single initial radiograph with diffuse bilateral alveolar infiltrates may present a diagnostic problem for the radiologist. Adult respiratory distress syndrome (ARDS), edema, and pneumonia can all present with this radiographic pattern. Occasionally aspiration and hemorrhage can also present in this fashion. Historical information, physical examination, and laboratory data must be used to increase the diagnostic ability of the single radiograph. The lack of prior films prevents the radiographic depiction of the evolvement of the chest radiographic abnormalities. Clinicians usually choose to treat the patient for several different possible diagnoses that could cause the diffuse radiographic alveolar infiltrates. As they start empirical treatment, they investigate the patient further. Patient response to the treatments and changes in the radiographs help the physicians and the radiologist make the correct diagnosis.

Adult Respiratory Distress Syndrome

ARDS is characterized by the development of hypoxemia, pulmonary infiltrates, stiff lungs, and noncardiogenic pulmonary edema, all of which usually occur within 72 hours after the onset of a definable risk factor. ARDS occurs when lung endothelial cell permeability increases and pulmonary edema ensues. Pulmonary involvement can occur in several ways. A primary lung process such as pneumonia can be the inciting event. Secondary pathologic changes can result from a variety of nonpulmonary events like sepsis and shock. Pathologically ARDS is characterized by endothelial cell injury and destruction, deposition of platelet and white blood cell aggregates in clots of fibrin and cellular debris, destruction of type I alveolar pneumocytes, and an acute inflammatory response. Clinically ARDS causes decreased lung compliance, ventilation/perfusion mis-

matches, arterial hypoxemia, and frequently pulmonary hypertension. Resolution of ARDS and survival are contingent on the ability to maintain adequate tissue oxygenation, allowing the lungs to repair endothelial and epithelial defects before fibrosis permanently alters the parenchyma. The cardiovascular response in ARDS is a high cardiac output and low systemic vascular resistance caused by a high peripheral demand for oxygen (10).

Radiographically ARDS presents with diffuse alveolar infiltrates that cannot reliably be differentiated from diffuse pneumonia and pulmonary edema. Radiographically ARDS has all the signs of alveolar filling, including air bronchogram and the obscuration of normal mediastinal contours. In ARDS the heart and vascular pedicle

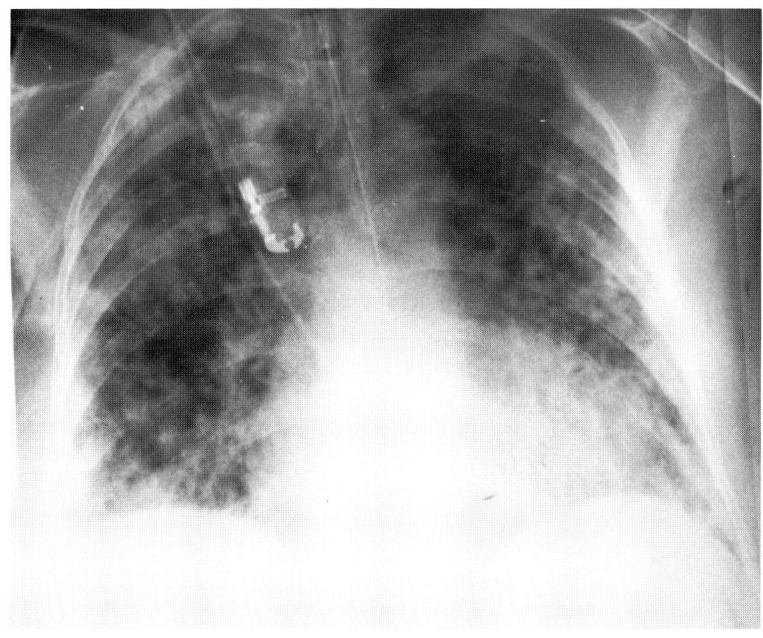

A

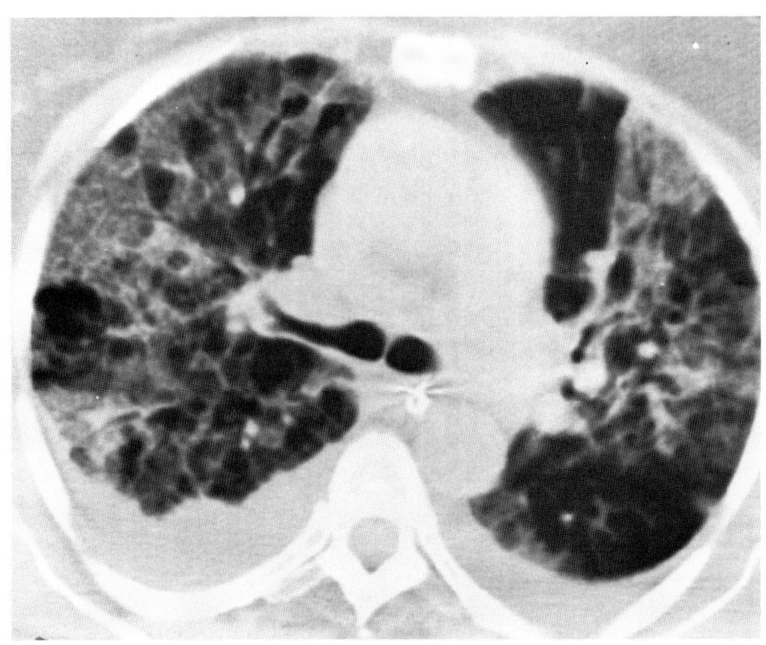

B

FIG. 10. (A) Portable chest radiograph with patchy alveolar infiltrates in a patient with sepsis. The radiographic findings are consistent with ARDS. **(B)** A CT scan was performed to rule out cavitary infiltrates. CT shows the early appearance of ARDS with patchy areas of alveolar infiltrates with intervening areas of normal lung.

width are usually normal and there is an absence of Kerley's B lines or pleural effusions. The radiographic abnormalities in ARDS usually become manifest within 24 hours of a defining insult. Initially there are patchy alveolar infiltrates in a perihilar distribution that progress rapidly to confluent alveolar infiltrates (Fig. 10). The radiographic abnormalities change very little over the following days. Complications of ARDS are common, including barotrauma, nosocomial infections, sepsis, pulmonary hemorrhage, and multisystem failure. Concurrent pneumonia is very hard to diagnose radiographically in patients with ARDS because of the preexisting bilateral diffuse infiltrates. Asymmetry of the diffuse infiltrates may be caused by superimposed pneumonia. However, this is not a reliable sign for discriminating between patients with and without pneumonia. Recovery from ARDS occurs in approximately 50 percent of patients and is a long process that takes weeks to months. The lungs are left with extensive interstial fibrosis and scarring (11,12).

Diffuse Pneumonia

Diffuse pneumonia is manifest by diffuse pulmonary alveolar infiltrates and is usually accompanied clinically by fever, leukocytosis, and purulent secretions. Radiographic signs of pneumonia include air bronchogram, alveolar infiltrates, the lack of visualization or normal mediastinal contours, and abutment of the infiltrate against a fissure. These signs are not very helpful in diagnosing diffuse pneumonia because ARDS and edema both may have air bronchogram, alveolar infiltrates, and obscuration of normal mediastinal contours. In addition, identifying an infiltrate against a fissure is not possible when all lobes are involved. It is not usually possible on one radiograph to distinguish the diagnosis of diffuse pneumonia from ARDS or edema with enough certainty that the clinicians can treat the patient only for pneumonia. Fever, leukocytosis, purulent tracheal secretions, and radiographic findings—developed to describe community-acquired pneumonia—may be nonspecific findings in intubated, mechanically ventilated patients. Therefore, more accurate diagnostic methods, such as bronchoscopy with quantitative cultures of protected specimen brushes, may be needed to establish the diagnosis of diffuse pneumonia (13).

Pulmonary Edema

Alveolar pulmonary edema can present with diffuse alveolar infiltrates that can be difficult to differentiate from ARDS or diffuse pneumonia. Fortunately, the patient's history, physical examination, or laboratory values can often point to the diagnosis of pulmonary edema. In patients with an acute myocardial infarction, acute shortness of breath, and an S3 gallop, the diagnosis of pulmonary edema can be made with some certainty on a radiograph with diffuse infiltrates. Additional radio-

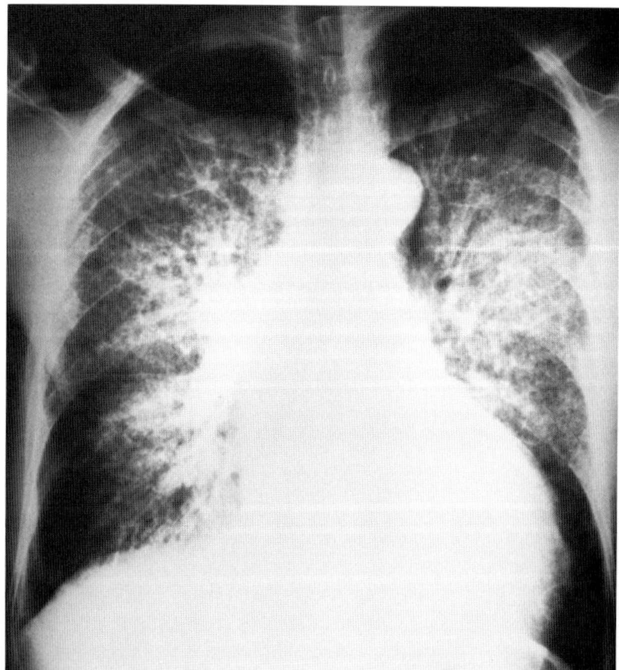
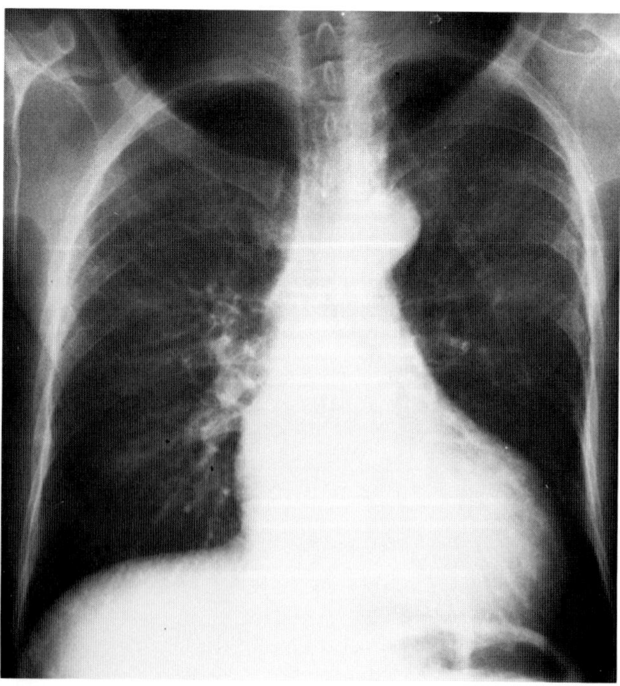

A   B

FIG. 11. **(A)** Portable chest radiograph with diffuse bilateral alveolar infiltrates. Clinically the patient had pulmonary edema due to a cardiac arrhythmia. **(B)** Follow-up radiograph 12 hours later after treatment with a diuretic showing complete clearing of the edema.

graphic findings, such as Kerley's B lines, small effusions, new cardiac enlargement, prominent pulmonary vascularity, and a widened vascular pedicle all make the diagnosis of edema more certain. However, quite often many of these additional findings are not present. Noncardiogenic pulmonary edema can also occur and may be differentiated from cardiogenic edema by the usual lack of cardiomegaly, Kerley's lines, and effusions. Follow-up films, Swan–Gantz catheter measurements, and the patient's response to treatment are often necessary to confirm the diagnosis of pulmonary edema (14) (Fig. 11).

TUBES, LINES, AND ERRORS

One of the most important functions of portable chest radiographs is to check on the position of tubes and lines. Often these devices end up in unexpected locations that cannot be suspected or determined without radiographs.

Endotracheal tube tips should lie approximately halfway between the vocal cords and the carina. This usually places the endotracheal tube 4–6 cm above the carina. Flexion of the neck can move the tip of the endotracheal tube 2 cm inferiorly and extension can move the tip 2 cm

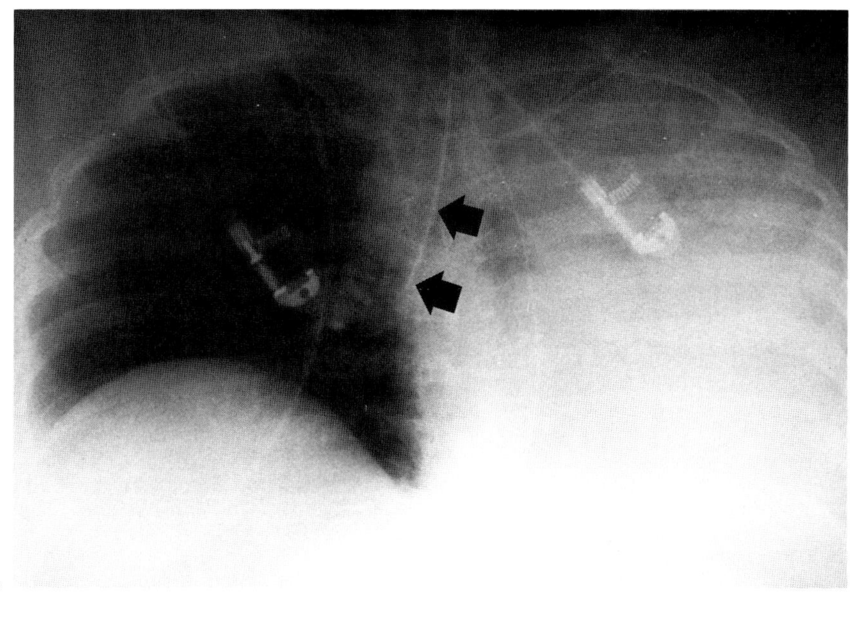

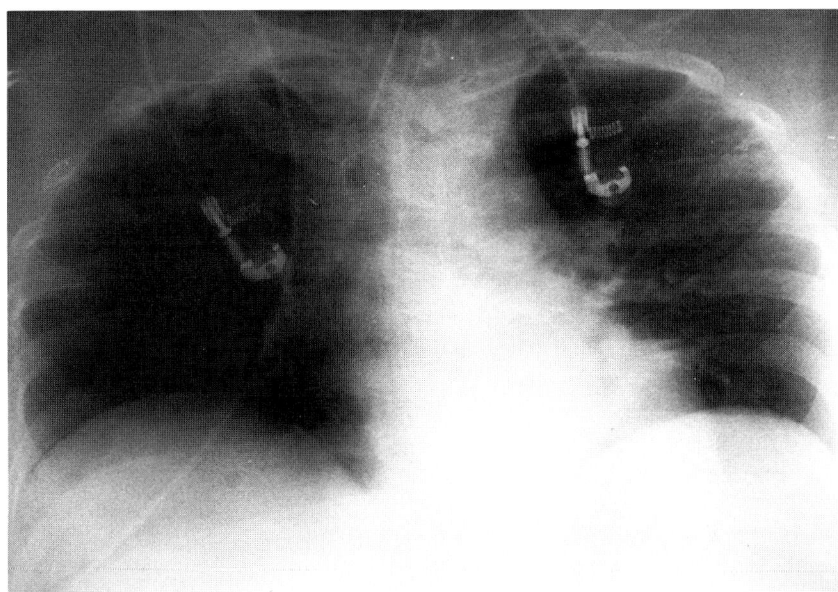

FIG. 12. **(A)** Portable chest radiograph of a right mainstem intubation (*arrows*) with collapse of the left lung. Collapse can occur rapidly when patients are on 100 percent oxygen, because all of the oxygen is absorbed whereas in patients on room air the 21 percent oxygen content is absorbed quickly but the nitrogen remains longer, keeping the lung aerated. **(B)** Repeat chest radiograph 1 hour later after the endotracheal tube has been pulled back.

superiorly (15). The carina can usually be seen on portable films and is usually at the level of the sixth thoracic vertebra. The position of the vocal cords is usually at the fifth or sixth cervical vertebral level. A method for approximating the position of the carina is to follow the course of the left mainstem bronchus back to the midline. Inadvertent intubation of the right mainstem bronchus is the most common malposition, because the right is a nearly straight continuation of the trachea. Right mainstem intubation often causes obstruction of the right upper lobe bronchus and right upper lobe partial atelectasis (Fig. 12). If the endotracheal tube is too high, even though the tip may be several centimeters below the vocal cords, the inflation cuff can press on the cords. This can cause irritation and edema of the cords, which can lead to postintubation hoarseness or stridor. Esophageal intubation usually is recognized by the clinicians at the bedside (Fig. 13). However, if unrecognized clinically, it may be difficult to identify radiographically. Ancillary signs, such as a large stomach bubble, hypoinflation of the lungs, and endotracheal tube tip below the carina, may all be important signs in diagnosing esophageal intubation. A slight oblique film will show the non-intubated trachea anterior to the esophageal placed tube. Other complications of endotracheal intubation include aspiration, tracheal rupture, tracheal stenosis, tracheomalacia, tracheoesophageal fistula, and dislodging of teeth (15).

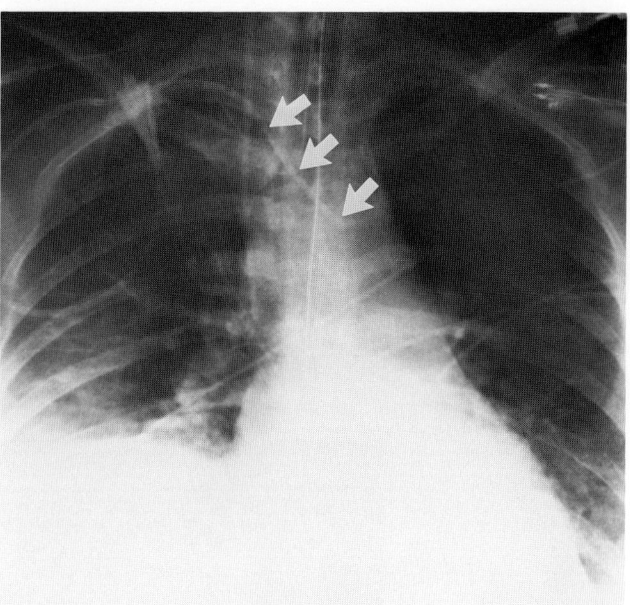

FIG. 14. Portable chest radiograph showing a right subclavian catheter tip in the aortic arch (*arrows*). The normal course of a right subclavian venous catheter is downward, in the right bracheocephalic vein and superior vena cava, along the right border of the mediastinum. Occasionally a right-sided venous catheter can pass into the left bracheocephalic vein, but its course is slightly higher than seen in this case.

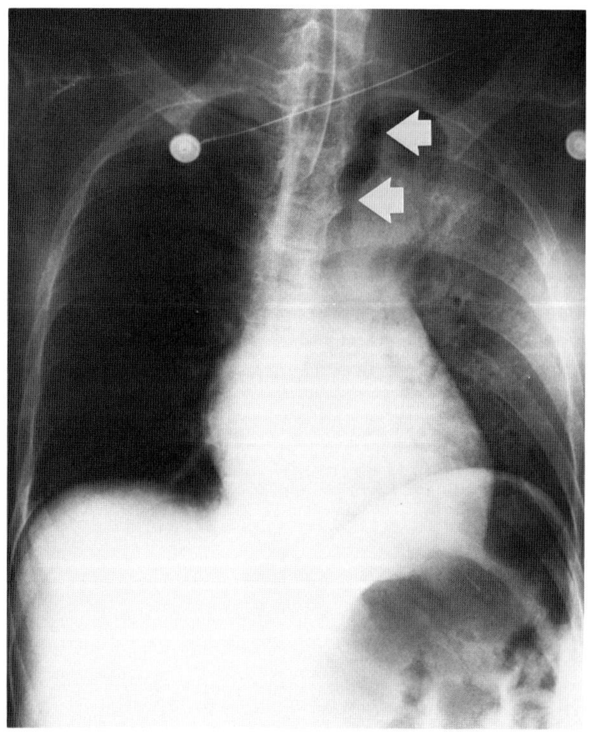

FIG. 13. Portable chest radiograph demonstrating an esophageal intubation. The trachea is to the left of the endotracheal tube (*arrows*).

Central venous catheters usually enter the internal jugular or subclavian veins. The tips should be located in the high-flow, large diameter superior vena cava that extends from the confluence of the right and left brachiocephalic veins to the top of the right atrium. Radiographically the superior vena cava begins just above the right upper lobe bronchus and ends at the top of the right atrial shadow. Several common complications can occur during the placement of central venous catheters (16). Common positions of misplaced venous catheters are to remain in the jugular or brachycephalic veins where they were placed, to pass from the right-sided great veins into the left-sided veins, or to enter the right atrium. Intraarterial placement can unknowingly occur, if the patient is hypotensive or there is a high-grade stenosis at the origin of the great vessel. Intravascular misplacements can usually be identified on the AP portable film, but occasionally a lateral film or injection of contrast into the errant catheter may be needed (Fig. 14). Pneumothorax is another complication of central venous catheter placement and should always be searched for on a postcatheter placement film. Pneumothorax rates vary with the experience of the person placing the catheter and are slightly higher when the subclavian approach is used. The Swan–Ganz catheter tip should be in the right or left pulmonary arteries usually within 1–2 cm of the thoracic spine. When the balloon on the tip is inflated, it is carried several centimeters into a more peripheral artery where

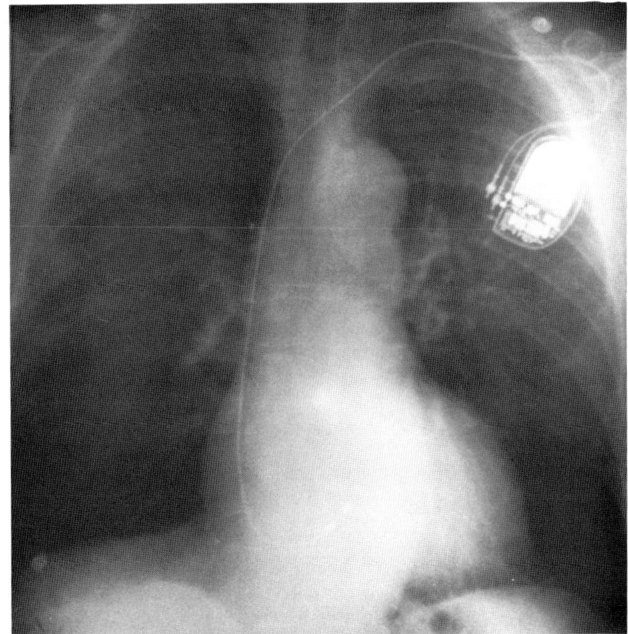
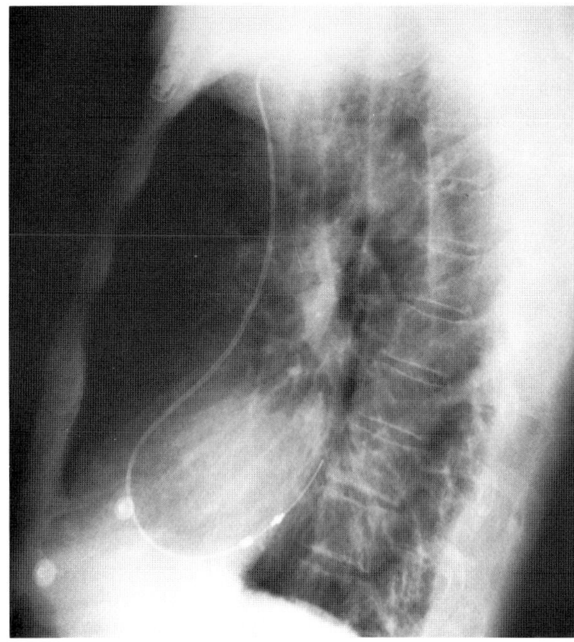

FIG. 15. (**A**) PA and (**B**) lateral chest radiograph showing a pacemaker tip in the coronary sinus.

the balloon occludes the pulmonary artery and a wedge reading can be obtained. When the balloon is deflated the natural recoil of the Swan–Ganz catheter brings the end of the catheter back to its original position in the proximal left or right pulmonary artery. If the catheters are too far out in the segmental arteries, thrombi may form or pulmonary infarctions can occur.

Pacemaker tip locations must be properly identified on portable films. Pacemaker patients usually get a post-placement portable film to check the position of the pacemaker tip. On an AP view the correct location can usually be determined. The usual tip location is in the right ventricle. However, occasionally it may be in the right atrial appendage or the coronary sinus (Fig. 15). Rarely, it may perforate the right ventricle. If the exact location cannot be determined from the single AP view a portable lateral view will help. On the lateral film, the coronary sinus is posterior, and the right atrial appendage is retrosternal in location.

Checking the position of nasogastric and feeding tubes is an important function of portable chest radiography (17). A chest film is usually taken after these tubes are inserted to check their position. Additional films are obtained if any difficulty or malfunction of the tubes is suspected (Fig. 16).

Many other catheters, tubes, and devices are inserted into patients. Radiologists must be familiar with the radiographic appearance and proper anatomic location of each device. In addition many confusing wires, monitoring devices, and tubes are on the outside of the patient, which must not be confused with tubes inside the patient.

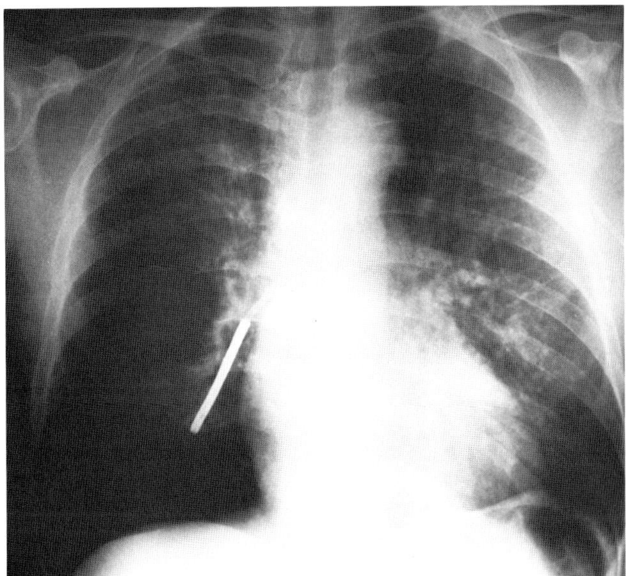

FIG. 16. Portable chest radiograph showing a feeding tube tip in the right lower lobe bronchus.

CHEST COMPUTED TOMOGRAPHY (CT) IN ICU PATIENTS

Historically, CT of ICU patients began with head scanning and continued with abdominal imaging. It became clear that the advantages of abdominal scanning outweighed the risks and trouble of bringing the patients to the scanner. However, chest CT scanning was not initially utilized, because the portable radiograph usually gave a fairly good representation of the thoracic pathology. In addition, the inability of the patients to stop breathing or the difficulty of halting the respirators during each scan slice was felt to limit the diagnostic ability of the scan. With faster scanners, diagnostic chest CTs can now be obtained despite patient breathing and movement.

Chest CT in ICU patients is utilized in several situations. The most common situations are to define further complex parenchymal densities and to check for occult abscesses or fluid collections. Despite the lack of adequate breathholding a diagnostic study can usually be obtained. The CT can identify the presence or absence of cavities, whether infiltrates are patchy versus diffuse, and whether there are discrete parenchymal nodules or just patchy alveolar infiltrates. CT can guide open lung biopsies by identifying which segments of lung are abnormal. CT can detect suspected pleural fluid collections and loculations. In patients with chest tubes CT can identify where the chest tubes are located and what pleural fluid collections are not being drained by the tubes. Some loculated pleural fluid collections may require CT guidance for aspiration and drainage. CT can also identify mediastinal abnormalities suspected on the portable radiographs. Paramediastinal fluid collections can usually be correctly identified without intravenous contrast. However, contrast can be used to help delineate masses or loculated fluid from normal mediastinal structures. Chest CT in ICU patients has proven to be a useful method for further evaluation of abnormalities seen on the portable radiographs (18,19).

ULTRASOUND OF THE CHEST IN ICU PATIENTS

Ultrasound of the chest is used in ICU patients to evaluate pleural effusions. Patients who are too ill to come to the radiology department can be evaluated at the bedside, because the ultrasound machines are portable. The presence of pleural fluid collections suspected on portable radiographs can be confirmed with ultrasound. The amount of fluid and the presence of loculations can also be determined. Ultrasound can guide bedside aspiration

of pleural fluid collections and aid in the placement of pleural drains. Overall, ultrasound's portability and excellent ability to depict pleural fluid have made chest ultrasound a common ICU procedure.

REFERENCES

1. Goodman LR, Putman CE. A radiologist's perspective of critical care imaging. In Putman CE, Goodman LR, eds. *Critical care imaging,* 3rd ed. Philadelphia: WB Saunders, 1992;3–12.
2. Bekemeyer WB, Crapo RO, Calhoon S, et al. Efficacy of chest radiography in a respiratory intensive care unit: a prospective study. *Chest* 1985;88:691–696.
3. MacMahon H. A new approach to bedside chest radiography: early clinical experience with a fixed geometry mobile system. Proceedings of the Society of Thoracic Radiology, Annual Meeting and Postgraduate Course, San Diego, 1989.
4. MacMahon H, Yasillo NJ, Carlin M. Laser alignment system for high-quality portable radiography. *Radiographics* 1992;12:111–120.
5. Aberle DR, Hansell D, Huang HK. Current status of digital projectional radiography of the chest. *J Thorac Imag* 1990;5:10–20.
6. Sagel SS, Jost G, Glazer HS, et al. Digital mobile radiography. *J Thorac Imag* 1990;5:36–48.
7. Fraser RG, Sanders C, Barnes GT, et al. Digital imaging of the chest. *Radiology* 1989;171:297–307.
8. Thompson MJ, Kubicka RA, Smith C. Evaluation of cardiopulmonary devices on chest radiographs: digital vs analog radiographs. *Am J Roentgenol* 1989;153:1165–1168.
9. Light RW. *Pleural diseases.* Philadelphia: Lea and Febiger, 1983;1–6.
10. Bone RC, Balk R, Slotman G, et al. Adult respiratory distress syndrome sequence and importance of development of multiple organ failure. *Chest* 1992;101:320–326.
11. Putman CE. Cardiac and noncardiac edema: radiological approach. In Putman CE, Goodman LR, eds. *Critical care imaging,* 3rd ed. Philadelphia: WB Saunders, 1992;116–119.
12. Greene R. Adult respiratory distress syndrome: acute alveolar damage. *Radiology* 1987;163:57–66.
13. Wunderink RG, Woldenberg LS, Zeiss J, et al. The radiologic diagnosis of autopsy-proven ventilator-associated pneumonia. *Chest* 1992;101:458–463.
14. Milne ENC. A physiological approach to reading critical care unit films. *J Thorac Imag* 1986;1:60–90.
15. Swenson SJ, Peters SG, LeRoy AJ, et al. Radiology in the intensive-care unit. *Mayo Clin Proc* 1991;66:396–410.
16. Henry DA, LeBolt S. Invasive hemodynamic monitoring: radiologist's perspective. *Radiographics* 1986;6:535–572.
17. Woodall BH, Winfield DF, Bisset GS. Inadvertent tracheobronchial placement of feeding tubes. *Radiology* 1987;165:727–729.
18. Peruzzi W, Garner W, Bools J. Portable chest roentgenography and computed tomography in critically ill patients. *Chest* 1988;93:722–726.
19. Mirvis SE, Tobin KD, Kostrubiak I, Belzberg H. Thoracic CT in detecting occult disease in critically ill patients. *Am J Roentgenol* 1987;148:685–689.

Thoracic Radiology, edited by
J.D. Newell, Jr., and R.D. Tarver,
Raven Press, Ltd., New York © 1993.

CHAPTER 10

Interventional Radiology of the Chest

Robert D. Tarver

Interventional chest radiology presently involves a number of procedures used for both diagnosis and therapy of thoracic disease. Invasive chest procedures initially consisted of needle biopsies of peripheral lung and rib lesions, or aspirations of small or loculated pleural effusions (1–5). Computed tomography (CT) has provided a much better display of thoracic and mediastinal anatomic detail and relationships than previous modalities. This improvement in imaging allowed needle biopsy of hilar and mediastinal lesions to be performed with increased accuracy and confidence. CT was also important in the development of therapeutic chest radiology. As the success of CT-guided abdominal aspiration and drainage techniques became apparent, these types of procedures were applied to the chest, resulting in the refinement of small tube percutaneous drainage of mediastinal and lung abscesses and empyemas. Today, the radiologist not only can biopsy formerly inaccessible areas of the chest, but also can perform therapeutic procedures. In this chapter, we shall review interventional chest radiology procedures. These include fine needle aspiration of lung nodules, pneumonias, hilar masses, mediastinal masses, and rib lesions, as well as drainage procedures for pneumothoraces, empyemas, and mediastinal and lung abscesses. For each procedure, indications, patient selection, technical aspects, and complications will be discussed. As with other interventional procedures, the radiologist undertaking these chest interventions must assume an active role in care of the patient, cooperating closely with the patient's primary and consulting physicians (6). Additionally, the radiologist should not hesitate to confer with other physicians skilled in the treatment of thoracic disease, such as the pulmonologist and thoracic surgeon. Careful attention

to technical aspects, knowledge about complications, and, most importantly, utmost concern for each patient's well-being help to optimize the outcome of all interventional chest procedures.

PERCUTANEOUS FINE NEEDLE ASPIRATION OF LUNG NODULES

Fine needle aspiration has an important role in the evaluation of patients with pulmonary nodules. It is the most common interventional chest procedure performed by the radiologist. Fine needle aspiration is important because it may provide a definitive tissue diagnosis and may obviate unnecessary surgical procedures (7–10). Percutaneous fine needle aspiration of lung nodules is a safe and simple procedure with a high diagnostic yield. In the diagnosis of malignant nodules, the procedure has a 90 to 95 percent true positive rate (1,2,11–16). The diagnosis of benign lesions has a slightly lower true positive rate due to the nonspecific nature of such cytologic specimens (1,17). However, when a specific benign diagnosis can be made from the aspirated material, the true positive rate also exceeds 90 percent (13,15–19).

Successful utilization of fine needle aspiration requires the availability of an expert cytologist. The importance of a cytologist cannot be overemphasized. Cytologists are now able to make an accurate diagnosis from a monolayer of cells. This accuracy is the product of special cytopathology training. Surgical pathology training alone will not provide the expertise needed to evaluate needle biopsy material properly. The correct interpretation of aspirated cellular material is difficult and requires the cytologist and radiologist to work together closely. The best situation occurs when the cytologist is present at the time of the biopsy procedure. The cytologist can give immediate preliminary interpretations about the adequacy of specimens and the presence or absence of malignancy (20). If the cytologist cannot attend the proce-

R. D. Tarver: Department of Radiology, Indiana University Medical Center, and Wishard Memorial Hospital, Indianapolis, Indiana 46202.

dure, then quick staining of specimens in the pathology department is helpful in planning further biopsies.

Indications

Fine needle aspiration biopsy has many applications in the evaluation of patients with pulmonary lesions. The basic indication for needle biopsy of the lung is an undiagnosed pulmonary lesion. A patient whose management would be affected by definitive tissue diagnosis of a pulmonary lesion is a candidate for needle biopsy. Fine needle aspiration biopsy of chest lesions is useful in many clinical situations, including:

1. Inoperable patient with suspected bronchogenic carcinoma.
2. Solitary pulmonary nodule suspected to be the source of metastatic disease.
3. Known extrapulmonary malignancy and a solitary pulmonary nodule.
4. Probable pulmonary carcinoma in a patient who refuses operation.
5. Multiple pulmonary nodules.
6. Two nodules in different lobes or lungs.
7. Undiagnosed solitary pulmonary nodule.
8. Superior sulcus tumor.
9. Immunocompromised patient with an infiltrate or nodule.

Patient Selection and Evaluation

Most patients are referred for transthoracic fine needle aspiration of lung nodules detected on their chest radiographs. Before biopsy, every effort should be made to establish identity of the lesion. Old radiographs should be reviewed. The presence of benign-appearing calcifications should be sought using thin section CT or the reference phantom. In central lesions, sputum cytology should be obtained. Physical, historical, or laboratory evidence for prior granulomatous infection or extrapulmonary malignancy is helpful. CT of the chest and liver prior to aspiration biopsy provides an adequate survey for occult lung nodules, mediastinal adenopathy, and liver metastases. Once noninvasive methods of determining the etiology of a pulmonary nodule have been exhausted, the patient may be considered for a transthoracic fine needle aspiration.

Several laboratory evaluations should be performed before each biopsy. Pulmonary function tests should be obtained prior to the aspiration because a biopsy-induced pneumothorax will alter the test results. Pulmonary function test will also determine if the patient is operable and, if a pneumothorax should occur, what type of pulmonary reserve the patient has. Prothrombin time, partial thromboplastin time, and platelet count should be obtained to ensure that adequate clotting exists. Hemoglobin and hematocrit will determine if the patient is anemic and, therefore, is prone to hypoxia in the event of a pneumothorax. These studies also provide a baseline in the event of actual or suspected hemorrhage. In any procedure, abnormal laboratory findings are relative contraindications, and risk versus benefit must be weighed.

Several contraindications to percutaneous fine needle biopsy of lung nodules are well accepted (1–3). Common to all laboratory studies, these following contraindications are relative, and patients must be evaluated individually. Patients who will not or cannot suspend respiration for a few seconds at a time are not candidates for percutaneous lung biopsy. Coagulopathies and bleeding disorders are contraindications. These conditions can be corrected by platelet transfusion, vitamin K administration, or the temporary discontinuation of anticoagulants. Pulmonary hypertension is a contraindication because of the danger of persistent pulmonary hemorrhage. Areas of severe emphysematous bullae or blebs, in the planned biopsy route, increase the risk of pneumothorax and should be avoided if possible. In these patients, provisions for immediate chest tube placement should be made. Severe pulmonary disease (forced expiratory volume less than 1.0 liter) is a relative contraindication; however, these patients may be biopsied if a chest tube can be placed immediately in the event of a clinically significant pneumothorax. Contralateral pneumonectomy is a relative contraindication unless a prophylactic chest tube is placed or immediate placement of a chest tube is available. Positive pressure ventilation increases the risk of air embolism (1). Suspected echinococcal cysts should not be biopsied because of the possibility of an anaphylactic reaction to spilled intracystic material. Suspected vascular lesions should be evaluated with CT or angiography before biopsy, and atriovenous malformations (AVM) should not be biopsied.

Prior to each biopsy, the radiologist should thoroughly discuss the risks and possible benefits with the referring physicians. All parties should agree that the biopsy is indeed indicated and that the potential information provided by the biopsy must be worth the risk to the patient. If the biopsy results will not change the patient's clinical course or management, the biopsy should not be performed.

Before each biopsy, the radiologist must discuss the procedure with the patient, making sure the patient understands the benefits and risks. Patients are told that the complications include a 30 percent chance of pneumothorax, a 10 percent chance they will need a small chest tube, a 10 percent chance they will experience a small amount of blood-streaked sputum, a theoretical chance they could get an infection, and a less than 1 in a 1000 chance they could die from the procedure. Alternative methods of making the diagnosis should be presented. At our institution, an informed consent is signed by the patient, a witness, and the radiologist performing the biopsy.

Percutaneous lung nodule aspiration can be performed on an outpatient basis. The safety of the procedure has been shown (4,21–23), and outpatient aspiration is less costly than admitting the patient solely for the biopsy. Most pneumothoraces occur within a few hours after the procedure. Patients may wait in a designated area within the radiology department or outpatient surgery area for a few hours after the biopsy. If after this time they have no pneumothorax or only a small, unchanged pneumothorax, the patients may be discharged to a nearby hotel or residence. Patients are carefully instructed about the signs and symptoms of pneumothorax and are told to return to the hospital, if these occur. Patients selected for outpatient biopsy must be reliable and cooperative, and they must have readily available transportation back to the hospital, should complications arise. They should also have a telephone to call for help and have another responsible person staying with them. Patients with severe underlying lung disease should not be biopsied as outpatients because of their inability to tolerate pneumothoraces.

Percutaneous lung biopsy is usually performed with little prebiopsy physical preparation. Most patients require no systemic analgesia or sedation. It is desirable for the patients to be fully alert and cooperative so that they can help with positioning and inform the radiologist about complaints that could signify a complication. However, if the patient is particularly anxious, small amounts of diazepam or meperidine may be used just prior to the procedure. It is preferable for the patient to be NPO for 3 hours before the biopsy because, although vomiting during the procedure is rare, this precaution lessens the chance of aspiration of gastric contents. Placement of an intravenous line may be helpful, should complications arise that require analgesia or supportive care.

Technical Aspects

Planning the biopsy site and route is an important aspect of any fine needle aspiration. In nearly all cases, the nodule is visible on routine chest radiographs, allowing the radiologist to determine the approach. Usually, the pathway selected is the one that involves the shortest distance through the lung parenchyma. Additional factors include avoiding passage through a fissure, needling the lesion from a posterior approach (posterior ribs move less than anterior ribs during respiration), and entering the chest over superior rib margins to avoid intercostal vessels. The posterior approach often decreases the patient's anxiety, because the individual cannot watch all of the procedure.

If the lesion is seen on only one view of the routine radiograph, using fluoroscopy or CT should allow accurate depth determination of the nodule. Most nodules are biopsied under fluoroscopic guidance and, therefore, must be well visualized on a fluoroscopic screen. Equipment that allows the operator to view the lesion in two planes, such as a C-arm fluoroscope, should be used if available. In the absence of such equipment, depth determination may be made from a prior CT scan or from the chest radiographs. If the nodule cannot be seen on fluoroscopy, then CT guidance may be used (24).

A variety of needles are available for percutaneous fine needle aspiration of chest lesions. Each has its proponents, particular attractions, and possible drawbacks. The needles can be broken down into two basic types: ones that are used to obtain cells for cytology and ones that take a small core sample for histology. The best approach to needle selection is frequent use of the smallest possible variety of needles. This approach avoids unfamiliarity with the needles and works well for the radiologist/cytologist team. If a cytologist is present at the biopsy, a coaxial system with an outer guide needle and an inner fine aspirating needle is desirable. This system allows multiple samples of the lesion, with just one pass through the pleura. However, if the material is sent to the pathology department for later staining and review, only a thin needle and one successful pass should be attempted at each biopsy (25).

The procedure should be performed in a room equipped to handle any emergency that may occur. A blood pressure cuff and stethoscope, saline and intravenous administration sets, and a crash cart with materials and drugs for a full resuscitation should be available. A chest tube set-up must be present for immediate use, if needed.

The patient is placed on the fluoroscopic table in the position determined prior to the start of the procedure. Small adjustments in position are usually required to place the ribs or scapula away from the proposed biopsy route. A preparation tray, such as those used for arthrography, provides proper skin preparation materials. The patient's skin is marked under fluoroscopic guidance, prepped, draped, and locally anesthetized. A skin nick is made with a #11 blade or an 18 gauge needle. At this time, the needle selected for the aspiration is checked for flaws in the hub, shaft, and point, and for smooth movement between the inner and outer components. Next, fluoroscopic observation of the patient's respiration is used to check the changing relationship between skin surface, ribs, and nodule. The needle pathway to the lesion should be parallel to the x-ray beam and in the center of the fluoroscopic field to avoid parallax errors. While the needle point is held on the entry site, the patient practices suspending respiration, and the needle point and lung nodule are superimposed on the fluoroscopic image. The phase of suspended respiration should be in midinspiration rather than deep inspiration or expiration. This allows the needle to be perpendicular to the chest wall during most of the procedure, because most of the time during a coaxial biopsy the needle is in the patient and biopsies are not being taken. If the biopsy is made in deep inspiration or expiration, the needle is severely angled most of the time and may exert more traction on the pleura. With the fluoroscope off, the needle is then placed upright and advanced straight downward into the chest wall. Its position should be fluoroscopically checked as often as needed. When the needle is about to enter the pleural space, the patient's respirations are suspended at the point of needle and nodule superimposition. The needle is advanced through the parietal and visceral pleura with one motion, then advanced within the parenchyma in serial steps while respirations are suspended. Frequent stops during needle advancement allow the patient to breathe and the radiologist to check needle position. The needle is advanced until it is just within the lesion. With a coaxial needle system, the outer guide needle is positioned just outside the lesion; the inner aspirating needle goes into the nodule. Adequate depth can be determined by lateral or angulated fluoroscopy (26), or predetermined from CT or chest radiographs. When the needle is in the lesion, the tip of the needle moves in conjunction with the lesion on the fluoroscopic screen as the patient breathes. Needle tip position can be confirmed by moving the needle hub during suspended respiration and watching the nodule move with the needle tip.

If a C-arm fluoroscopic unit is available, axial aiming may be used. This technique is useful when the lesion to be biopsied is under a rib. The fluoroscope is angled so that the lesion is not overlying the rib. The needle is placed in the extrapleural soft tissues above the rib and angled toward the target lesion. If the needle is superimposed over the lesion, it is advanced in a stepwise fashion as described previously. If the needle is not superimposed, further adjustments of both the needle angulation and fluoroscope are made until the needle and lesion are projected over one another.

Next, the aspirating needle stylet is removed, and a 10–20 ml syringe is attached with 1–2 ml of air within the syringe. Any time the needle is held, the patient should suspend respiration to minimize the traction on the pleura. The specimen is then obtained by aspirating on the syringe and making several up, down, and rotating motions (27,28). Cytologists at our institution prefer that the first two samples be obtained without aspiration. Often excellent specimens can be obtained in this fashion, with very little blood within the specimens. A tissue core sometimes may be obtained by advancing the needle with a rotational motion. Samples should be taken from the edge of large lesions because the center often contains only necrotic material. The needle and syringe are now removed with no suction being applied during removal, as the goal is to aspirate tissue only into the needle tip. If a cytopathologist is in attendance, and a

coaxial system is used, then the samples are reviewed as they are obtained. When more material is needed, further samples are taken until the cytopathologist has adequate material. In a coaxial system, a final specimen can be obtained through the guide needle by advancing it the short distance into the lesion and aspirating in the same fashion.

Aspirated material is handled differently by different pathology departments. If a cytopathologist is present at the procedure, the specimens can be ejected onto microscope slides, and immediate staining and interpretation can take place. In the absence of a cytologist, the specimens can be placed on slides, fixed, and stained later. Also, the specimens can be placed in vials of saline or fixative. If infectious etiology of the lung mass is suspected, specimens can also be placed into appropriate culture media and smeared on slides for microbiologic staining.

Throughout the procedure, the patient is asked if he/she is experiencing any dyspnea or pain away from the biopsy site. The welfare of the patient is the primary concern; success of the biopsy is secondary. After the biopsy, the patient's pulse and blood pressure are obtained, and the individual is allowed to lie quietly for 10 minutes of observation. Then the patient is asked to sit up and breathe quietly for a few minutes. Specific inquiries about dyspnea and chest pain are made, and the chest is examined by auscultation. Sharp pain in the biopsied hemithorax often indicates pneumothorax. If the patient has tolerated sitting in the fluoroscopy room, then a chest radiograph is obtained. If the film shows no pneumothorax, an inpatient may leave the x-ray department. The patient should be reminded to notify appropriate staff immediately of any chest pain, dyspnea, or persistent or severe hemoptysis. A follow-up chest radiograph is obtained at 4 hours or sooner if the patient begins to have dyspnea or pain. Outpatients, with no postbiopsy pneumothorax, are required to remain in the department until their 4-hour film is obtained after an immediate postbiopsy film shows no pneumothorax.

If a pneumothorax is present on the postbiopsy film, and no treatment is immediately necessary, another chest film is obtained in 1 hour. Four to 6 hours after this film, another follow-up radiograph is obtained.

Complications

Pneumothorax is the most common complication of needle aspiration of lung nodules (29). In most series, the incidence of pneumothorax is about 25 percent (1,3,4). Most of the pneumothoraces are present on the initial postbiopsy chest film; rarely do pneumothoraces solely manifest on a later radiograph (1). However, the size of the pneumothorax may increase on later films. Less than one-third of the pneumothoraces require treatment

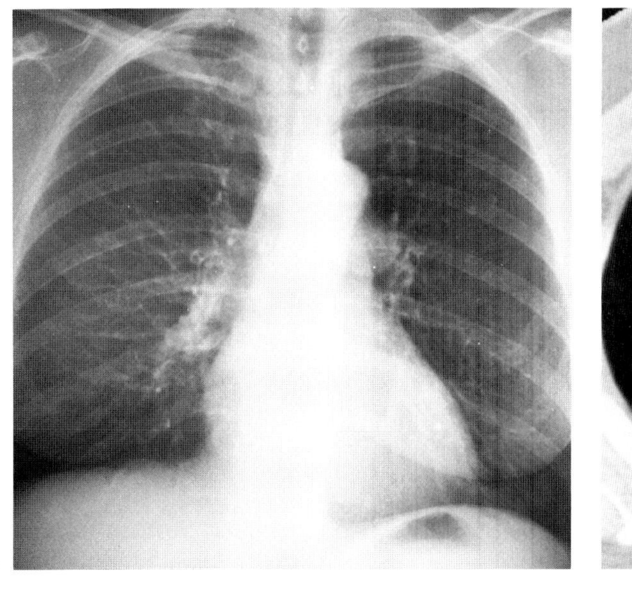

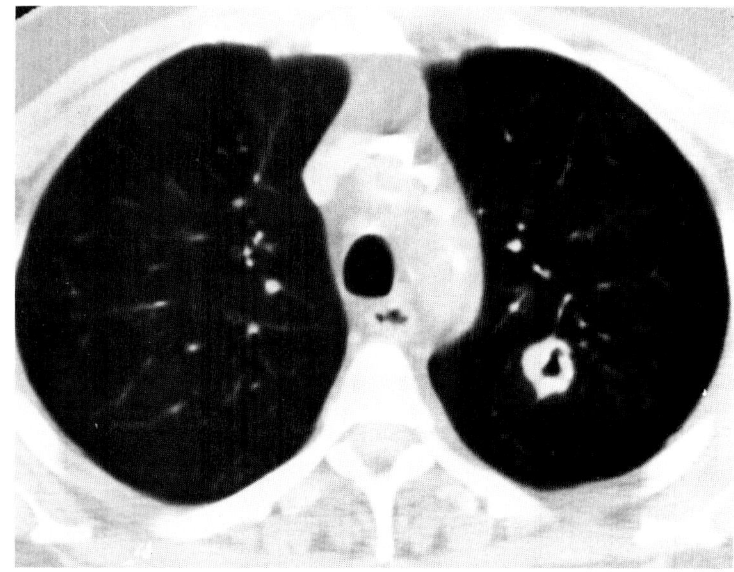

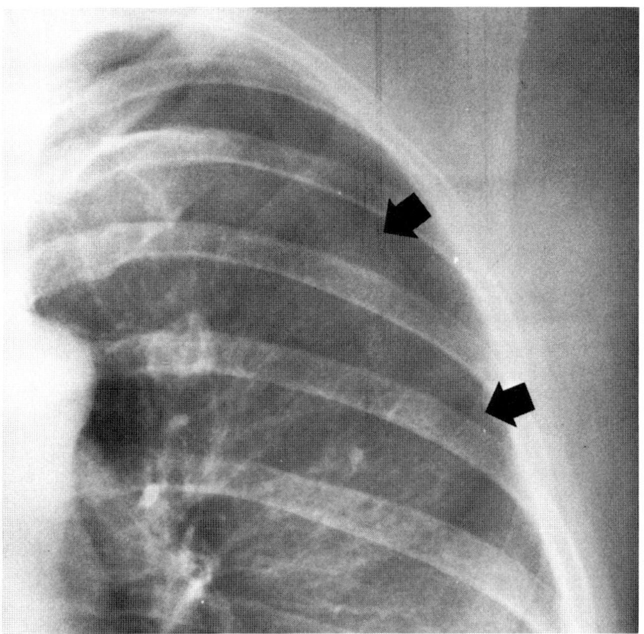

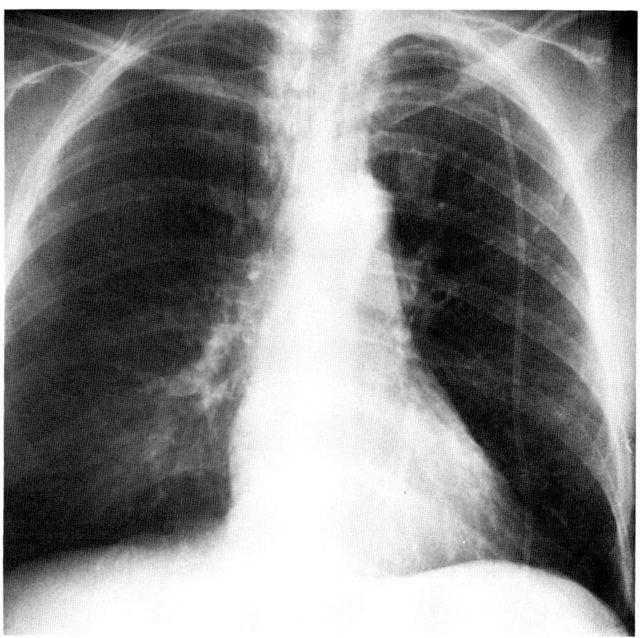

FIG. 1. Case demonstrating the use of fine needle aspiration biopsy showing the planning sequence and treatment of a complication. (**A**) Chest radiograph showing a left upper lobe cavitary mass. (**B**) CT of the same mass used for staging and determining biopsy pathway. (**C**) Enlargement of the left hemithorax showing a pneumothorax (*arrows*). (**D**) Chest radiograph after the placement of a small caliber chest tube and a Heimlich valve showing sucessful treatment of the pneumothorax.

(1,2). Positioning the patient with the puncture site down for 1 hour after the biopsy does not reduce the incidence of pneumothoraces but may decrease the number of patients who need chest tubes (30).

The decision to treat a pneumothorax is made jointly by the radiologist and referring physician. Small and asymptomatic pneumothoraces may be followed with daily radiographs and close clinical follow-up. It is helpful to distinguish whether the patient's dyspnea is caused by actual compromise of pulmonary function or by the pleuritic pain often associated with a small pneumotho-

rax. This difference is important because chest tube insertion should not be undertaken for chest pain alone. The purpose of a chest tube is to alleviate a decrease in pulmonary function secondary to the partially collapsed lung.

If the patient develops a large (25 percent or greater) pneumothorax or is dyspneic, treatment is required. Pneumothorax can be treated by one of three methods. First, the air in the pleural space can be aspirated with an 18 gauge needle connected to a 50 ml syringe by a three-way stopcock. An angiocath also can be used to aspirate a pneumothorax; the advantage is that the plastic sheath will not lacerate the surface of the lung as reexpansion occurs (31). Often, the pneumothorax resolves after aspiration, but the patient must be followed closely for evidence of recurrence. The second form of treatment is the placement of a small caliber chest tube (Cook Catheter, Bloomington, IN, or Arrow, Reading, PA) (32) (Fig. 1). The pneumothorax may then be aspirated immediately, and the tube can later be attached to a Heimlich valve or wall suction. A third type of treatment for pneumothorax is placement of a standard thoracostomy tube.

Hemoptysis is another complication of percutaneous needle biopsy. The incidence is usually less than 10 percent (1,2). Hemoptysis, which is usually minimal, manifests itself as bloodstreaked sputum for less than 1 hour. Occasionally, hemoptysis can be massive. Although quite rare, massive hemoptysis has been responsible for some of the deaths associated with fine needle lung biopsies (2). The radiologist and referring physician should be aware of the complication and prepared to control the bleeding with bronchial artery embolization or pulmonary resection. Hemorrhage around a lesion without hemoptysis is fairly common and is manifest as slight obscuration of the nodule's borders on follow-up chest radiographs.

The reported fatality rate for lung aspiration biopsies is about 0.02 percent (1,33). The causes of death have been tension pneumothorax, air embolism, and pulmonary hemorrhage (2,34). The invasive radiologist must recognize these possibilities and be prepared to treat them emergently. If close attention is paid to the technical performance of the procedure and to the patient's welfare, the chance of drastic complications is decreased, and excellent results can be obtained.

PERCUTANEOUS FINE NEEDLE ASPIRATION OF OTHER THORACIC ABNORMALITIES

Using the techniques of lung nodule aspiration, biopsy of rib and pleural abnormalities, as well as pulmonary infiltrates, can be accomplished. Slight modification of nodule aspiration techniques is necessary to obtain satisfactory results.

Percutaneous needle aspiration of rib lesions is a simple and quick method for determining etiology. The usual question to be answered is whether the lesion is malignant or not. Benign bone lesions and primary bone tumors other than plasmacytoma may require more tissue, for a definitive diagnosis, than a fine needle aspiration provides. The only alteration of the previously described lung fine needle technique required to biopsy rib lesions is that a shorter needle can be used. A small 20 or 18 gauge standard hypodermic needle can be used successfully. Using a short 18 gauge hypodermic needle as a guide for a 20 gauge spinal needle makes a good rib biopsy set. Cook Catheter (Bloomington, IN) has coaxial

sets available in shorter lengths that are useful in rib biopsies. The greater the degree of rib destruction, the easier it is to pass the biopsy needle through the bone cortex. Care must be taken not to pass the needle into the pleural space. Complications of this procedure include pneumothorax and hemorrhage.

Pleural masses are easily biopsied by the percutaneous route. The biopsies can be accomplished under fluoroscopic or CT control, depending on which modality best demonstrates the lesion. Usually, a standard length 18 or 20 gauge hypodermic needle can be used. If thick pleural lesions are to be biopsied, or if the patient has thick subcutaneous tissue, a spinal needle may be employed. The advantage of short needles is that they can be manipulated more easily than the longer lung biopsy needles. When the pleural mass is very thick, and there is almost no chance of encountering lung tissue, a 14 or 16 gauge liver biopsy needle can be used (35). These needles give a large tissue sample that can be sent for histologic interpretation. If CT guidance is used, the needle can be angled to produce tangential entry into the lesion, thus increasing the thickness of the tissue to be sampled. Large tissue specimens are helpful, because fine needle aspirations can often be nondiagnostic in the case of mesotheliomas. Complications of pleural aspiration are the same as for rib biopsy: pneumothorax and hemorrhage.

Focal pulmonary parenchymal infections can be evaluated by fine needle aspiration (36,37). Patients referred for this procedure are usually immunocompromised from malignancies, chemotherapy, organ transplantation, or other immunodeficiency states. Diagnosing pneumonia and identifying the causative organisms in these patients is important for two reasons. First, the patient may be infected with any of a number of organisms that require specific antibiotic coverage. Second, pneumonias in these patients spread rapidly and have a high mortality, if not treated promptly and appropriately.

These patients are often considerably more ill than the usual patients undergoing needle biopsy of lung nodules. Particular attention must be given to the status of clotting functions, the degree of underlying respiratory embarrassment, and ability to cooperate with breathholding. Also, careful attention must be given to sterile technique.

Technically, aspiration of inflammatory masses is similar to biopsy of lung nodules. If no material is aspirated on initial passes, then 2 to 5 ml of sterile saline, without preservative, is rapidly injected and aspirated in an attempt to lavage the lesion. Material collected is then placed in anaerobic, aerobic, fungal, and tuberculous culture media; specimens are also stained for organisms that infect immunocompromised hosts. Complication rates are similar to those for aspiration of lung nodules (36,37). However, the radiologist must be aware that these patients are quite ill and that any complications must be treated without delay. Needle aspiration of inflammatory lesions is an alternative to bronchoscopic

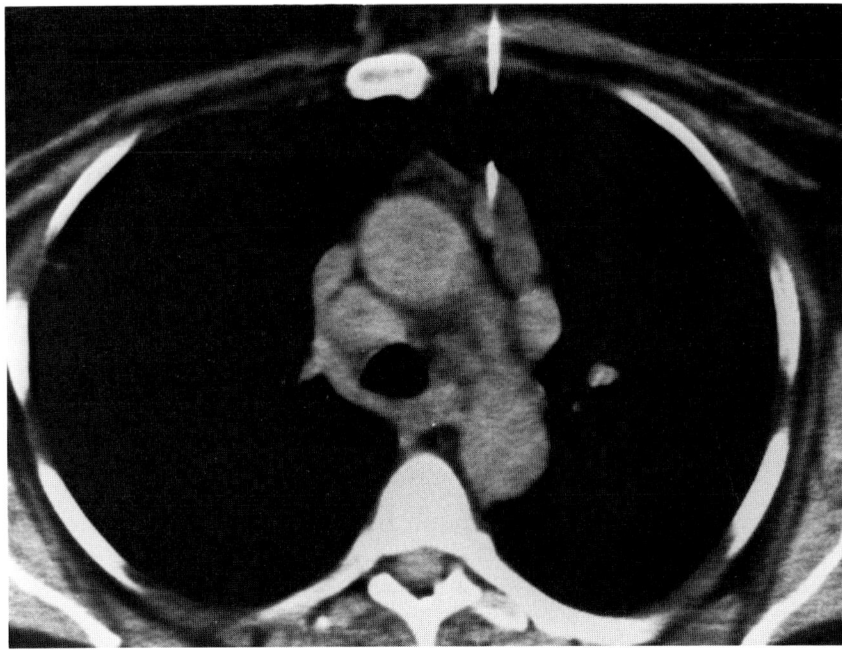

FIG. 2. CT scan of a biopsy of nodes adjacent to the aortic arch. CT allowed for the exact placement of the needle, and a diagnosis of sarcoid was made on biopsy.

evaluation or open lung biopsy. The diagnostic yield for this procedure is reported to be in the 70 percent range (36).

PERCUTANEOUS FINE NEEDLE ASPIRATION OF MEDIASTINAL AND HILAR MASSES

CT has increased the use of percutaneous biopsy of mediastinal and hilar masses. CT offers a better display of the anatomic detail and relationships of both normal structures and abnormal masses within the thorax than do plain radiography and conventional tomography. Once the anatomic relationships between lesion and normal structures are established, a biopsy route, which avoids major blood vessels, can be planned.

Technical Aspects

Fluoroscopically guided biopsy of hilar and mediastinal masses is possible. If a prior CT scan demonstrates a portion of the mass to be away from vascular structures, and that portion of the mass can be seen on the image intensifier, fluoroscopy may be used. Again, the technique is similar to that used for aspiration of lung nodules. However, if the relationship between the mass and hilar and mediastinal blood vessels is such that accurate placement of the needle is not possible with fluoroscopy, the biopsy should be done under CT guidance. The advantage to CT guidance is that difficult, often angulated, approaches to the lesion can be undertaken with com-

plete confidence, because CT clarifies needle course and tip location (Fig. 2).

Fluoroscopic needle guidance offers immediate information on needle location. With CT guidance, the progress of the needle tip can be visualized only after each

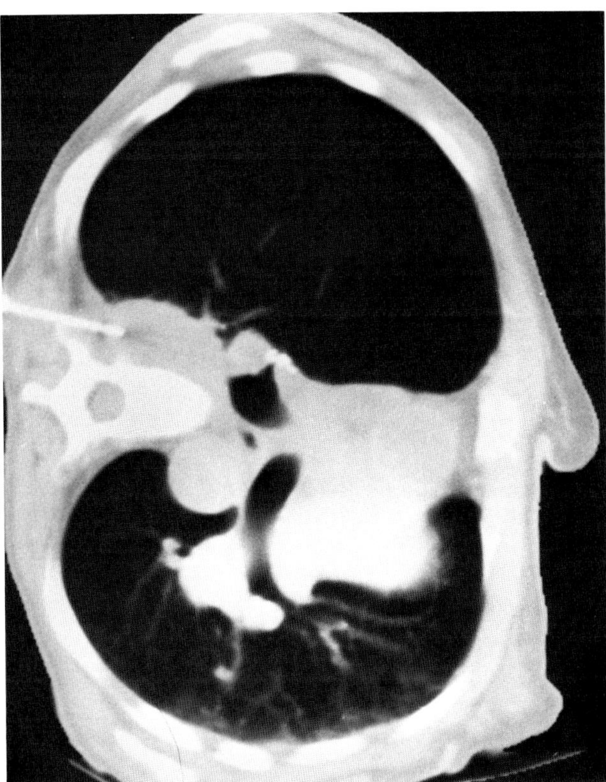

FIG. 3. CT scan of a biopsy of a pleural mass. CT guided the biopsy path so that it remained extrapulmonary.

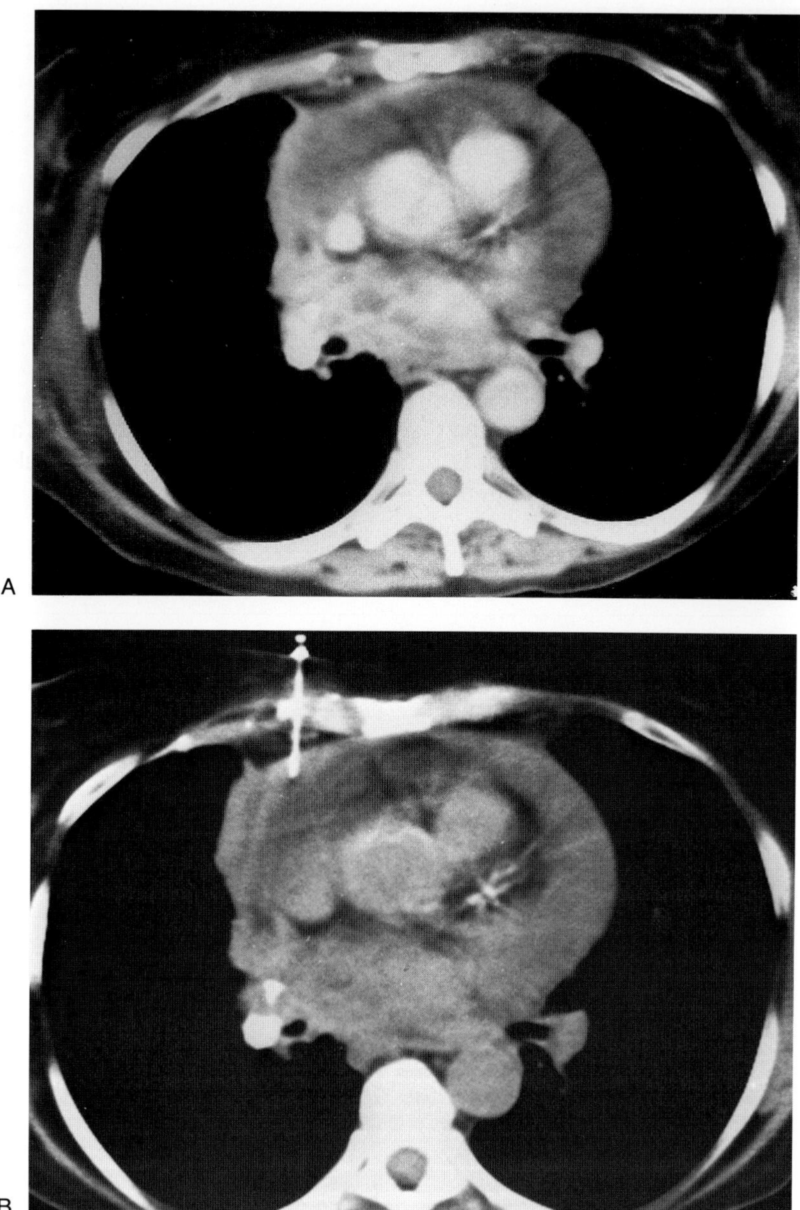

FIG. 4. CT-directed aspiration biopsy of a malignant pericardial effusion. (**A**) CT with contrast identified the exact location of the great vessels, and (**B**) a safe biopsy path was chosen.

tomographic slice has been processed. Because this procedure is time consuming, a coaxial needle system is advantageous, because multiple samples can be obtained from only one needle insertion.

A CT scan through the area of the planned biopsy should be performed with contrast bolus injection to ensure accurate identification of all vascular structures. Next, a biopsy pathway that avoids blood vessels and passes through the least amount of lung parenchyma is chosen. Occasionally, the biopsy route can be entirely extrapleural, and the potential for pneumothorax is minimized (38) (Fig. 3). However, most mediastinal or hilar biopsy approaches require that the needle pass through both parietal and visceral pleura twice, once as the lung is entered and once as the hilar or mediastinal mass is entered. Although, intuitively, this factor would seem to increase the risk of pneumothorax, the true incidence of this complication is no higher than for lung parenchymal biopsies (39–42).

Once the approach is determined, the patient is placed on the scanner table in a position that puts the entry site in a location convenient for both the radiologist and patient. Usually, placing the proposed needle tract perpendicular to the table top allows for easiest placement of drapes and offers the maximum amount of working space. A pilot scan is then obtained and compared to the chest radiograph. Then a limited CT scan through the lesion is taken. If the patient is not lying in the same position as in the original CT scan, the relationship between the mass and the mediastinal or hilar structures may change. This occasionally necessitates a new biopsy approach. If there is any doubt about the relationship between the new biopsy route and intrathoracic blood vessels, a new CT scan with a bolus of intravenous contrast material should be performed (Fig. 4).

From the limited CT scan, a level for the biopsy site is determined. A single slice is taken at this level with the table index set to zero. Using the measurement scale on the CT cathode ray tube, the distance between a surface landmark (such as sternum, spinous process, or arbitrarily placed metal marker) and desired entry site is measured. This distance is transferred to the patient's skin surface, and a thin metal object (e.g., a paper clip, covered needle, or metal shot) is attached to the patient's skin at this site. The marker indicates the proposed entry site. A repeat scan is obtained to see if the metal marker corresponds to the desired entry area on the CT screen. If these areas do not superimpose, the marker is moved, and the scan is repeated. Once the marker and entry site correspond, two lines are drawn on the patient's skin: one corresponds to the scan plane (defined by the laser or light indicator), and the other is perpendicular to the scan plane and passes through the intersection of the marker and scan line. Next the patient is removed from the gantry. At the intersection of the two lines, an impression is made on the patient's skin with a needle hub.

This mark should persist throughout skin preparation, draping, and anesthetization. The exact distance from the entry site to the lesion is measured on the CT screen. After the needle is inserted, it is advanced in increments, and its position is checked with repeat scans. Sometimes it is necessary to scan just above and below the selected level to find a needle tip that has veered from the biopsy plane. When the needle tip has reached the mass, samples are taken.

After the biopsy samples are taken and the needle has been removed, a repeat scan in the area may be done to look for pneumothorax or hemorrhage. Postbiopsy chest physical exam and upright expiratory radiograph are done. The types of complications and complication rates are similar to those of lung nodule aspiration (40–42).

PERCUTANEOUS PLACEMENT OF SMALL CHEST TUBES AND HEIMLICH VALVES

Percutaneous placement of small chest tubes may be used by interventional radiologists for the treatment of pneumothoraces (43–45). Pneumothoraces are a frequent complication of percutaneous intrathoracic fine needle aspiration biopsies. Pneumothoraces from other sources can also be treated with small chest tubes. Small chest tubes are most effective in treating pneumothoraces without associated pleural fluid. Pleural fluid can obstruct the small diameter of the tube.

Technical Aspects

The pneumothorax drainage kits we use are available from Cook Catheter in Bloomington, IN, or Arrow in Reading, PA. The Cook system is a straight 31 cm, 9 Fr. angiographic catheter with an end hole and 20 side holes. The distal 8 cm of the tube is stiffened with the end of a 21 cm trocar, which is inserted through the most proximal side hole and protrudes through the end hole. Included in the kit is a Heimlich valve, a one-way airflow device constructed from a rubber sleeve housed in a plastic casing. The valve is connected to the chest tube by a flexible plastic tube and stopcock. During expiration, the positive intrapleural pressure forces excess air through the rubber sleeve. During inspiration, negative intrapleural pressure causes the sides of the rubber sleeve to collapse, thus not permitting air to reenter the pleural space. The Arrow system is similar, except that the 8 Fr. chest tube is inserted entirely on a trocar. A one-piece chest tube and one-way valve system—the Tru-Close Thoracic Vent (UreSil Corporation, Skokie, IL)—has recently become available and has had favorable reviews (46,47).

The patient with a pneumothorax is placed on a fluoroscopic table, and the skin entry site is chosen. Areas of pleural adhesion should be avoided, because the chest tube could injure the tethered lung parenchyma. The usual skin entry site is in the midclavicular line between the second and third intercostal space or between the third and fourth. The tube should be placed over the superior border of a rib to avoid piercing the intercostal neurovascular bundle. Actual skin entry site should be about 1 cm below the top margin of the selected rib. The skin is marked, prepped, draped, and anesthetized. A skin nick with a #11 blade is made. At this time, a check of the fluoroscopic field of view should be obtained to ensure that the entry site and hemithorax are visible. Prior to insertion, the chest tube is connected to a three-way stopcock that is turned onto the chest tube. The patient is warned that, when the tube enters the pleural space, there will be some pleuritic pain, even though the skin has been anesthetized. Next, the chest tube and trocar are inserted into the skin nick perpendicularly to the chest wall; the tip should not be advanced farther than the subcutaneous tissue in this position. Then, the skin and entry site are moved together cephalad until the tip is at the level of the superior border of the rib (the chest tube and trocar are still perpendicular to the chest wall). Under a steady pressure, the trocar and tube are then advanced into the pleural space. Rapid advancement should be avoided until intercostal soft tissue resistance has been overcome. When the resistance lessens, the trocar and tube are quickly advanced 2 or 3 cm into the pleural space; less distance is traversed if the separation of visceral and parietal pleura is less than 3 cm. Now the trocar is withdrawn 5 mm back into the tube. This configuration allows for good control of the chest tube while eliminating the danger of piercing the pleura or parenchyma with the sharp trocar tip. Next, the tube and trocar are angled cephalad and advanced until the tip is at the level of the clavicle. The tube is angled to make sure that the tip goes toward the apex. All side holes must be within the pleural space, or there will be an antegrade air leak into the subcutaneous tissues or a retrograde leak into the pleural space. Next, the trocar is removed, and a 50 ml syringe is attached to the three-way stopcock. Intrapleural air is aspirated into the syringe and then expelled through the third hub of the stopcock through the Heimlich valve. In patients with large pneumothoraces or acute symptoms, the tube can be attached to wall suction for rapid evacuation of the pneumothorax. Alternatively, the patient can be asked to cough with the stopcock turned to allow egress of air out the Heimlich valve. Most pneumothoraces will rapidly evacuate using this later method.

Pneumothoraces can thus be treated in most patients. Pneumothorax removal restores vital capacity quickly and decreases dyspnea. However, when the pneumothorax has been reduced enough so that the pleural surfaces are in apposition, the patient begins to experience pain. This pain should not be confused with that of worsening pneumothorax.

When intrapleural air can no longer be aspirated the valve is turned to the Heimlich valve and the syringe is removed. The Heimlich valve is working properly when the walls of the rubber sleeve separate during expiration or coughing. Next the chest tube is sewn to the skin near the entry site. Three milliliters of topical antibiotic ointment are placed on the entry site, and an occlusive dressing with gauze bandages and tape is applied. The stopcock should be secured with tape so that its valve is not accidentally turned off. The tube and valve are then taped to the chest, while care is taken to avoid kinks in the tubing. Positioning the Heimlich valve so that moisture will drain from the system is important, because moist intrapleural pneumothorax air will condense in the system. If not allowed to drain, the moisture will clog the system, thus stopping the free egress of pneumothorax air. A postprocedure chest radiograph is taken to check the adequacy of pneumothorax drainage and the position of the tube.

Attending physicians, ward personnel, and the patient are instructed on the function of the Heimlich valve and chest drain. The radiologist should visit the patient twice a day to check for proper system function and possible complications. After 24 hours, a chest radiograph is obtained to check for residual pneumothorax. Should there be a persistent pneumothorax, the system is checked for malfunction. If the system is working properly, it is left open to drain for another 24 hours before rechecking for pneumothorax. The stopcock may be turned off, if the pneumothorax has resolved. Another chest radiograph is obtained approximately 2 hours after turning off the valve. When the tube has been turned off for 24 more hours, another radiograph is obtained. If there is no residual pneumothorax, the chest tube can be removed. Removal is accomplished by cutting the skin sutures to the tube and then pulling the tube out in one quick motion while holding another occlusive dressing on the entry site. This new dressing is taped to the patient, who is then checked for signs or symptoms of recurrent pneumothorax.

Complications

Small chest tube insertion carries the same types of risks as do large thoracostomy tubes. Laceration of an intercostal artery may cause a hemothorax or chest wall hematoma. If bleeding is persistent, transfusion and surgical ligation of the bleeding vessel may be required. Although perforation of the heart or great vessels can occur, usually it can be avoided with the use of fluoroscopic guidance. Laceration of the lung or inadvertent placement of the tube into the lung parenchyma may produce a large air leak and lead to a bronchopleural fistula. Any time a foreign body such as a chest tube enters the pleural space, there is risk of infection. However, the risk is small enough so that systemic antibiotic prophylaxis is not necessary either before or after placement of a small chest tube. A small sympathetic effusion may occur as a result of pleural irritation. If the effusion becomes large, fluid may enter the chest tube when the patient is supine, causing it to malfunction. As the warm, moist intrapleural air leaves the chest and enters the cooler tubing connecting the chest tube to the Heimlich valve the moisture in the air condenses. This condensate can fill the small connecting tubing and prevent the normal egress of the pneumothorax.

Persistent pneumothorax can be a problem with any method of treatment. If the small chest tube and Heimlich valve are functioning properly, but the pneumothorax is not decreasing in size, the chest tube should be connected to low pressure continuous suction. The Heimlich valve does not have to be removed; the suction tube can be attached directly to the distal end of the valve housing. Suction is continued for 24 hours before rechecking for residual pneumothorax. Should the pneumothorax persist, a second small chest tube may be placed. A large thoracostomy tube placed by the surgeon or pulmonary physician is an alternative. Some air leaks are so large that successful treatment by a small chest tube is not possible. Patients on mechanical ventilation who develop pneumothoraces usually require treatment with a standard thoracostomy tube. If a small tube is used in such patients, it should be placed on wall suction. Inadvertent backward connection of the Heimlich valve is a possible complication that can quickly result in a tension pneumothorax (48).

PERCUTANEOUS DIAGNOSIS AND DRAINAGE OF PLEURAL FLUID COLLECTIONS

Pleural effusions often require aspiration and analysis for diagnosis. Although aspiration of large free pleural effusions usually can be accomplished on the ward, small, loculated, or inaccessible pleural effusions may have to be aspirated with radiologic guidance.

Radiographic evaluation of a pleural effusion begins with the posteroanterior, lateral, and appropriate decubitus chest films. These studies help determine the size and position of the fluid collection. They also demonstrate whether the effusion is free or loculated.

Ultrasound or CT can be used in the localization and aspiration of effusions. Ultrasound is the procedure of choice for aspirating small mobile effusions. CT can accurately delineate small effusions, but if they are mobile, it is difficult to position the patient properly for aspiration. Loculated effusions may require either CT or ultra-

sound for localization. Occasionally, fluoroscopy may be used in the aspiration of loculated effusions.

Technical Aspects

Aspiration of pleural effusion with CT or fluoroscopic guidance involves the same techniques described for CT or fluoroscopically guided aspirations of lung or mediastinal masses. However, larger gauge needles than those used for aspiration biopsies are often needed for effusion aspiration to ensure successful removal of a viscous fluid.

Ultrasound is the most frequently used imaging modality for aspirating pleural fluid. It can be used in both free and loculated collections. With free effusions the patient is usually scanned in the sitting position, which causes effusions to collect in the (dependent) lateral and posterior costophrenic sulci. Loculated effusions should be scanned with the patient placed in the optimum position for visualization of the fluid, as determined by the chest films. Once the effusion is visualized, its change in position during respiration is observed. The patient then practices halting respiration at the point in which the effusion is easiest to aspirate. The skin is marked at a site that will allow the needle to pass over the superior aspect of a rib and then is prepped, draped, and anesthetized. For an initial diagnostic aspiration of the effusion, a 20 gauge spinal needle or angiocath is used. The needle is attached to a two-way stopcock and 20 ml syringe. With the patient suspending respiration at the predetermined point, the needle is advanced into the pleural space, with an aspirating force applied to the syringe. When fluid enters the syringe, needle advancement is stopped, and the diagnostic tap is then completed. The patient should use shallow breaths when the needle is within the thorax. Enough fluid for all diagnostic tests should be removed; these tests include cytology, culture, and various chemical analyses, including pH. The needle is then removed during breath-holding.

Occasionally during the initial pass, fluid cannot be obtained, even after the needle has entered to the maximum planned depth. The most common cause for this phenomenon is that the patient has suspended respiration at the wrong phase. Rescanning with additional practice at breath-holding helps to solve this problem. Another reason for an unsuccessful first tap is that the effusion is too viscous to be aspirated with a 20 gauge needle. Switching to a larger gauge needle may help.

A therapeutic pleural tap can be a one-stage procedure, if the effusion is small. A large effusion that compresses the lung should be aspirated in several separate procedures. Otherwise, rapid expansion of lung could result in reexpansion pulmonary edema. Two or three taps of 500 to 1000 ml over several days will usually suffice. Also, large or recurrent effusions can be managed with small percutaneously placed pleural drains. The technique is discussed in the following section.

After each tap, the patient is examined for complications. A chest radiograph is used to check for pneumothorax. The overall risk of pneumothorax after pleural tap is less than 10 percent (49). There is less risk with large effusions than small ones, because the needle remains farther away from the visceral pleura with large effusions. Bleeding from an intercostal artery and infection of the pleural space are two additional potential complications. Sonography-guided thoracentesis has a significantly lower risk of pneumothoraces than conventional techniques. In a recent study the ability to localize accurately the effusion and the use of thin needles allowed a pneumothorax rate of only 3 percent (50).

PERCUTANEOUS CATHETER DRAINAGE OF PLEURAL EFFUSIONS

After a diagnostic tap has been performed, many pleural effusions require catheter drainage. Traditionally, large thoracostomy tubes are used. However, smaller percutaneous drains offer an alternative with some advantages (51) (Fig. 5). These small tubes are better tolerated by the patient. Also, use of CT or ultrasound allows very accurate positioning of such drains. Small drainage tubes can be used in conjunction with large

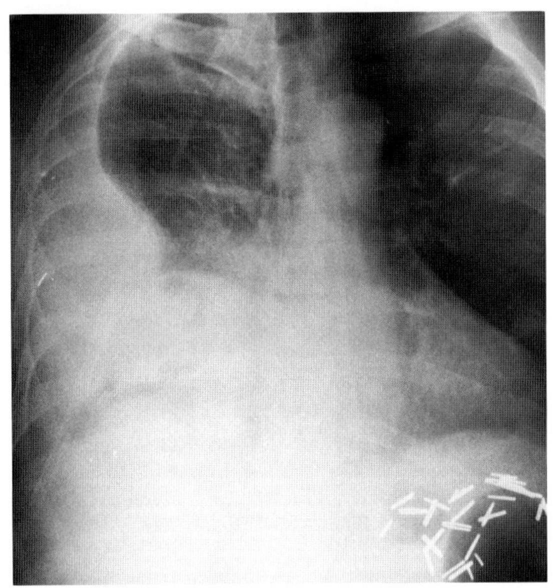

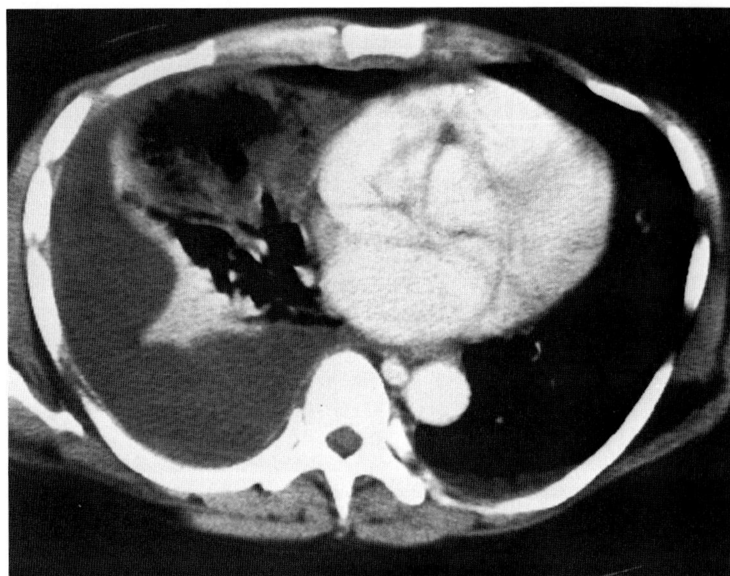

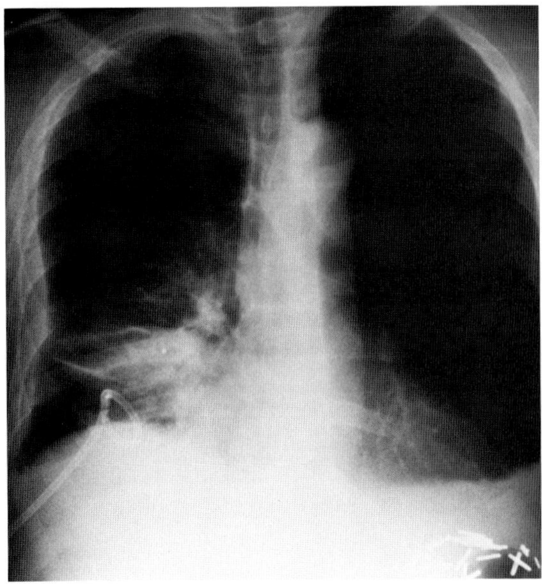

FIG. 5. (A) Chest radiograph showing a large right effusion. **(B)** CT scan demonstrating the right effusion and partial collapse of the right lung. On CT there are no apparent loculations. Ultrasound showed the effusion to be fixed but have no internal loculations. **(C)** Chest radiograph after successful removal of 900 ml of bloody malignant effusion with a small pig-tail drainage catheter.

thoracostomy tubes to remove any loculated fluid collections that are not effectively drained by the large chest tube.

Technical Aspects

The pleural effusion is located with fluoroscopy, CT, or ultrasound. Accuracy of localization is important; therefore, the modality that best demonstrates the effusion should be used. Ultrasound can often help predict which effusions can be adequately drained with small catheters. If the ultrasound demonstrates thick-walled loculations, single catheter drainage may not be successful (Fig. 6). Actual catheter insertion is best performed under fluoroscopic control, because guidewire and catheter manipulations during placement can be monitored

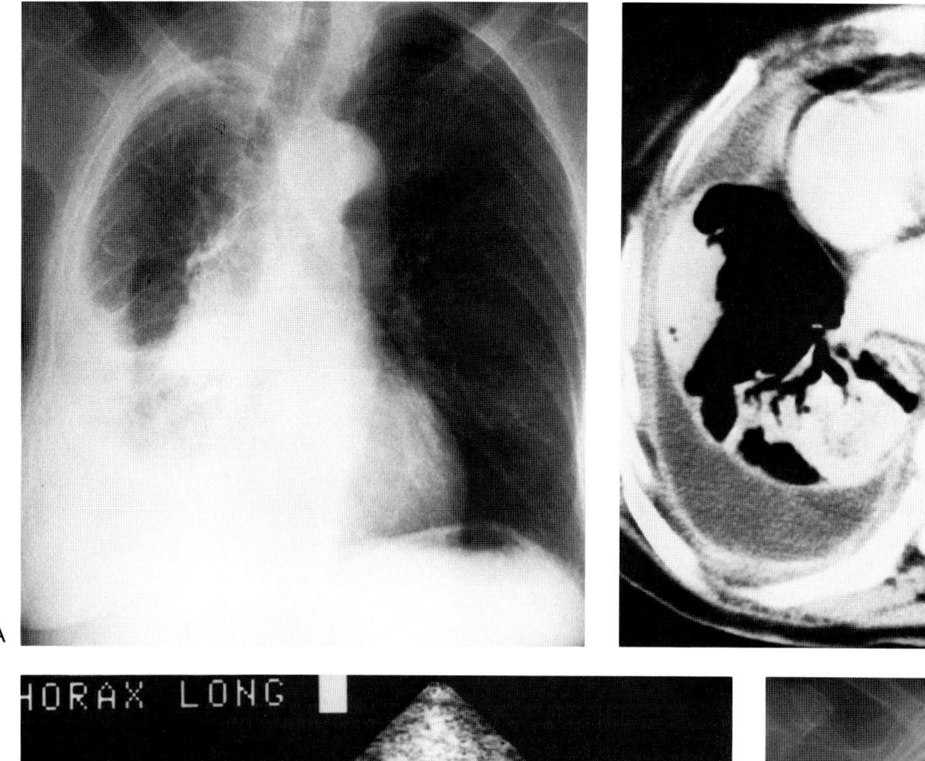
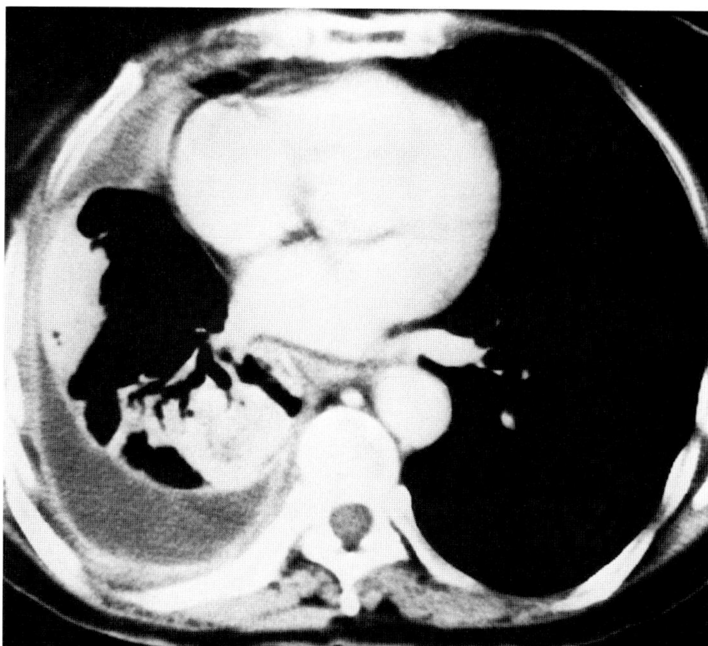
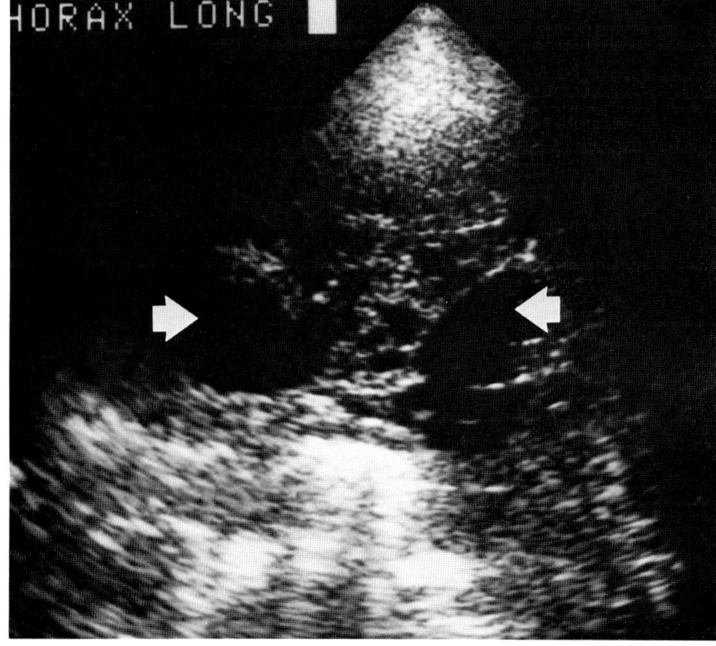

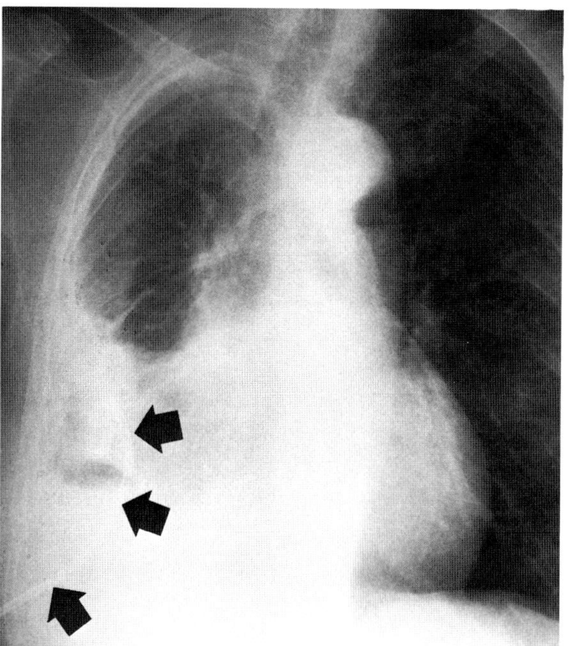

FIG. 6. (**A**) Chest radiograph of a patient with a nonflowing right effusion. (**B**) CT showing a right effusion with no apparent internal loculations. (**C**) Ultrasound of the right chest demonstrating that the effusion has many internal loculations (*arrows*). (**D**) Chest radiograph after the placement of a small pig-tailed drainage catheter (*arrows*) showing that little effusion has been removed. The tube was not successful in draining the multiloculated effusion as the appearance of the ultrasound had suggested.

most easily with fluoroscopy. The entire procedure may be performed under CT guidance, if fluoroscopic visualization of the effusion is poor. This process is more time consuming than fluoroscopy, because each manipulation requires that a new scan be taken and processed before viewing the catheter position. Occasionally, the needle may be placed under CT or ultrasound guidance, and a guidewire may be advanced and left in the pleural space. With just a guidewire in the pleural space, the patient can be transported to fluoroscopy for catheter placement.

Once the pleural fluid is accurately located, a skin entry site should be chosen and marked. If the effusion is free, the skin entry site is in the posterior axillary line at an intercostal level above the diaphragm and below the uppermost level of the effusion. The supine patient is positioned with the involved side elevated 20°–30°. If the fluid is loculated, a skin entry site is chosen directly over the largest portion or the most dependent portion of the loculated effusion and the patient is placed with this site up. The entry site is over the superior portion of a rib to avoid the intercostal vessels. The skin is prepped, draped, and anesthetized. A diagnostic tap with a 22 or 20 gauge needle is performed, if one has not yet been done. Examination of the fluid is often useful to determine its viscosity and help influence what size drainage catheter may be required.

Next, a 10 cm, 18 gauge Pott's needle is inserted into the pleural effusion through a small skin incision. Withdrawing fluid through the 18 gauge needle with a syringe proves proper positioning of the tip within the fluid. A "J" tip guidewire is then passed into the pleural effusion. If the effusion is loculated, the wire is seen to curl within the loculation pocket. However, if the effusion is free, the wire follows the normal pleural margin and extends into the normal pleural space. Enough wire should be maintained in the pleural effusion to prevent its removal during catheter placement or dilator exchanges. Next the 18 gauge needle is removed, and the tract dilated with increasing size dilators until a dilator one Fr. size larger than the catheter to be used. Choice of catheters depends on the viscosity of the fluid. Six or 7 Fr. pigtail angiographic catheters are sufficient for uncomplicated pleural effusions. Eight to 10 Fr. drainage catheters with multiple side holes are used for viscous effusions. The catheter should drain the most dependent portion of the effusion. All side holes should be within the pleural space. The catheter is secured to the skin surface by sutures and occlusively dressed. A chest radiograph at this time determines the exact position of the tube, and follow-up radiographs determine the adequacy of drainage. The drainage tube can be attached to an external drainage bag or aspirated several times a day through a stopcock. If certain areas of the effusion are not drained by the initial catheter, additional ones may be placed. An effusion should be drained slowly over more than a day if it is large (greater than 1500 ml). Once the effusion has been drained and follow-up radiographs show that there is no recurrence, the percutaneous drainage catheter can be removed. Pleural sclerotherapy can be performed through a sonographically placed small-bore catheter with results comparable to those of large-bore, surgically placed catheters. Success rates of 70 percent have been reported using bleomycin or tetracycline as a sclerosing agent through 7- to 24-Fr. catheters (52).

Complications

Pneumothorax, intercostal artery laceration, and infection are possible complications with this procedure. Obstruction of the catheter requires that it be irrigated with 10–20 ml of sterile saline to reestablish flow. Passing a guidewire through an occluded catheter often reestablishes flow. Repeat CT or ultrasound examination may be necessary to detect loculated areas not adequately drained by the initial catheter. These areas may require treatment with additional catheters. If the fluid is too viscous or the catheter is plugged, larger or new catheters can be placed by catheter exchange over a guidewire.

PERCUTANEOUS CATHETER DRAINAGE OF EMPYEMAS

Empyema is defined as purulent, inflammatory exudate in the pleural space. It may be loculated or may involve the entire pleural space. *Staphylococcus aureus* is the most common organism in empyema (53), but a variety of Gram-negative organisms may also be found. Acute empyemas usually result from pneumonias or abscesses of the lung extending into the pleural space. Effective antimicrobial therapy has reduced the incidence of postpneumonic empyemas to less than 1 percent. The

FIG. 7. (A) Chest radiograph of a patient with empyema after the placement of a large-bore chest tube (*arrows*) that removed 800 ml of pus. The radiograph shows that there is still a large amount of undrained empyema. **(B)** CT showing the chest tube (*curved arrows*) surrounded by the right middle lobe. The tube was either within the parenchyma or enveloped by it. A large fluid collection is present posteriorly (*arrows*). **(C and D)** PA and lateral chest radiographs demonstrating the pig-tail catheter within the empyema (*arrows*) after 500 ml more pus was removed. **(E)** CT of the chest several days later showing a marked reduction in the amount of empyema (*arrows*). The right middle lobe is still consolidated, but the right lower lobe is now aerated.

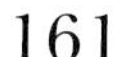

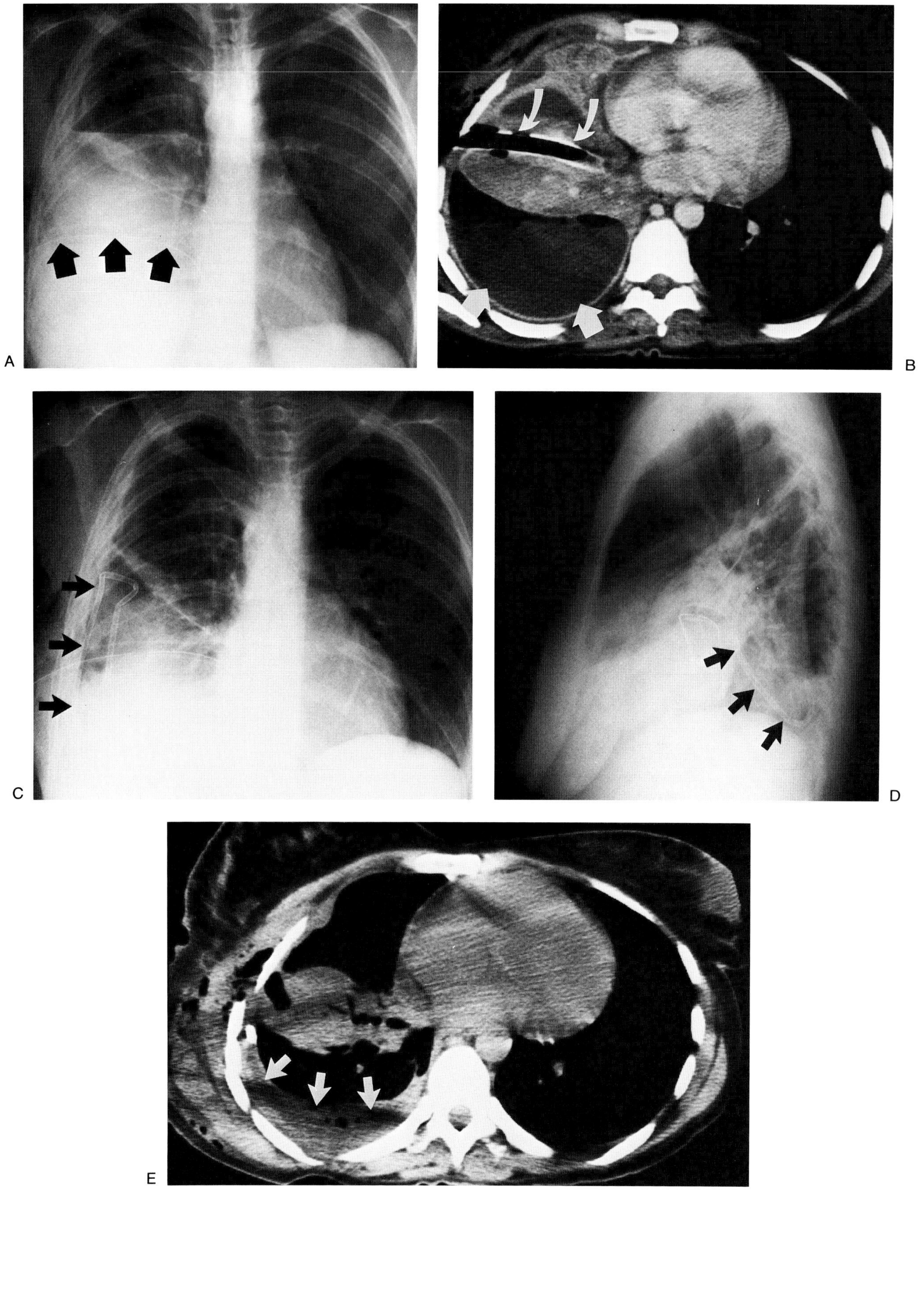

incidence is higher with necrotizing pneumonias (53). Other sources of empyema include infections extending into the pleural space from contiguous sources, such as the mediastinum, ribs, or abdomen. Empyema may also occur following thoracic surgery or instrumentation of the pleural space. Chronic empyemas are the result of untreated or inadequately healed acute empyemas.

There are three stages in the development of empyema that have a direct bearing on the timing and proper selection of drainage therapy (53,54). *Exudative empyema* is an early phase characterized by watery fluid with a low cell count. *Fibrinopurulent empyema* is characterized by large numbers of polymorphonuclear leukocytes and fibrin depositions coating the pleural surfaces. Loculations develop at this stage. *Organizing empyema* is the last stage; fibroblasts appear in the fibrin coating, and the exudate is thick.

These distinctions are important, as therapy differs with the stage of empyema. Exudative empyemas may be treated with needle aspiration. If thoracentesis does not completely drain the empyema, if the fluid reaccumulates, or if the patient is not improving clinically, continuous intercostal tube drainage is indicated. Fibrinopurulent empyemas require closed tube drainage. Several large bore tubes may be required to drain all collections adequately. Open drainage and possible resection of a portion of rib may be required, if closed tube thoracostomy is ineffective in removing thick or loculated pus. Occasionally, decortication of the lung is required to remove the fibrinopurulent pleural peel.

Percutaneous drainage of empyemas can be performed during the exudative and fibrinopurulent stages of an empyema (55,56). Exudative empyema can be treated with a percutaneously placed pleural drain in much the same manner as a pleural effusion is drained (see previous section). The pleural drain must be placed in the most dependent portion of the empyema to ensure complete drainage. The drainage catheter must be large enough so that the empyema fluid can pass easily. The catheter is connected to water seal suction or an external drainage bag. Daily chest radiographs and close patient follow-up are necessary until drainage is complete. If loculations are suspected or residual fluid is difficult to localize on daily frontal and decubitus films, ultrasound or CT examinations may be used to localize residual collections accurately. Additional catheters may be necessary to drain loculations.

Fibrinopurulent empyemas are difficult to drain because of the high incidence of loculations. CT or ultrasound is helpful in localizing all loculations. Once localized, each loculation is entered using the same technique utilized for draining a pleural effusion. When the guidewire is inserted into the loculation, it will coil around the periphery of the loculation rather than pass freely into the pleural space. If the catheter becomes plugged, flushing with 15–20 ml of sterile saline often will reestablish

drainage. If not, a new or larger catheter is needed. The drainage catheter should remain in place as long as it is functioning. It may take several weeks to drain an empyema adequately. Intrapleural urokinase at an average dose of 400,000 IU has proven successful in treating multiloculated empyemas (57). Often percutaneous drainage catheters are used in conjunction with larger thoracostomy tubes to drain loculations not reached by the thoracostomy tube (58) (Fig. 7). The radiologist should not hesitate to ask the surgeon to place a large thoracostomy tube if the percutaneous drainage catheters fail to evacuate the empyema. Occasionally, large bore thoracostomy tubes with suction are necessary to expand the lung and obliterate the pleural space left empty by the removal of the empyema.

PERCUTANEOUS ASPIRATION AND DRAINAGE OF LUNG ABSCESSES

A lung abscess is an area of necrotic lung parenchyma containing purulent material. Most lung abscesses are caused by necrotizing pneumonias from anaerobic bacteria. These bacteria enter the lung parenchyma through aspiration of contaminated oropharyngeal contents; less frequently, lung abscesses arise from hematogenous spread to the lung parenchyma from distant infections or endocarditis. Lung abscesses also can occur with fungal and tuberculous infections or from cavitation of an inflammatory site behind an endobronchial obstruction such as a neoplasm. Most lung abscesses occur in the posterior segments of the upper lobes or superior segments of the lower lobes, because they are the ones most often infected during aspiration. Patients who develop lung abscesses often have predisposing factors, such as poor dentition, alcoholism, general anesthesia, epilepsy, stroke, or esophageal motility disorders (59).

The radiographic diagnosis of a lung abscess involves demonstration of the cavity. This cavity may have an air fluid level within it, indicating that some drainage of the purulent necrotic material into the bronchi has occurred. The air fluid level should be visible in two projections to ensure it is indeed within a cavity. (An area of normal parenchyma visualized projecting through a consolidated area may appear as an abscess in one projection.) CT demonstrates the abscess to be an area of enhancing parenchyma surrounding a central low density that may contain an air fluid level. Chest radiographs, CT, and the use of decubitus films allow for accurate detection and localization of lung abscesses.

The incidence of lung abscesses has declined in recent years, because of rapid and effective treatment of pneumonias with broad spectrum antibiotics. Before antibiotics, lung abscesses were a serious complication of pneumonia and carried a high mortality. With the advent of surgical drainage of abscesses, the mortality was reduced

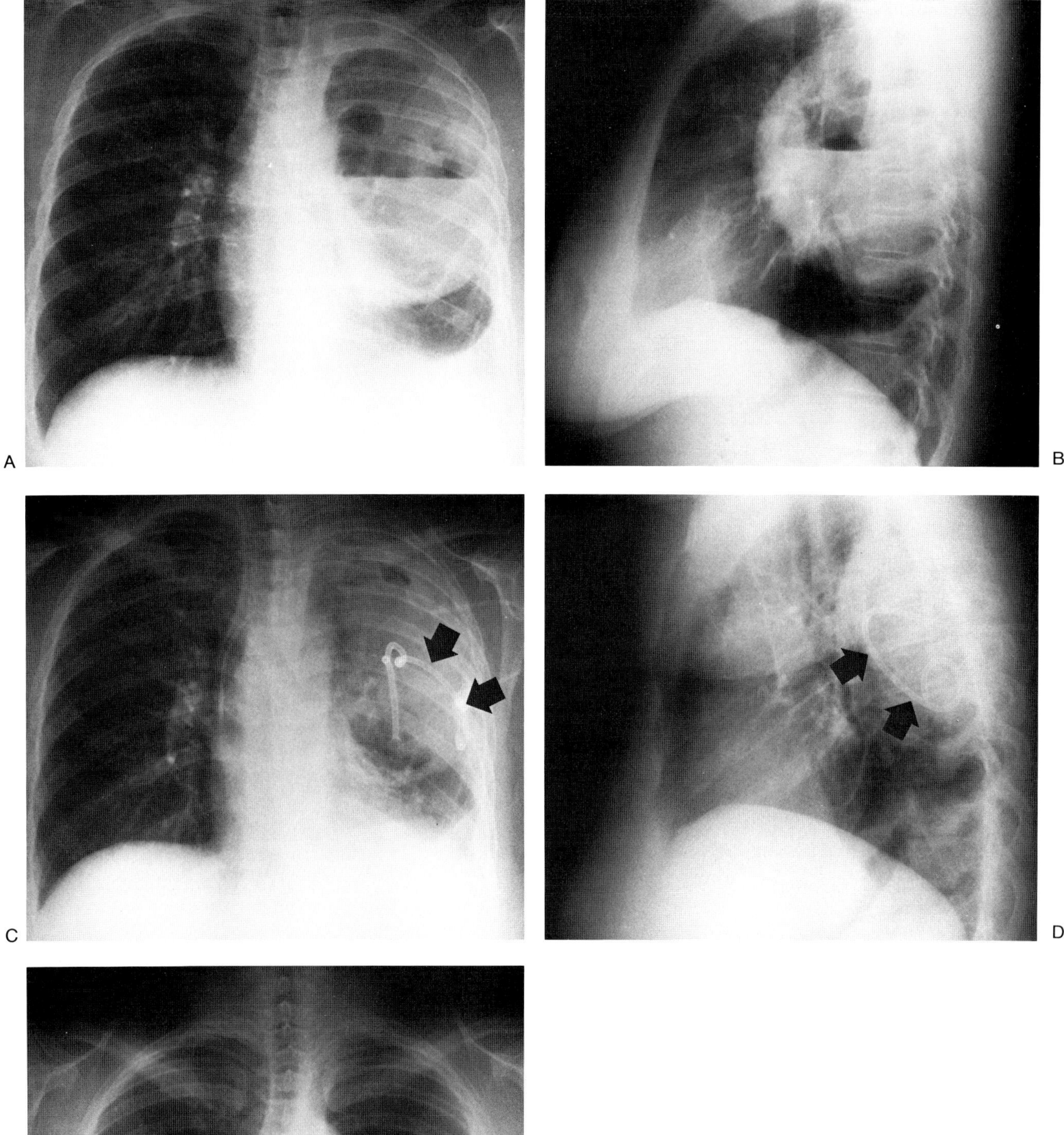

FIG. 8. (**A** and **B**) PA and lateral chest radiograph of a patient with a left upper lobe abscess. The patient remained febrile after appropriate antibiotic treatment. CT scan (not shown) showed a large abscess with fluid within it. (**C** and **D**) PA and lateral chest radiograph after the placement of a 10 Fr. catheter within the abscess and removal of 300 ml of pus (*arrows*). The tube remained in for 6 weeks as the patient cleared up the infection. Much of the time the patient was an outpatient. The tube was aspirated three times a day by the patient's family. (**E**) PA chest radiograph 2 months after the removal of the tube showing complete resolution of the abscess.

(60,61). The use of antibiotics has markedly reduced the need for surgical treatment of lung abscesses (54). In patients who are not responding well to therapy, or in whom the risk of the purulent material spreading throughout the lung is great, a drainage or aspiration procedure may be indicated. Also, these patients may need a diagnostic needle aspiration or bronchoscopy to make a definitive microbiological diagnosis.

Percutaneous Aspiration

In patients with lung abscesses who are not responding well to antibiotics, a diagnostic percutaneous aspiration is often helpful (62). The technique for needle aspiration is the same as that for lung nodule or pneumonia aspiration and can be performed under CT or fluoroscopic guidance. Aspiration with a 21 or 22 gauge needle should be attempted first. However, if the purulent material cannot be withdrawn, a larger gauge aspiration needle must be used. All of the aspirated material should be handled with sterile technique and sent for microbiological processing, including anaerobic, fungal, and tuberculous cultures. It is helpful to withdraw as much of the infected purulent material as possible by placing the patient so that the needle will reach the most dependent portion of the abscess. The number of bacteria and amount of contaminated material the patient may aspirate into an uninfected area of lung are thereby substantially reduced.

Percutaneous Drainage

In patients who are not responding well to antibiotic treatment, percutaneous catheter drainage of lung abscesses is an effective treatment alternative to lobectomy (63–67). Percutaneous lung abscess drainage was effectively utilized during the preantibiotic era with excellent results (60,61). The decision for drainage should be made with the pulmonary, infectious disease, and thoracic surgical consultants. The abscess should be accurately localized by plain films or CT, whichever is most helpful. Transversing normal lung and the pleural space during the drainage has not resulted in excess complications in our hands. However, a catheter course through abnormal lung is preferred. Abscess drainage is not effective, if there is no fluid within the cavity. Percutaneous lung abscess drainage is an effective method to treat lung abscesses refractory to conventional therapy with 100 percent cure rate and an 84 percent rate of avoiding surgery in one study (68) (Fig. 8).

Under fluoroscopic or CT guidance, an 18 gauge biopsy needle capable of accepting a 0.038 inch "J" tip guidewire is inserted into the cavity. Fluid may be aspirated and sent for analysis and culture, if this has not been performed. Next the guidewire is threaded into the cavity. The needle is removed from the cavity and a small skin incision is made with a #11 blade. At this point, the patient should be moved to fluoroscopy if the initial procedure is being done with CT guidance. With the wire in the abscess cavity, the tract through the chest wall is dilated until a dilator has been passed that is one French size larger than the drainage catheter to be used. Next, the drainage catheter is inserted into the abscess cavity. An 8 to 10 Fr. pigtail nephrostomy catheter is used for the drainage.

With the catheter in position, as much fluid as possible is aspirated. The catheter is sewn in place and connected to an underwater seal or to a small syringe for intermittent aspiration. Immediate chest radiographs should be obtained to check for catheter position and for the presence of a pneumothorax.

The radiologist should follow the patient and catheter at least daily. Radiographs taken daily permit checking for complications, the drainage progress, and position of the tube. Occasionally, decubitus views or CT may be needed to check for fluid. The catheter can be under constant low suction or aspirated intermittently with a syringe. Moving the patient in different positions often helps with drainage by permitting the catheter tip to be submerged in the remaining abscess fluid. The catheter should be irrigated intermittently, with small volumes of sterile saline to prevent obstruction. Rinsing the cavity with sterile saline to remove infected material and prevent loculation is not possible as it often is with abdominal abscesses because the pulmonary abscess communicates with the bronchial tree, and washing would put the remaining lung at risk for further aspiration. If the catheter becomes obstructed, a new one may be placed. The catheter may remain in place from 1 week to greater than 1 month. Occasionally, the percutaneously placed drain can be used to shrink the abscess so that its surgical removal can be performed.

Complications

Complications of percutaneously placed abscess drainage catheters and abscess aspirations include pneumothorax and bleeding. Infection of the pleural space is a possibility but has not been a significant problem (69). Close attention to the patient's course, position of the catheter, and frequent communication with the consultants are required to ensure success of the procedure.

ASPIRATION AND DRAINAGE OF INFECTED BULLAE

Patients with bullae occasionally present with air fluid levels within the bullae. If the patient is not symptomatic, the air fluid level is generally felt not to represent an infected bulla; if followed, most of these air fluid levels resolve. However, if the patient is symptomatic, the air fluid level in the bulla may indeed represent an infection. The presence of an air fluid level does not indicate that the infected bulla is connected with the bronchial tree. Fluid can accumulate within the normally air-filled bullae from inflammatory exudate caused by an infection. The patient with an infected bulla is treated with appropriate antibiotics. If the patient remains symptomatic despite adequate antibiotic treatment, intervention may be necessary. Aspiration and drainage of an infected bulla are performed in the same manner described for abscesses.

Aspiration of fluid in a bulla provides an accurate microbiological diagnosis. Culture and stains for fungi, tuberculosis, and anaerobic and aerobic bacteria should be performed. Accurate identification of the infecting organism is often all that is needed to treat the infected bulla. When the diagnostic aspiration is performed, and the material is obviously infected or purulent, as much fluid as possible is withdrawn at that time. If the patient remains symptomatic after aspiration has provided a chance for the correct antibiotic treatment, drainage may be necessary. Infected bullae are drained in the same manner as lung abscesses. The risks and complications are similar as well.

ASPIRATION AND DRAINAGE OF MEDIASTINAL ABSCESSES

Mediastinal abscesses are usually caused by penetrating trauma, thoracic operation, rupture of the esophagus, or infection spread from adjacent structures, such as lung, neck, or abdomen. Infection of the mediastinum is a serious problem, with a high mortality and morbidity. Success enjoyed by treatment of intraabdominal abscesses with percutaneous aspiration and drainage has prompted similar intervention in the mediastinum (69–74).

The diagnosis of the abscess is made with the use of CT-guided fine needle aspiration. Once the diagnosis has been made, the decision to perform a percutaneous catheter drainage is made with close consultation with the thoracic surgeons.

Percutaneous catheter drainage of mediastinal abscess is a CT-guided procedure. CT is used for the entire procedure because it allows for accurate localization of the abscess and precise placement of the needle, guidewire, and drainage catheter. The accuracy available with CT is a compromise for the real-time visualization of guidewire and catheter manipulations available with fluoroscopy. The patient is positioned to facilitate catheter placement along a tract that avoids cardiovascular and tracheobronchial structures. Secondary consideration is given to keeping the catheter entirely outside the pleural space. A catheter can be placed through the lung parenchyma as long as no drainage holes are in the lung parenchyma.

Once a drainage tract is chosen, the skin is marked, prepped, and draped at a site just above a superior rib margin. A skin nick is made with a #11 blade. An 18 gauge biopsy needle is advanced into the abscess, using CT to check the needle tip position. Fluid is aspirated to confirm the needle tip location. A 0.035 inch "J"-tipped guidewire is advanced into the cavity until resistance is felt, and its position is checked with CT before the needle is removed. Enough guidewire should be within the abscess so that accidental withdrawal from the abscess does not occur while the tract is being dilated. The chest wall tract is dilated to one French size larger than the drainage catheter to be used. Next, a 10 Fr. pigtail nephrostomy catheter is advanced over the wire until the pigtail and all the side holes are within the abscess cavity. The catheter position and tract are then checked with CT scans. Following aspiration of as much fluid as possible, the catheter is connected to underwater seal and suction or a syringe for intermittent suction. The catheter is then sewn in place, the skin site is dressed, and a chest film is obtained. As with lung abscess drainage, daily monitoring of patient and tube is required.

CT-directed drainage of mediastinal abscesses is a more difficult procedure than lung abscess or empyema drainage because of the proximity of major cardiovascular and tracheobronchial structures. These structures can be avoided by careful CT guidance during the initial catheter placement. Although catheter erosion into mediastinal vessels or trachea is a theoretical possibility, this complication has not been reported. The excellent experience of abdominal abscess drainage with catheters near major structures will lead to more acceptance of mediastinal drainage procedures. Percutaneous catheter drainage of mediastinal abscesses may allow patients to stabilize before major mediastinal surgical treatment is performed. As with all interventional chest procedures, the radiologist must work closely with the pulmonary, infectious disease, and thoracic surgery consultants in order to achieve the desired outcome.

REFERENCES

1. Green RE. Transthoracic needle aspiration biopsy. In: Athanasoulis CA, Green RE, Pfister RC, Roberson GH, eds. *Interventional radiology.* Philadelphia: WB Saunders, 1982;587–634.
2. Feldman PS, Covell JL. Fine needle aspiration, cytology and its clinical applications, breast and lung. Chicago: American Society of Clinical Pathologists Press, 1985;121–143.
3. Stitik FP. Percutaneous lung biopsy. In: Siegelman SS, Stitik FP, Summer WR, eds. *Multiple imaging procedures, pulmonary system, practical approaches to pulmonary diagnosis,* vol 1. New York: Grune and Stratton, 1979;181–220.
4. House AJS. Biopsy techniques in the investigation of diseases of the lung, mediastinum, and chest wall. *Radiol Clin North Am* 1979;17:393–412.

5. Bernardino ME. Percutaneous biopsy. *Am J Roentgenol* 1984;142:41–45.

6. Goldberg MA, Mueller PR, Saini S, et al. Importance of daily rounds by the radiologist after interventional procedures for the abdomen and chest. *Radiology* 1991;180:767–770.

7. Gobien RP, Bouchard EA, Gobien BS, Valicenti JF, Vujic I. Thin needle aspiration biopsy of thoracic lesions: impact on hospital charges and patterns of patient care. *Radiology* 1983;148:65–67.

8. Jereb M, US-Krasovec M. Thin needle biopsy of chest lesions: time saving potential. *Chest* 1980;78:288–290.

9. Perlmutt LM, Johnston WW, Dunnick NR: Percutaneous transthoracic needle aspiration: a review. *Am J Roentgenol* 1989;152:451–455.

10. Westcott JL. Percutaneous transthoracic needle biopsy. *Radiology* 1988;169:593–601.

11. Thornbury JR, Burke DP, Naylor B. Transthoracic needle aspiration biopsy: accuracy of cytologic typing of malignant neoplasms. *Am J Roentgenol* 1981;136:719–724.

12. Greene R, Szfelbein WM, Isler RJ, Stark P, Jantsch H. Supplemental tissue-core histology from fine-needle transthoracic aspiration biopsy. *Am J Roentgenol* 1985;144:787–792.

13. Khouri NF, Stitik FP, Erozan YS, et al. Transthoracic needle aspiration biopsy of benign and malignant lung lesions. *Am J Roentgenol* 1985;144:281–288.

14. Poe RH, Tobin RE. Sensitivity and specificity of needle biopsy in lung malignancy. *Am Rev Respir Dis* 1980;122:725–729.

15. Westcott JL. Direct percutaneous needle aspiration of localized pulmonary lesions: results in 422 patients. *Radiology* 1980;137:31–35.

16. Stanley JH, Fish GD, Andriole JG, Gobien RP, Betsill WL, Laden SA, Schabel SI: Lung lesions: cytologic diagnosis by fine-needle biopsy. *Radiology* 1987;162:389–391.

17. Gobien RP, Valicenti JF, Paris BS, Daniell C. Thin-needle aspiration biopsy: methods of increasing the accuracy of a negative prediction. *Radiology* 1982;145:603–605.

18. Hamper UM, Khouri NF, Stitik FP, Siegelman SS. Pulmonary hamartoma: diagnosis by transthoracic needle aspiration biopsy. *Radiology* 1985;155:15–18.

19. Nahman BJ, VanAman ME, McLemore WE, O'Toole RV. Use of the rotex needle in percutaneous biopsy of pulmonary malignancy. *Am J Roentgenol* 1985;145:97–99.

20. Davenport RD: Rapid on-site evaluation of transbronchial aspirates. *Chest* 1990;98:59–61.

21. Lalll AF, McCormack LJ, Zeich M, Reich NE, Belovich D. Aspiration biopsies of chest lesions. *Radiology* 1978;127:35–40.

22. Stevens GM, Jackman RJ. Outpatient needle biopsy of the lung: its safety and utility. *Radiology* 1984;154:301–304.

23. Poe RH, Kallay MC. Transthoracic needle biopsy of lung in non-hospitalized patients. *Chest* 1987;92:676–678.

24. vanSonnenberg E, Casola G, Ho M, Neff CC, Varney RR. Difficult thoracic lesions: CT-guided biopsy experience in 150 cases. *Radiology* 1988;167:457–461.

25. Johnsrude IS, Silverman JF, Weaver MD, McConnell RW. Rapid cytology to decrease pneumothorax incidence after percutaneous biopsy. *Am J Roentgenol* 1985;144:793–794.

26. Smith DF, Doust BD. Angulated fluoroscopy for needle biopsy localization. *Am J Roentgenol* 1982;138:765–767.

27. Kreula J. Effect of sampling technique on specimen size in fine needle aspiration biopsy. *Invest Radiol* 1990;25:1294–1299.

28. Kreula J, Virkkunen P, Bondestam S. Effect of suction of specimen size in fine-needle aspiration biopsy. *Invest Radiol* 1990;25:1175–1181.

29. Poe RH, Kallay MC, Wicks CM, Odoroff CL. Predicting risk of pneumothorax in needle biopsy of the lung. *Chest* 1984;85:232–235.

30. Moore EH, LeBlanc, Montesi SA, et al. Effect of patient positioning after needle aspiration lung biopsy. *Radiology* 1991;181:385–387.

31. Bevelaqua FA, Aranda C. Management of spontaneous pneumothorax with small lumen catheter manual aspiration. *Chest* 1982;81:693–694.

32. Perlmutt LM, Braun SD, Newman GE, Cohan RH, Saeed M, Sussman SK, Dunnick NR: Transthoracic needle aspiration: use of a small chest tube to treat pneumothorax. *Am J Roentgenol* 1987;148:849–851.

33. Milner LB, Ryan K, Gullo J. Fatal intrathoracic hemorrhage after percutaneous aspiration lung biopsy. *Am J Roentgenol* 1979;132:280–281.

34. Baker BK, Awwad EE. Computed tomography of fatal cerebral air embolism following percutaneous aspiration biopsy of the lung. *J Comput Assist Tomogr* 1988;12:1082–1083.

35. Goralnik CH, O'Connell DM, El Yousef SJ, Haaga JR. CT-guided cutting-needle biopsies of selected chest lesions. *Am J Roentgenol* 1988;151:903–907.

36. Castellino RA, Blank N. Etiologic diagnosis of focal pulmonary infection in immunocompromised patients by fluoroscopically guided percutaneous needle aspiration. *Radiology* 1979;132:563–567.

37. Palmer DL, Davidson M, Lusk R. Needle aspiration of the lungs in complex pneumonias. *Chest* 1980;78:16–21.

38. Williams RA, Haaga JR, Karagiannis E. CT guided paravertebral biopsy of the mediastinum. *J Comput Assist Tomogr* 1984;8:575–578.

39. Berquist TH, Bailey PB, Cortese DA, Miller WE. Transthoracic needle biopsy accuracy and complications in relation to location and type of lesion. *Mayo Clinic Proc* 1980;55:475–481.

40. Gobien RP, Skucas J, Paris BS. CT-assisted fluoroscopically guided aspiration biopsy of central hilar and mediastinal masses. *Radiology* 1981;141:443–447.

41. Rosenberger A, Adler O. Fine needle aspiration biopsy in the diagnosis of mediastinal lesions. *Am J Roentgenol* 1978;131:239–242.

42. Wescott JL. Percutaneous needle aspiration of hilar and mediastinal masses. *Radiology* 1981;141:323–329.

43. Heimlich HJ. Valve drainage of the pleural cavity. *Dis Chest* 1968;53:282–287.

44. Sargent LN, Turner AF. Emergency treatment of pneumothorax: a simple catheter technique for use in the radiology department. *Am J Roentgenol* 1970;109:531–535.

45. Peters J, Kubitschek KR. Clinical evaluation of a percutaneous pneumothorax catheter. *Chest* 1984;86:714–717.

46. Samelson SL, Goldberg EM, Ferguson MK. The thoracic vent, clinical experience with a new device for treating simple pneumothorax. *Chest* 1991;100:880–882.

47. Molina PL, Solomon SL, Glazer HS, et al. A one-piece unit for treatment of pneumothorax complicating needle biopsy: evaluation in 10 patients. *Am J Roentgenol* 1990;155:31–33.

48. Mainini SE, Johnson FE: Tension pneumothorax complicating small-caliber chest tube insertion. *Chest* 1990;97:759–760.

49. Fraser RG, Pare JAP. *Diagnosis of diseases of the chest,* 2nd ed. Philadelphia: WB Saunders, 1977;301–302.

50. Raptopoulos V, Davis LM, Lee G, et al. Factors affecting the development of pneumothorax associated with thoracentesis. *Am J Roentgenol* 1991;156:917–920.

51. Westcott JL. Percutaneous catheter drainage of pleural effusion and empyema. *Am J Roentgenol* 1985;144:1189–1193.

52. Morrison MC, Mueller PR, Lee MJ, et al. Sclerotherapy of malignant pleural effusion through sonographically placed small-bore catheters. *Am J Roentgenol* 1992;158:41–43.

53. Finegold SM. Empyema. In: Hoeprich PD, ed. *Infectious diseases,* 3d ed. Philadelphia: Harper and Row, 1983;503–505.

54. Takaro T. Lung abscess and fungal infections. In: Sabiston DC, ed. *Textbook of surgery.* Philadelphia: WB Saunders, 1981;2066–2068.

55. Crouch JD, Keagy BA, Delany DJ. "Pigtail" catheter drainage in thoracic surgery. *Am Rev Respir Dis* 1987;136:174–175.

56. Silverman SG, Mueller PR, Saini S, Hahn PF, Simeone JF, Forman BH, Steiner E, Ferrucci JT. Thoracic empyema: management with image-guided catheter drainage. *Radiology* 1988;169:5–9.

57. Lee KS, Im J, Kim YH, et al. Treatment of thoracic multiloculated empyemas with intracavitary urokinase: a prospective study. *Radiology* 1991;179:771–775.

58. VanSonnenberg E, Nakamoto SK, Mueller PR, et al. CT- and ultrasound-guided catheter drainage of empyemas after chest-tube failures. *Radiology* 1984;151:349–353.

59. Hirshmann JV, Murray JF. Lung abscess. In: Petersdorf RG, Adams RD, Braunwald E, Isselbacher KJ, Martin JB, Wilson JD. *Harrison's principles of internal medicine,* 10th ed. New York: McGraw-Hill, 1983;1537–1539.

60. Snow N, Lucas A, Horrigan TP. Utility of pneumonotomy in the treatment of cavitary lung disease. *Chest* 1985;87:731–734.
61. Weissberg D. Percutaneous drainage of lung abscess. *J Thorac Cardiovasc Surg* 1984;87:308–312.
62. Grinan NP, Lucena FM, Romero JV, et al. Yield of percutaneous needle aspiration in lung abscesses. *Chest* 1990;97:69–74.
63. Parker LA, Melton JW, Delaney DJ, Yankaskas BC. Percutaneous small bore catheter drainage in the management of lung abscesses. *Chest* 1987;92:213–218.
64. Aronberg DJ, Sagel SS, Jost RG, Lee JI. Percutaneous drainage of lung abscess. *Am J Roentgenol* 1979;132:282–283.
65. Cameron EWJ, Whitton ID. Percutaneous drainage in the treatment of *Klebsiella pneumoniae* lung abscess. *Thorax* 1977; 32:673–676.
66. Keller FS, Rosch J, Barker AF, Dotter CT. Percutaneous interventional catheter therapy for lesions of the chest and lungs. *Chest* 1982;81:407–412.
67. Vainrub B, Musher DM, Guinn GA, Young EJ, Septimus EJ, Travis LL. Percutaneous drainage of lung abscess. *Am Rev Resp Dis* 1978;117:153–160.
68. vanSonnenberg E, D'Agostino, Casola G, et al. Lung abscess: CT-guided drainage. *Radiology* 1991;178:347–351.
69. Gobien RP, Stanley JH, Gobien BS, Vujic I, Pass HI. Percutaneous catheter aspiration and drainage of suspected mediastinal abscesses. *Radiology* 1984;151:69–71.
70. Gerzof SG, Robbins AH, Johnson WC, Birkett DH, Nabseth DC. Percutaneous catheter drainage of abdominal abscesses. *N Engl J Med* 1981;305:653–657.
71. Mandel SR, Boyd D, Jaques PF, Mandell V, Staab EV. Drainage of hepatic, intraabdominal, and mediastinal abscesses guided by computerized axial tomography. *Am J Surg* 1983;145:120–125.
72. Mueller PR, vanSonnenberg E, Ferrucci JT, Jr. Percutaneous drainage of 250 abdominal abscesses and fluid collections. *Radiology* 1984;151:343–347.
73. Sones PJ. Percutaneous drainage of abdominal abscesses. *Am J Roentgenol* 1984;142:35–39.
74. vanSonnenberg E, Ferrucci JT, Mueller PR, Wittenberg J, Simeone JF. Percutaneous drainage of abscesses and fluid collections: technique, results and applications. *Radiology* 1982; 142:1–10.

Subject Index

171